Handbook of Physical Medicine and Rehabilitation Basics

Handbook of Physical Medicine and Rehabilitation Basics

■ Susan J. Garrison, MD

Associate Professor
Department of Physical Medicine and Rehabilitation
Baylor College of Medicine
Medical Director, Rehabilitation Center
The Methodist Hospital
Houston, Texas

with 30 contributors

J. B. Lippincott Company   Philadelphia

Acquisitions Editor: James D. Ryan
Associate Editor: Wendy Greenberger-Czarnecki
Indexer: Anne W. Cassar
Production Service: Caslon, Inc.
Cover Designer: Tom Jackson
Production Manager: Janet Greenwood
Production Editor: Mary Kinsella
Compositor: The Composing Room of Michigan, Inc.
Printer/Binder: RR Donnelly & Sons Company, Crawfordsville

6 5 4 3

Library of Congress Cataloging in Publication Data
Handbook of physical medicine and rehabilitation basics / [edited
by] Susan J. Garrison : with 30 contributors.
    p. cm.
    Includes bibliographical references and index.
    ISBN 0-397-51336-4
    1. Medicine, Physical—Handbooks, manuals, etc.
        2. Medical rehabilitation—Handbooks, manuals,
etc. I. Garrison, Susan J.
    [DNLM: 1. Physical Medicine—handbooks.
    2. Rehabilitation—   handbooks. WB 39 H23654 1995]
RM700.H15   1995
617'.03—dc20
DNLM/DLC
for Library of Congress   94-3795
                                         CIP

The authors and publisher have exerted every effort to ensure that
drug selection and dosage set forth in this text are in accord with
current recommendations and practice at the time of publication.
However, in view of ongoing research, changes in government regula-
tions, and the constant flow of information relating to drug therapy
and drug reactions, the reader is urged to check the package insert for
each drug for any change in indications and dosage and for added
warnings and precautions. This is particularly important when the
recommended agent is a new or infrequently employed drug.

This book is dedicated to all students of
Physical Medicine and Rehabilitation.

Acknowledgments

Martin Grabois, MD, Professor and Chairman, Department of Physical Medicine and Rehabilitation, Baylor College of Medicine, Houston, Texas

Administrative and Clinical Services Committee Members, 1987–1990
Betty Bacha, David X. Cifu, MD, Steve Gnatz, MD, David Hirsh, MD, Katie Irani, MD, Michael Krebs, MD, Janusz Markowski, MD, Anthony O'Callaghan, MD, Henry Ostermann, PhD, Barry Smith MD, Charlotte Stelly-Steitz, MD, and James Williams, MD
Susan J. Garrison, MD, Chair

Emily Linkins, J. B. Lippincott Company
Wendy Greenberger-Czarnecki, J. B. Lippincott Company
Ann Saydlowski
Becca Gruliow, Caslon, Inc.
Chris Robinson
Greg, Grant, and Gwen Gerber

Contributors

Susan Linder Blair, MD
Former Resident in Physical Medicine and Rehabilitation
Baylor College of Medicine
Houston, Texas
Associate Medical Director
Harris Methodist Fort Worth
Fort Worth, Texas

Catherine F. Bontke, MD
Associate Professor
Clinical Physical Medicine and Rehabilitation
Baylor College of Medicine
Houston, Texas

Barry L. Bowser, MD
Medical Director Brain Injury Program
Rio Vista Rehabilitation Hospital
El Paso, Texas

John C. Cianca, MD
Assistant Professor of Physical Medicine and Rehabilitation
Baylor College of Medicine
Director of Sports and Human Performance Medicine
Human Performance and Rehabilitation Center
Houston, Texas

David Xavier Cifu, MD
Assistant Professor
Department of Physical Medicine and Rehabilitation
Director, Rehabilitation Consultation Service
Medical Director, Rehabilitation and Research Center
Director, Brain Injury Rehabilitation Program,
Rehabilitation and Research Center
Medical College of Virginia Hospital
Richmond, Virginia

William H. Donovan, MD
Professor and Chairman, Department of Physical Medicine
and Rehabilitation
The University of Texas - Houston Medical School
Executive Vice President for Medical Affairs
The Institute for Rehabilitation and Research
Houston, Texas

Susan L. Garber, MA, OTR, FAOTA
Assistant Professor
Department of Physical Medicine and Rehabilitation
Baylor College of Medicine
Assistant Director for Research and Education
Department of Occupational Therapy
The Institute for Rehabilitation and Research
Houston, Texas

Fae Garden, MD
Assistant Professor
Physical Medicine and Rehabilitation
Baylor College of Medicine
Assistant Chief
Physical Medicine and Rehabilitation Service
St. Luke's Episcopal Hospital
Houston, Texas

Susan J. Garrison, MD
Associate Professor
Department of Physical Medicine and Rehabilitation
Baylor College of Medicine

Medical Director, Rehabilitation Center
The Methodist Hospital
Houston, Texas

Terrence P. Glennon, MD
Assistant Professor
Department of Physical Medicine and Rehabilitation
Baylor College of Medicine
The Methodist Hospital
Houston, Texas

Steve M. Gnatz, MD
Associate Professor of Clinical Physical Medicine and
Rehabilitation
University of Missouri
Rusk Rehabilitation Center
Columbia, Missouri

Martin Grabois, MD
Professor and Chairman
Department of Physical Medicine and Rehabilitation
Baylor College of Medicine
Chief of Service
Physical Medicine and Rehabilitation
The Methodist Hospital & The Harris County Hospital
District
Executive Vice President
The Institute of Rehabilitation and Research
Houston, Texas

S. Ann Holmes, MD
Assistant Professor
Baylor College of Medicine
Spinal Cord Injury Service
Veterans Affairs Medical Center
Houston, Texas

Katie D. Irani, MBBS
Assistant Professor Physical Medicine and Rehabilitation
Baylor College of Medicine

Chief of Physical Medicine and Rehabilitation
Harris County Hospital District
Ben Taub General Hospital, Quentin Mease Community
Hospital and L. B. Johnson Hospital
Houston, Texas

Cindy B. Ivanhoe, MD
Assistant Professor
Department of Physical Medicine and Rehabilitation
Baylor College of Medicine
Co-Director, Brain Injury Program
The Institute for Rehabilitation and Research
Houston, Texas

Anjali Jain, MD
Medical Director of Physical Medicine and Rehabilitation
and Electromyography
Twelve Oaks Hospital
Houston, Texas

C. George Kevorkian, MD
Assistant Professor
Baylor College of Medicine
Chief, Physical Medicine and Rehabilitation Service
St. Luke's Episcopal Hospital
Houston, Texas

Thomas A. Krouskop, PE, PhD
Professor, Department of Physical Medicine and
Rehabilitation
Baylor College of Medicine
Director, Rehabilitation Engineering
The Institute for Rehabilitation and Research
Houston, Texas

Indira S. Lanig, MD
Formerly Co-Chief Resident and Assistant Professor
Departments of Physical Medicine and Rehabilitation
Baylor College of Medicine and
Chief, Spinal Cord Injury Service, Veterans Affairs Medical
Center

Houston, Texas
Assistant Clinical Professor, Department of Rehabilitation
Medicine
University of Colorado Health Science Center
Denver, Colorado
Staff Physician, Craig Hospital
Rocky Mountain Regional Spinal Injury System
Engelwood, Colorado

Janusz Markowski, MD
Assistant Professor
Department of Physical Medicine and Rehabilitation
Baylor College of Medicine
Chief, Spinal Cord Injury Service
Veterans Administration Medical Center
Houston, Texas

Maureen R. Nelson, MD
Assistant Professor
Departments of Physical Medicine and Rehabilitation and
Pediatrics
Baylor College of Medicine
Chief, Physical Medicine and Rehabilitation
Texas Children's Hospital
Houston, Texas

Madhura V. Patel, MD
Clinical Instructor, Baylor College of Medicine
Medical Director, Center for Rehabilitation
San Jacinto Methodist Hospital
Houston, Texas

Shahzadi Saleem, MD
Assistant Professor
Department of Physical Medicine and Rehabilitation
Baylor College of Medicine
Staff Physician
Veteran Administration Medical Center
Houston, Texas

Donna Marie Schramm, MD
Assistant Professor
Baylor College of Medicine
Houston, Texas

Itzel S. Solis, MD
Clinical Assistant Professor of Physical Medicine and
Rehabilitation
Clinical Assistant Professor of Pediatrics
Affiliated with Baylor College of Medicine
Medical Director for Muscular Dystrophy Clinic at The
Institute for Rehabilitation and Research
Houston, Texas
Medical Director, BayCoast Rehabilitation Unit
Baytown, Texas

Barry S. Smith, MD
Clinical Associate Professor
Department of Physical Medicine and Rehabilitation
The University of Texas Southwestern Medical Center at
Dallas
Chief of Physical Medicine and Rehabilitation
Baylor University Medical Center
Dallas, Texas

Carlos Vallbona, MD
Distinguished Service Professor
Chairman, Department of Community Medicine
Baylor College of Medicine
Houston, Texas

Jon VanDeventer, MD, PhD
Assistant Professor
Department of Physical Medicine and Rehabilitation
Baylor College of Medicine
Houston, Texas
Private Practice
Harrison-Methodist Hospital
Fort Worth, Texas

Michael J. Vennix, MD
Assistant Professor
Baylor College of Medicine
Director, Electromyography Laboratory
Methodist Hospital
Houston, Texas

Foreword

The conception and birth of this special book was inevitable. Only two questions remained: who would be the lucky parents, and what would be the result? We now know the impeccable parentage but would we now greet a lusty offspring to match that heredity with a marvellous future?

The interested onlooker will ask if the newcomer can compete in the burgeoning field of Physical Medicine and Rehabilitation textbooks. Indeed, it can and it will because it possesses brilliant and healthy qualities that place it immediately into a successful class of useful books. In a game that is becoming dominated by three-hundred-pound linebackers, it clearly will become an inspired and unbeatable quarterback.

All this is no accident. The editor, Dr. Garrison, was designed as though by nature to produce such a handbook. Her illustrious team of authors are an American Who's Who of practical physiatrists with skills to complement hers. This little book will bring to the ponderous game of giants a clarity and zip that has been missing, even though it was neither designed to replace nor will it replace the ponderous textbooks. They, of course, provide the muscle and weight that rehabilitation also requires.

So now the team is complete. Every important maneuver is stored in essential form within this handbook, ready for practical application. Medical students, interns, and residents will quickly find in its pages the fundamental game plans for both the most common and uncommon situations they meet in Rehabilitation.

As an author of rehabilitation books, naturally I am envious of the easy success this handbook will achieve, but I am proud to be asked to be its godfather by my writing this Foreword. With sincere thoughts and emotions, I welcome this lovely creation to the family. Long may it thrive!

John Basmajian, O.Ont,
MD, FRCPC, FRCP (Glasgow),
FACA, FSBM, FABMR, FAFRM
(Australia), Hon Dip (St L C)
Professor Emeritus, Medicine
and Anatomy
McMaster University

Preface

The idea for compiling a basic written approach to the practice of Physical Medicine and Rehabilitation was conceived in response to a need frequently vocalized by medical students, residents, and attending faculty for a quick, handy, reliable pocket-type guide to be used in the hospital or office setting, literally outside of the patient's door. Here in the nationally renowned Department of Physical Medicine and Rehabilitation at Baylor College of Medicine, Houston, we have easy access to a number of diverse, academically and clinically astute physiatrists who could readily put their practice management techniques into writing, so the task began.

The cookbook-type format and the chapter template emerged from the 1987–1988 Administrative Committee of the department. After a basic introduction to Physical Medicine and Rehabilitation (PM&R), topics are listed alphabetically by general diagnosis, such as fractures, stroke, and spinal cord injury. The chapters follow the outline of definition, anatomy, epidemiology, etiology/pathophysiology, assessment, treatment, complications, prognosis, and outcome/follow-up. They include both general information and specifics as related to various age groups. Each chapter is complete but also directs the reader to related information in other chapters. In order to keep the text practical, each chapter includes a reading list, rather than specific references. The index serves as a quick guide to common PM&R terms and topics.

The Administrative Committee was also responsible for selecting the original 14 chapter topics, subsequently revised and expanded to the current 20. Many of these committee members, in addition to writing chapters, served as informal second editors for review of initial chapter drafts. Other members reviewed and revised subsequent chapters.

As the project progressed, some faculty members left and others joined the department. Although all the chapter authors at one time in their respective careers were faculty at Baylor, the total of 30 authors were educated at 10 different PM&R training programs and now represent 7 different academic programs.

I am grateful to Dr. Martin Grabois for his permission to undertake the project through the auspices of the Administrative Committee, as well as his assistance in leading me to J. B. Lippincott Company. Others who were helpful include Mr. Tony O'Callaghan, who read and commented on all initial chapters, Dr. David Cifu, who critically reviewed additional chapters, and Dr. Henry Ostermann, who converted various software formats into a final form. Artist Ann Saydlowski created line drawings, and Lippincott editors, Emily Linkins and Wendy Greenberger-Czarnecki, were always helpful.

This project could not have been completed without the unwavering daily effort of my secretary, Chris Robinson. I will be forever grateful for her many creative ideas and tenacity in completing this project. I also appreciate the patience of my husband, Dr. Greg Gerber, and children, Grant and Gwen, for enduring the seemingly never-ending interruptions in their lives during the completion of this book.

It is my sincere hope that we have met our initial objectives in providing a clear, concise, basic approach to the ever-expanding field of Physical Medicine and Rehabilitation. The person who will most benefit from the handbook will use the basic points presented to guide independent study, beginning with the suggested readings. Use this book to learn enough to ask more questions.

Susan J. Garrison, MD, Editor
Associate Professor
Department of Physical Medicine and Rehabilitation
Baylor College of Medicine
Houston, Texas

Contents

1

David X. Cifu
Janusz Markowski

Physical Medicine and Rehabilitation: Philosophy, Patient Care Issues and Physiatric Evaluation

▮ Philosophy

Physical medicine and rehabilitation (PM&R) involves the diagnosis and treatment of physical and functional disorders. The rehabilitation model differs from the traditional medical model in several ways. Management of disability, rather than treatment of disease, is emphasized. The physician is considered a teacher or facilitator rather than merely a "knower" or a "doer"; the patient is an active, rather than passive, participant. PM&R employs an interdisciplinary team approach, wherein specialists exchange information and ideas about various problems. The traditional model utilizes a more fragmented multidisciplinary approach of multiple specialists working independently on specific problems. The goals of the rehabilitation model are improvement of function and adjustment to disability, rather than disease cure.

Commonly used terms in PM&R include impairment, disability, and handicap. Impairment signifies the residual limitation resulting from disease, injury, or a congenital defect, such as loss of motor strength of the legs after a spinal cord injury. Disability signifies the inability to perform a functional skill, such as walking. Handicap signifies the interaction of a disability with the environment, such as being unable to enter a restaurant because it is not wheelchair accessible.

Susan J. Garrison (Ed.): *Handbook of Physical Medicine and Rehabilitation Basics*. First Edition. Copyright © 1995 J. B. Lippincott Company

History

The origins of physical medicine can be traced to the centuries-old tradition of employing physical agents such as heat, cold, and water for medical benefit, and specifically to the 1890 introduction of therapeutic diathermy, a type of deep heating using shortwaves. The principles of medical rehabilitation were initially formulated during treatment of soldiers in 1919 following World War I. The merging of PM&R into a single field began in the 1920s, gained momentum in the 1930s, and was spurred on by World War II; by 1947 PM&R was officially sanctioned as a specialty by the American Board of Medical Specialties. Physiatry, from the Greek "physio," or nature, is the shortened name of the specialty, and the physiatrist (pronounced fizz-ee-at' trist) is a specialist in PM&R.

Board qualification in PM&R requires a 1 year medical, surgical, or pediatric internship followed by 3 years of PM&R residency. Fellowships in PM&R are generally 1 year in duration, and include pediatrics, head injury, spinal cord injury, sports medicine, electrodiagnosis, and research. Board certification requires successful completion of both a written and oral examination. Currently, there are approximately 1200 PM&R residents in over 75 accredited residency programs nationwide. Since 1947, over 4300 physicians have been certified as Diplomates of the American Board of Physical Medicine and Rehabilitation; over half of these have been certified in the last 10 years.

Patient Care Issues

Interdisciplinary Team

Use of the interdisciplinary team in patient management distinguishes PM&R practice from other medical specialties. The team works together to evaluate and identify problems, set therapeutic goals, and provide intervention. The patient's diagnosis and the therapeutic setting, such as inpatient or outpatient, determines the degree of interdisciplinary in-

volvement as well as the specific team members who comprise the team. These may include the following:

Dietician.   The dietician evaluates nutritional status; recommends appropriate diet based on personal and team assessments; and counsels patient/family on dietary modifications.

Occupational Therapist (OT).   The OT emphasizes fine motor
skills; evaluates and trains patient in activities of daily living
(ADL) skills (dressing, hygiene, bathing, eating); provides
range of motion (ROM), strengthening, endurance, and coordination exercises for the upper extremities and cervical area;
assesses driving skills; and recommends orthoses (braces) for
the upper extremities, adaptive equipment (modified utensils, reachers), and home modifications as needed.

Physiatrist.   The physiatrist evaluates medical/functional
status, manages medical care, orders therapies, and usually
coordinates total rehabilitation/physical medicine efforts.

Physical Therapist (PT).   The PT emphasizes gross motor
skills; evaluates and trains patient in mobility, such as wheelchair and gait; teaches balance and transfer skills involving
moving from one fixed position to another, such as from bed
to chair; provides ROM, strengthening, endurance and coordination exercises for limbs and trunk; provides physical modalities including superficial and deep heat, cold, hydrotherapy, electrical stimulation, and traction; and recommends
specific orthoses and adaptive equipment such as wheelchairs
and gait aides.

Prosthetist/Orthotist.   The prosthetist/orthotist designs, fab-
ricates, and fits prostheses (artificial limbs) and orthoses
(braces and splints).

Psychologist.   The psychologist assesses emotional, intellectual and perceptual functioning; counsels and provides psychotherapy to patient and family; and provides the team with
recommendations for care.

Recreational Therapist (RT).   The RT assesses the patient's
interests and skills; incorporates leisure time activities into
the rehab program; and assists in the patient's community
reintegration.

Rehabilitation Nurse.   The rehabilitation nurse manages the
nursing care team, serves as an educational resource to other
(non-rehabilitation) nursing personnel, instructs patient/

family in functional skills, and reinforces skills learned in therapy.

Social Worker.   The social worker evaluates the patient's living situation; discusses financial and living arrangement options; provides emotional support to patient, family and team; and serves as a liaison between patient/family and the team.

Speech Pathologist.   The speech pathologist evaluates and treats problems with communication and swallowing, and assists with cognitive retraining.

Vocational Counselor.   The vocational counselor evaluates vocational interests, training and skills; provides counseling concerning returning to work; and serves as a liaison between the patient and prospective employers.

Others.   Professionals who may be a part of the team (depending on the clinical milieu) include: respiratory therapist, child life specialist, horticultural therapist, music therapist, dance therapist, animal-assisted therapy specialist, chaplain, rehabilitation dentist, audiologist, and pharmacist.

Rehabilitative Care Settings

PM&R is involved in the care of patients with a variety of diagnoses. These include amputation, arthritis, traumatic brain injury (TBI), burns, cancer, cardiopulmonary disease, chronic pain, fractures, pressure ulcers, sports injury, stroke, musculoskeletal (acute) pain, neuromuscular disease, congenital deformities, childhood onset disabilities, peripheral and central nervous system dysfunction, osteoporosis, disabilities related to aging, polytrauma, spinal cord injury, and generalized deconditioning due to any factors. The settings in which each of these is typically managed and the interdisciplinary team members usually involved can be summarized as follows in Table 1-1.

Future Trends

The future of physiatry, while difficult to predict, will certainly include a greater emphasis on the rehabilitation con-

Table 1-1. Rehabilitative Care Settings

Setting	Rehabilitation Category	Team Members
Inpatient Rehabilitation • Free-standing facility, general or specialized • Unit within an acute care hospital, usually general rehabilitation	Amputation, arthritis, brain injury, cancer, cardiopulmonary, musculoskeletal, CNS dysfunction, fractures, geriatrics, neuromuscular, pediatrics, peripheral neuropathy, polytrauma, SCI, stroke. Patient demonstrates lack of independence in mobility, ADLs, and/or communication.	Physiatrist, OT, PT, social worker, psychologist, dietician, RT, speech pathologist, pharmacist, prosthetist/orthotist, nurse, vocational counselor, and other specialty therapists
Inpatient Consultation • Acute care facility including psychiatry • Skilled nursing facility • Nursing home	Same as above, as well as chronic pain, and generalized deconditioning. Patient may not yet be a candidate for inpatient rehabilitation due to medical/surgical instability.	Physiatrist, consulting physician, appropriate therapists, social worker, prosthetist/orthotist, pharmacist, and dietician
Outpatient rehabilitation • Free-standing comprehensive outpatient rehab facility • Affiliated with acute care facility (PT/OT/speech departments)	Same as above, and chronic pain, industrial injuries, and sports medicine. Patient has progressed through inpatient rehab or does not require inpatient hospitalization for treatment.	Physiatrist, social worker, therapists, prosthetist/orthotist, vocational counselor

cerns of the geriatric population and the severely disabled. This is due to a number of factors:

- Overall increased life expectancy—the proportion of elderly individuals 65 years and older in this society is projected to increase from 12% in the 1990s to 20% in 2030.
- The percentage of so-called "old-old" individuals, 75 years and over, in the geriatric population will increase from 39% at present to 50% in the year 2030.
- The population of "oldest-old," 85 years and older, by the year 2050 will have increased nearly 7 times compared to 1920. Individuals of these advanced age groups are more prone to have multiple diseases and require more functional support. In order to allow an enhanced quality of life, more extensive and comprehensive interventions are required.
- Survivability of even the severely disabled has vastly increased in recent years, due to technological advances in care. This has resulted in an increasing proportion of dependent individuals, capable of living near-normal life-spans, who will require extensive intervention.

▉ Physiatric Evaluation

Chief Complaint

Record the chief complaint in the patient's own words. This gives important clues in assessing the patient's perceptual status, intellectual level, and concerns regarding existing illness and dysfunction.

Medical History and the Review of Systems

Regardless of medical specialty, the basic elements of medical history taking are the same. In PM&R, the history should also reflect upon the extent to which the chief complaint affects the patient's physical and functional independence. In

Table 1-2. Medical Rehabilitation Patient Problem List

1. Left hemiplegia secondary to right CVA, thrombotic, on *(date)*

2. Functional dependence secondary to #1

3. Urinary incontinence secondary to #2

4. History of hypertension, medication controlled

5. History of coronary artery disease with angina pectoris

6. History of glaucoma with decreased visual acuity

7. History of urinary tract infection (resolved)

8. Status post cholecystectomy (inactive)

certain situations, this information may require the corroboration of the patient's primary caregiver.

In reviewing organ systems, remember that any illness or disability affects multiple areas. Carefully address each of these. Create a comprehensive problem list, listing active and inactive problems. (See Table 1-2).

Use patience in taking a history from a patient with a communication disorder, such as a stroke, cerebral palsy, or head injury. Speech difficulties are far more frustrating to the patient than to the physician. Assistance from a speech therapist or a family member may be helpful.

Vocational and Social History

Document the patient's social and vocational history in detail. The social history gives insight into social dynamics and available support systems which will affect the patient's reintegration into society. The vocational history provides a guideline for possible retraining to return the patient to the workforce or to assist in vocational or recreational activities. See Table 1-3.

Functional History and Evaluation

When loss of function results from an illness or an injury, the disability must be assessed in terms of the patient's indepen-

Table 1-3. Social/Vocational History

> Support system
>
> Premorbid personality
>
> Premorbid life style
>
> Educational level
>
> Substance abuse
>
> Work history (type, place, abilities)
>
> History of avocational (recreational) interests

dent functioning at home, at work, or at school, and compared to premorbid functioning. The key functions include:

- Self-Care (feeding, grooming, bathing, dressing, and toileting).
- Sphincter control (bladder and bowel).
- Mobility/transfers (bed, chair, toilet and shower).
- Locomotion (wheelchair, ambulation and stair-climbing).
- Social cognition (social interaction, problem solving and memory).
- Communication.

Degrees of dependence/independence can be briefly described as follows:

- Fully independent.
- Independent with an assistive device or modification of the environment.
- Stand-by assistance required (supervision by another person) in some, or most, of daily functioning.
- Physical assistance required in some, or all, of daily functioning.
- Fully dependent.

Various scales have been developed for a more uniform evaluation of function. The Functional Independence Measure (FIM) assesses activities of self-care, mobility, locomotion, communication and social cognition on a 7-point scale from fully independent to fully dependent. It is the most widely used global (general) scale of function. There are more task specific scales which can be utilized, including the Barthel Index, the Katz Index, the Kenny Index, and the Klein-Bell ADL Scale.

Physical Examination

The physical examination in its key elements (inspection, palpation and auscultation) does not differ from that of any other specialty. It is, however, more problem-focused in its attempt to determine how the existing disability affects the functioning of other organ systems, and to what extent the body compensates for impaired or lost function of any organ systems.

The physical examination should include:

1. Vital signs.
2. Mental status exam.
   a. Alertness.
   b. Logical thinking.
   c. Understanding and following instructions.
   d. Recent and immediate recall.
   e. Hostile or threatening behavior.
   f. Confabulations.
3. Neuromuscular examination: DOCUMENT PATIENT POSITION! (lying, sitting, or standing).
   a. Inspection.
      1. Joint alignment (contractures, hypomobility or deformity).
      2. Muscle bulk (atrophy or hypertrophy).
      3. Muscles' activity (clonus or increased tone at rest).
      4. Body posture (leaning, imbalance).
      5. Cranial and peripheral nerve assessment (muscle asymmetry, posturing).
   b. Palpation.
      1. Range of motion (active and passive).
      2. Joint stability.
      3. Muscle tone (both active movement and passive stretch).

Table 1-4. Muscle Strength*

Grade	Assessment
0/5 (absent)	No evidence of muscle contraction
1/5 (trace)	Visible contraction but no joint movement
2/5 (poor)	Full range of motion with gravity eliminated
3/5 (fair)	Full range of motion against gravity
4/5 (good)	Full movement against moderate resistance
5/5 (normal)	Full movement against strong resistance

*This does not apply to the strong antigravity muscles, which are too powerful to be assessed by manual examination. Tiptoe or heel walking is a better way of assessing the gastrocnemius and tibialis anterior muscles, respectively.

    4. Muscle strength (see Table 1-4).
    5. Altered perception of touch, pain, temperature, and proprioception.
    6. Deep tendon reflexes (on scale 0–4+).
    7. Presence of abnormal reflex (Babinski, Kernig, Bulbocavernosus).
    8. Cerebellar exam (synchronous action of muscle groups with volitional movement, nystagmus, imbalance).
4. Functional examination.
    a. Bed mobility (turning from side to side).
    b. Sitting.
      1. Coming from supine to sit.
      2. Static (supported) vs. dynamic (unsupported).
    c. Transfers.
      1. From sit to stand.
      2. From bed to other surface.
      3. Type, *i.e.,* standing pivot.
      4. Document equipment, such as sliding board.
    d. Gait.
      1. Document assistive device, if any:
        Hand used.
        Appropriate sequencing.
        Condition of device.

2. Observe ambulation from front, side, and rear.
3. Note abnormalities such as wide or narrow base of support, prolonged or shortened stance phase, hip hiking, circumduction, Trendelenburg gait (indicating pelvic stabilizer weakness).

Electrodiagnosis

Electrodiagnosis is a diagnostic tool which augments the clinical examination, specifically with regard to the neuromuscular system. It consists of needle examination of a muscle (electromyography), which determines the presence of any involuntary muscle activity at rest, (fibrillations, sharp waves, fasciculations), reflecting a muscle membrane's instability; the presence or absence of motor units, action potentials, and their recruitment patterns; and quantification and configuration of motor unit action potentials.

Nerve conduction studies (NCS) are performed to evaluate the conductibility of a peripheral nerve, including proximal and distal nerve segments; functional integrity of the neuromuscular junction; a quantitative reflex evaluation; and sensory/visual/auditory parameters (evaluating peripheral and control nerve pathways).

The most important points to remember are that the electrodiagnostic study is only an adjunct to the clinical examination, not a substitute; and it is much easier for the electromyographer to assist in making a diagnosis if the referral includes a tentative diagnosis and the reason for requesting the study.

▉ Suggested Readings

Delisa JA, Martin GM, Currie DM. Rehabilitation Medicine: Past, Present and Future. *In* Delisa JA, ed. *Rehabilitation Medicine: Principles and Practice.* Philadelphia: J.B. Lippincott, 1988, pp. 3–24.

Erickson RP, McPhee MC. Clinical Evaluation. *In* Delisa JA, ed. *Rehabilitation Medicine: Principles and Practice.* Philadelphia: J.B. Lippincott, 1988, pp. 25–65.

Grabois M. Evaluation of Disability. *In* Halstead LS, Grabois M eds. *Medical Rehabilitation.* New York: Raven Press, 1985, pp. 13–32.

Halstead LS. Philosophy of Rehabilitation Medicine. *In* Halstead LS, Grabois M eds. *Medical Rehabilitation.* New York: Raven Press, 1985, pp. 1–6.

Halstead LS, Grabois M: Rehabilitation Specialists. *In* Halstead LS, Grabois M eds. *Medical Rehabilitation.* New York: Raven Press, 1985, pp. 7–12.

Itoh M, Lee MHM. The Epidemiology of Disability as Related to Rehabilitation Medicine. *In* Kottke FJ, Stillwell GK, Lehmann JF, eds. *Krusen's Handbook of Physical Medicine and Rehabilitation.* Philadelphia: W.B. Saunders, 1982, pp. 199–217.

2

Steve M. Gnatz

Acute Pain

▦ Definition

Pain is the most common reason patients seek treatment by physicians. Biologically, the pain signal represents potentially dangerous tissue damage. Pain is a warning to the organism to stop or escape from damaging activity and allow regenerative processes to work. However, pain is a complex interplay of peripheral nerve, spinal cord, and brain processes which are incompletely understood. If, for unknown reasons, the pain signal continues despite the removal of the painful stimulus, pain loses its adaptive value and may result in significant physical and psychosocial disability.

Most acute pain can be eliminated by discontinuing the source of tissue damage, resting the damaged part, and using simple analgesia. Physical medicine techniques enhance physical recovery from many painful conditions, particularly if simple measures have not eliminated the pain or significant loss of function has occurred.

▦ Neuroanatomy and Neurophysiology of Pain Pathways

Most nociceptor afferent input is transmitted from the peripheral pain sensors through the small (0.1–1.0 μm diameter) unmyelinated C-fibers to the central nervous system

Susan J. Garrison (Ed.): *Handbook of Physical Medicine and Rehabilitation Basics*. First Edition. Copyright © 1995 J. B. Lippincott Company

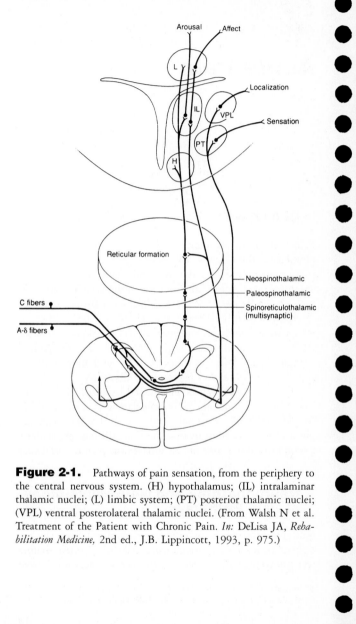

Figure 2-1. Pathways of pain sensation, from the periphery to the central nervous system. (H) hypothalamus; (IL) intralaminar thalamic nuclei; (L) limbic system; (PT) posterior thalamic nuclei; (VPL) ventral posterolateral thalamic nuclei. (From Walsh N et al. Treatment of the Patient with Chronic Pain. *In:* DeLisa JA, *Rehabilitation Medicine,* 2nd ed., J.B. Lippincott, 1993, p. 975.)

(CNS). Some pain impulses, particularly thermal and mechanical pressure stimuli, reach the CNS through myelinated A-delta-fibers (1–4 μm diameter). Peripheral stimuli enter the dorsal horn of the spinal cord where most of the C fibers synapse in the substantia gelatinosa (lamina II). Pain impulses ascend the spinothalamic and spinoreticular tracts to project on the lateral and medial thalamic nuclei and the brainstem, respectively (see Figure 2-1). Projection of these impulses to the sensory cortical areas brings the pain to consciousness and makes locating it in the body possible. Substance P, an 11-amino acid peptide, has been identified as a peripheral neurotransmitter in the dorsal horn of the spinal cord. Endogenous opioids such as beta endorphin and enkephalins in the CNS and periphery inhibit pain.

▇ Epidemiology

Pain is a universal phenomenon. Everyone will experience pain during his/her lifetime. At least 80% of the population at some time will have low back pain, the most common cause of worker absence and loss of productivity in industrialized countries. Neck pain may be present in up to 50% of the population at some time in life, and up to 20% of the female population experiences fibromyalgia. About 1.6% of the population has an ongoing problem with temporomandibular joint pain. See Table 2-1 for common symptoms of craniomandibular dysfunction.

▇ Etiology and Pathophysiology

Acute pain can usually be linked to a precipitating event, usually traumatic. Possible etiologies are in Table 2-2.

   Assume that all pain is real. However, remember that pain is subjective; there can be no objective measurement of it. Pain that is incapacitating to one may be inconsequential to another, or to the same person under different circumstances. All pain perception is individual.

   In general, the longer pain persists, the less likely complete resolution becomes. This assumes that adequate work-

Table 2-1. Common Symptoms of Craniomandibular
Dysfunction

- **Jaw Symptoms**
  Painful movement and limited opening

  Clicking, popping or other joint noise

  Locking open or closed

- **Headaches**
  Usually muscle-contraction type

  Areas involved: temporal, occipital, or generalized

  May present with vascular or migraine-like symptoms

- **Ear symptoms**
  Tinnitus, fullness in the ears, hearing loss

  Vestibular dysfunction, vertigo, dizziness, nausea

- **Eye symptoms**
  Pain behind the eyes, blurring of vision, photophobia

- **Facial, neck, and upper back pain**
  Generally described as tightness, soreness, stiffness

  May be sharp, hyperesthetic (can mimic neuralgia,
  radiculopathy)

- **Other**
  Sinus pressure, stuffiness

  Tooth and gum complaints

  Autonomic phenomena, sweating, lacrimation

  Swallowing difficulty

up for etiologic and contributing factors has been performed
and that perpetuating factors have been controlled as much as
possible. Patients who are adaptable, educable and willing to
take responsibility for aspects of treatment within their control generally have better outcomes than those with significant psychosocial issues, lack of insight, or secondary gain
motives.

Table 2-2. Etiologies of Acute Pain

Trauma

Overuse syndrome

Improper body mechanics

"Microtrauma"

Systemic or localized disease process
Degenerative
Inflammatory
Infectious
Malignant

General Guidelines for Assessment of the Patient with Pain

* Obtain a complete medication and treatment history. Do not repeat a previously unsuccessful treatment, unless it was implemented incorrectly.
* Review previous diagnostic tests, operative reports, therapists' notes, consultants' notes and recorded psychosocial information.
* Have the patient complete a pain diagram.
* Use a pain rating scale.
* Identify an acute traumatic event, if possible.
* Characterize pain using the mnemonic PQRST: Provocative and Palliative Factors, Quality, Region-Radiation, Severity and Temporal Characteristics. Pain can be diffuse and difficult for the patient to describe.
* Obtain pain descriptors which help identify a specific pain syndrome.
* Observe the patient walking, sitting, and moving both when unaware of being observed and when being directed. Assess what, if any, functional overlay is present.
* Organize the proper work-up for diagnosis.
* Develop a rational treatment plan, based on the established diagnosis. It is better to leave a patient undiagnosed than to make an erroneous diagnosis.

Table 2-3. Differential Diagnosis of Commonly Seen
Musculoskeletal Pain Problems

• **Bone**
  Fracture (acute traumatic, stress, compression)

  Dislocation

  Metastatic lesion

  Other intrinsic bone lesion (bone cyst, osteoma,
  hemangioma, etc.)

  Infection

• **Joint**
  Cartilaginous dysfunction (tear, degeneration, inflammation,
  dislocation)

  Synovial fluid (gout, pseudogout, infection, etc.)

  Ligaments (tear, stretch, contracture)

  Capsule, bursae (inflammation, contracture)

  Osteophytic spurring

• **Muscle, tendon**
  Overstretch, tear, rupture

  Contracture

  Weakness, fatigue

  Inflammation, intrinsic muscle disease

  Trigger points, tender points (myofascial pain)

  Inflammation of tendon sheath (tenosynovitis)

• **Nerve**
  Compression (nerve roots, peripheral entrapments)

  Stretch (brachial plexus, etc.)

  Direct Trauma

  Inflammation

  Neuropathy (diabetic, EtoH etc.)

Table 2-3. (*continued*)

• **Biomechanical, kinesiologic**
  Postural abnormality

  Overuse, unequal or imbalanced strength

  Gait abnormality

  Anatomical variation (unequal leg lengths, etc.)

Differential diagnoses of commonly seen musculoskeletal pain problems are listed in Table 2-3.

■ Functional Evaluation

Obtain a history of the patient's current and past social situation, including vocational, family and interpersonal stresses. Characterize the extent of disability by noting current functional limitations in activities of daily living, exercise endurance, and dependence on adaptive equipment. Record litigation status and other aspects of potential secondary gain which may impede recovery.

■ Physical Exam

The physical exam is a directed neuromuscular and joint exam. Identify the painful structures and document variations from the normal which may interfere with function. While details of the exam are specified by the history, certain elements are constant. Seek alterations in muscle strength, sensation, and deep tendon reflexes. Patients often cannot participate in manual muscle testing because of the resulting pain. "Give-way" weakness is not always associated with poor cooperation on the patient's part.

Search carefully for dermatomal or root level dysfunction of sensory and reflex systems. These hard neurologic signs are difficult to produce voluntarily. However, muscle atrophy due to immobility may contribute to decreased deep tendon reflexes.

Examine joint structures for effusion, decreased range of motion, and deformity; palpate tendons and ligamentous structures.

Palpate muscle to evaluate for trigger areas or tight bands of muscle that, when deeply palpated, cause referred pain. Figure 2-2 demonstrates common areas related to fibromyalgia (myofascial pain). Instruct the patient to perform specific maneuvers such as a straight leg raising test (patient

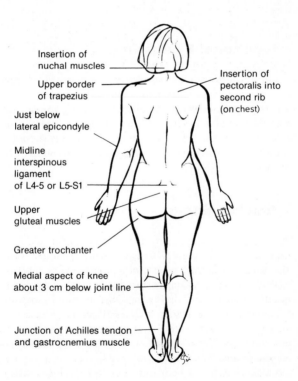

Insertion of
nuchal muscles

Upper border
of trapezius

Just below
lateral epicondyle

Midline
interspinous
ligament
of L4-5 or L5-S1

Upper
gluteal muscles

Greater trochanter

Medial aspect of knee
about 3 cm below joint line

Junction of Achilles tendon
and gastrocnemius muscle

Insertion of
pectoralis into
second rib
(on chest)

Figure 2-2. Typical locations of tender points in myofascial pain.

Table 2-4. Other Tests

Category	Uses/Examples
Physical quantitative testing	Cybex/Stress test
Diagnosis-specific laboratory data	Rheumatoid factor, ANA, CPK, sedimentation rate
Radiographic evaluation	
Routine	Identify fractures, bone and joint pathology
MRI	Identify muscle, tendon, ligament abnormalities
Electrodiagnostic testing (EMG/NCV)	Evaluation of the neuro-muscular system, nerve entrapments, radiculopathy, myopathy, or myositis

supine, leg raised from horizontal), Tinel's sign (tap over median nerves of wrist), or the Finkelstein test (thumb wrapped up in fist, wrist ulnar deviated) to aid in the clinical confirmation of the suspected diagnosis. Other tests are listed in Table 2-4.

Treatment

Treatment of acutely painful conditions differs from the treatment of chronic pain. In acute pain management, resting the damaged structure is essential for recovery. This contrasts with the management of chronic pain, where the patient usually needs mobilization due to underuse of affected areas. Contracture of collagenous structures, including tendon, ligament, and joint capsules, occurs rapidly in patients with painful range of motion. These may require gentle passive range of motion (PROM) to avoid the vicious cycle of pain to immobility to contracture to increased pain. Similarly, atrophy of immobilized muscle should be avoided, if possible, through the use of isometric exercise.

Physical Modalities

The physical modalities of heat, cold, electricity, sound, and water are used to accomplish the goal of increased function while minimizing pain. Both heat and cold provide analgesic effects. Heat is useful in both acute and chronic pain for analgesia, muscle relaxation, and enhancement of the stretchability of collagen. Cold may be more beneficial in acute pain for its ability to control edema; heat may exacerbate edema, if present. In general, use cold for the first 24 to 48 hours after an acute injury and heat thereafter.

Many forms of heat are available, including hot packs, shortwave and microwave diathermy, and ultrasound. Hydrotherapy provides heat, but is a much better debriding agent than a heating one. Such devices as moist air cabinets, paraffin baths, and fluidotherapy are indicated in some cases of arthritic pain.

The depth of penetration of heating modalities varies. Hot packs give superficial heat to the skin and subcutaneous tissue; microwave and shortwave diathermy provide deeper heat, warming some muscle layers. Ultrasound, working at the tissue/fluid interface, is the only heating modality which raises the intra-articular temperature of large joints significantly. Heating modalities are contraindicated in specific cases. See Table 2-5.

Electrical Modalities

Transcutaneous neuronal electrical stimulation (TENS) modulates pain by applying electrical impulses to the skin. There are two basic types: high frequency, low intensity TENS (conventional TENS), and low frequency, high intensity TENS (electro-acupuncture). Conventional TENS works due to the "gate" theory of pain. Presented simply, this involves incoming cutaneous sensory and proprioceptive impulses carried through larger myelinated nerve fibers, which inhibit pain impulses carried more slowly by unmyelinated nerve fibers at the level of the dorsal column of the spinal cord. The

Table 2-5. Contraindications for use of heat

Insensate areas (risk of burns)

Acute infection, inflammation or edema

Compromised vascular supply

Tumors

Unknown underlying pathology

faster impulses arrive at the dorsal column first and "close the gate," forestalling propagation of the slower pain impulses.

The second type of TENS, high voltage galvanic stimulation or electro-acupuncture, utilizes a more pronounced "jolt" of electrical stimulation, which increases endogenous opioid substances in the brain. Electro-acupuncture may be less useful in the treatment of some pain disorders because of the painful nature of the stimulus itself.

The advantage of TENS is that it is noninvasive. Several different electrodes and stimulator settings should be utilized before discontinuing it for failing to relieve pain. Individual response to TENS is the rule. There are a few contraindications to TENS. To avoid vagal stimulation, it should not be placed over the anterolateral aspect of the neck. Theoretically, it may cause malfunction of cardiac pacemakers. Hypersensitivity to the electrodes (skin irritation) occasionally necessitates discontinuation, but can be minimized if different electrodes are used.

Medications

Many patients will have been prescribed numerous medications by other physicians if they have had pain for any length of time. It is important to know which medications have been tried, which were effective, and how they were taken in order rationally to provide pharmacologic adjunct therapy in a rehabilitation program.

Narcotic analgesics are rarely indicated in the treatment

of pain, other than in emergency or very acute situations. However, some patients may be dependent on or frankly addicted to narcotic analgesic medications. Do *not* prescribe pain medications on a PRN basis; this reinforces pain behavior. Patients should take medication on a schedule, regardless of the level of pain. If they feel they do not need the prescribed amount of medication, they should reduce the dosage. If they feel they need more pain relief, they should be instructed to try nonpharmacologic techniques first. Failing these, new therapy should be planned with their physician.

Nonsteroidal anti-inflammatory drugs (NSAIDs) such as ibuprofen have both analgesic and anti-inflammatory properties. While there is significant variability between agents, usually the anti-inflammatory effect is obtained at 2 to 4 times the analgesic dose. Generally, those NSAIDs with a longer half-life allow better patient compliance, but do not afford as quick an analgesic effect after the dose is taken. Aspirin produces more gastrointestinal irritation and less anti-inflammatory effect than the other NSAIDs. Other side effects of NSAIDs include fluid retention and, rarely, renal or liver problems.

Muscle relaxants such as cyclobenzaprine HCl (Flexeril), methocarbamol (Robaxin), and carisoprodol (Soma) may be indicated for the short-term (10–day) treatment of acute muscle spasm. Drowsiness associated with these agents makes them potentially dangerous for certain patients such as machinery operators, whose mental alertness is required for safety. They should not be taken with alcohol.

Amitriptyline (Elavil) is a tricyclic antidepressant with excellent analgesic properties, probably based on CNS modulation of the serotenergic pathways. It can be effective for pain relief in doses much lower than those used for depression. Usually 25 to 100 mg at bedtime is sufficient for analgesia. The side effects include drowsiness, which is limited by use at bedtime, and anticholinergic effects.

The antiseizure medications phenytoin sodium (Dilantin) and carbamazepine (Tegretol) probably control pain through their membrane stabilizing effects. Monitor for side effects.

Other Treatments

Other treatment methods are listed in Table 2-6.

Exercise is an important adjunct therapy. Finding the ideal combination of rest and exercise is a challenging concept for patients and practitioners alike. When acute inflammation of the muscle or joint is present, rest is necessary to allow healing to occur. However, muscle weakness and joint contracture can take place very rapidly when there is complete immobility. The key is passive range of motion (PROM) up to, but not past, the point of pain. The power required to range the joint may be provided by a therapist or by the patient after proper training. Causing pain during the ROM of the joint will only restart the vicious cycle of pain to immobility to contracture to more pain.

Isometric exercise may be initiated even in the presence of acute joint inflammation. When combined with surface electromyographic (EMG) biofeedback techniques, isometric contraction and relaxation of the muscle can be coordinated easily.

Therapeutic exercise of a subacute joint begins with gentle PROM up to, but not past, the point of pain after application of a suitable heating modality, such as hot packs and ultrasound. This maximizes ROM and minimizes pain. As inflammation subsides, the patient becomes more active in the isotonic use of muscles around the joint. Therapy ultimately concentrates more on strengthening through resistive exercise. The timing of this program is highly variable, as it depends on the patient's tolerance, and requires close follow-up by both the therapist and the doctor.

It is difficult, if not impossible, to strengthen painful muscles. To develop a muscle training response requires forces applied to the muscle and other tissues which will not be tolerated by a patient in pain; no progress will be made. Refer to Figure 2-3 for stages of recovery from acute pain.

Specific details regarding evaluation and treatment of back, neck, and fibromyalgic (myofascial) pain are listed in Tables 2-7, 2-8, and 2-9.

Table 2-6. Other Treatment Methods

What	Why	How	Limitations
Trigger point injections	Spreading out muscle fibers can relieve pain	Palpate an isolated painful point in muscle with pain referral; inject with 1–2 cc of 0.5% Procaine or 1% Xylocaine without epinephrine; Normal saline works, but does not produce immediate effect; Use ultrasound immediately afterward	Trigger points may recur, fibrosis of muscle
Spray and stretch techniques	Counterirritant effect similar to TENS and topical agents (liniments)	Use Fluoromethane or other vapocoolant spray	Works best for large muscles (trapezius)
Massage	Decreases muscle tension	Various techniques	Labor-intensive, best for short term, acute problems
Manipulation	Realignment of abnormal musculo-skeletal positioning	Apply short-arm lever techniques appropriately	Remains controversial
Functional Electrical Stimulation (FES)	Used with surface EMG biofeedback, retrains/ strengthens muscles	Use of electrical current strengthens muscle	Burns, skin sensitivity

Stage I		Stage 2		Stage 3		
Pain relief through modalities	→	Regain normal resting muscle length through ROM and flexibility exercises	→	Gradual muscle strength-ening	→	Recovery

Figure 2-3. Stages of Recovery from Acute Pain

▪ Complications

Many patients are sensitive about the psychological overlay associated with pain. Allow the patient to gain some confidence in your ability to control acute pain using physical techniques. Then, educate about the usefulness of long-term lifestyle adjustment in the management of pain. Psychological support may help the patient handle pain which you cannot control medically. Never promise to eliminate all pain!

Secondary gain, both monetary and emotional, can be a persuasive and often totally subconscious motivating factor in continuing pain behaviors. Secondary gain must be eliminated before the patient can recover.

If not treated aggressively and effectively, acute pain may progress to a chronic pain syndrome. Recognize psychosocial/behavioral issues early in order to plan comprehensive acute pain management.

Table 2-7. Back Pain—Evaluation and Treatment

History
Trauma—mechanism of injury

Past history, prior episodes, surgery

Locking, pop, snap, inability to straighten up

Radiating pain or numbness in the legs

Weakness, bladder or bowel dysfunction

Prior exercise/fitness level

Physical
Observation—skin markings, posture, pain behaviors

Range of motion—flexion, extension, lateral bending, rotation

Palpation—muscle, facet joint and spinous process tenderness

Manual muscle testing—quadriceps (L4); extensor hallicus longus (L5); gastrocnemius (S1)

Sensory—L4–S1, dermatomes

DTRs—ankle jerk-S1, knee jerk L4

Straight leg raise—sitting versus supine

Other tests—Hips, sacroiliac joints

Differential diagnosis of acute back pain
Sprain—ligamentous, strain—muscle

Disc disease—degenerative, herniation, inflammatory

Arthritis

Spondylosis, spinal stenosis, spondylolysis, spondylolisthesis

Facet joint arthropathy, subluxation

Arachnoiditis, iatrogenic—"failed back syndrome"

Neurogenic, vascular—aortic aneurysm

Viscerogenic, gynecological

Osteoporosis—fracture, dislocation, subluxation

Psychogenic—malingering

Table 2-7. (*continued*)

Malignancy—multiple myeloma, metastasis

Infectious—AIDS, TB, abscess

Treatment
Acute—rest, analgesia, superficial heat

Subacute—mobilization, PT (modalities, ROM, stretching, gradual exercise), education, posture, +/− bracing

---

Table 2-8. Neck Pain—Evaluation and Treatment

History
Trauma—mechanism of injury

Locking, crepitation, noise, spasm

Headache, dizziness

Jaw pain

Arm symptoms—numbness, weakness, leg symptoms

Past history, episodes

Dysphagia—severe spondylosis

Stress related factors

Posture-related factors—computer terminal, phone

Physical
Observation

Range of motion, crepitation

Manual muscle testing upper extremities—deltoid C5, biceps C5–6, triceps C6–7, wrist extensors C6–7, intrinsics C8

Sensory—C4–T1 dermatomes

DTRs—biceps C5–6, triceps C7–8

Differential diagnosis of neck pain
Sprain—ligamentous, strain—muscle

Disc disease—degenerative, herniation, inflammatory

Table 2-8. (*continued*)

Arthritis

Spondylosis, spinal stenosis

Facet joint arthropathy, subluxation

Arachnoiditis, iatrogenic—"failed neck syndrome"

Neurogenic

Osteoporosis—fracture, dislocation, subluxation

Psychogenic—malingering

Maliganancy—multiple myeloma, metastasis

Infectious—AIDS, TB, abscess

Torticollis, antecollis, retrocollis, other movement disorder

Treatment
Acute—rest, analgesia, superficial heat

Subacute—mobilization, PT (modalities, ROM, stretching, gradual exercise traction), education, posture, +/− bracing

Table 2-9. Myofacial Pain (Fibromyalgia)—Evaluation and Treatment

History
Pain

Muscle stiffness

Tightness

Burning

Waxing and waning

Varies in location/intensity

Stress related

Sleep disorder

Headaches

Table 2-9. (*continued*)

Soft neurological symptoms—numbness, weakness—in a nondermatomal pattern

Tolerance for exercise
Usually low

Generalized fatigue

Nutrition

Other medical stressors

Psychosocial stressors

Anxiety

Depression

Autonomic symptoms—sweating, irritable bowel

Physical
Trigger points—latent, active—in characteristic locations

Normal neurological exam

Postural abnormalities—check head to toe—evaluate for leg length discrepancy

Differential diagnosis (rule these out before making diagnosis of primary fibromyalgia)
Intrinsic muscle disease—myositis, myalgias (viral infections, etc.), infections, trichinella

Rheumatologic disease

Hyothyroidism*

Anemia*

Mitral valve prolapse*

Treatment
Patient counseling—diagnostic and therapeutic reassurance, avoidance of aggravating factors, frequent follow-up

Physical modalities—stretching, flexibility, exercises; attention to posture, position, local anesthetic sprays or injection, aerobic conditioning, muscle massage, stretching, ultrasound

Table 2-9. *(continued)*

Medications—amitriptyline (Elavil) and cyclobenzaprine
(Flexeril) of significant benefit in controlled trials; start with
10 mg of either at bedtime and increase to 25–50 mg
depending on response and toxic effects; NSAIDS and simple
analgesics may be used in combination with above, but of no
demonstrable efficacy; prednisone and narcotics should not be
used

* May be a contributing factor

▌ Suggested Readings

Bennett RM. The fibrositis-fibromyalgia syndrome. *In*
Schumacher HR, ed. *Primer on Rheumatic Diseases.* 9th ed.
Atlanta: Arthritis Foundation, 1988, pp. 227–229.

Caillet R. *Soft Tissue Pain Disability.* Philadelphia: F.A. Davis,
1981.

Caillet R. *Low Back Pain Syndrome.* Philadelphia: F.A. Davis,
1981.

Campbell CD, Loft GH, Davis H, et al.. TMJ symptoms and
referred pain patterns. *J Prosth Dent* 1987;47:430–433.

Gelb H. Present day concepts in diagnosis and treatment of
craniomandibular disorders. *NY Dent J* 1985;51:266–271.

Gnatz SM. Referred pain syndromes of the head and neck.
Phys Med Rehabil: State of the Art Reviews 1991;5:585–
596.

Hoppenfeld S. *Physical Examination of the Spine and Extremities.* Norwalk: Appleton-Century-Crofts, 1976.

Lehmann JF, ed.. *Therapeutic Heat and Cold.* 3rd ed. Baltimore: Williams & Wilkins, 1982.

Manual of Orthopaedic Surgery. Chicago: American Orthopaedic Society, 1979.

Schmidt KL, Oh VR, Rocher G, et al. Heat, Cold and Inflammation. *Rheumatology* 1979;38:391–404.

Sola AE. Evaluation of the patient presenting with upper extremity pain. *In* Wall PD and Melzack R, eds. *Textbook of Pain.* 2nd ed. London: Churchill Livingstone, 1989, pp. 354–367.

Travell JG and Simons DG. *Myofascial Pain and Dysfunction, The Trigger Point Manual.* Baltimore: Williams & Wilkins, 1983.

Wall PD. The Gate Control Theory of Pain Mechanisms. A Re-examination and Re-statement. *Brain* 1978;101:1–18.

Wall PD, Melzack R, eds.. Textbook of Pain. Edinburgh: Churchill Livingston, 1984.

Yunis MB. Diagnosis, etiology, and management of fibromyalgia syndrome: An update. *Comprehensive Therapy* 1988;14:8–20.

Terrence P. Glennon
Barry S. Smith

3

Amputations

◼ General Information

Definition

An amputation is the loss of a body part or portion of a body
part. This can be as small as the tip of the nose or as large as
the entire body below the lower lumbar vertebrae. Amputations have multiple etiologies (see Table 3-1).

This chapter focuses on the basic physiatric approaches to
the most commonly occurring amputations: below knee amputation (BKA), above knee amputation (AKA); and, in the
upper limb, below elbow (BE), and above elbow (AE). Following general comments about anatomy, clinical assessment,
treatment (including preprosthetic training), prosthetic fitting and prescription writing, complications, and outcome,
each amputation level is discussed in detail.

Anatomy

The most important aspect of an amputation is the anatomy
of the residual limb, the portion of a limb that remains after
an amputation. Important considerations are the remaining
skeletal structures; "covering" tissue, such as skin, muscle,
and subcutaneous tissue; and range of motion (ROM) and
strength of the limb. Most important is how these anatomic

Susan J. Garrison (Ed.): *Handbook of Physical Medicine and Rehabilitation
Basics.* First Edition. Copyright © 1995 J. B. Lippincott Company

Table 3-1. Causes of Amputations

Congenital

Traumatic

Dysvascular

Malignant

features relate to the residual function of the limb. This will determine how, with prosthetics or by other means, the physiatrist can assist the patient in returning to a state of maximal physical function.

Epidemiology

Amputations affect individuals in all age groups. Congenital limb deficiencies are present at birth. Amputations are necessary for treatment of some bone tumors in adolescents. Traumatic amputations result from accidents, particularly in the active young population. Vascular insufficiencies from various disease processes may result in limb loss in the older population.

Incidence/Etiology

In 1990, there were an estimated 1.23 million individuals in the United States with major limb loss. Disease of the lower limb is the most common cause of amputation in all age groups. This may result from arteriosclerotic disease, diabetes mellitus, venous dysfunction, or a combination of these as well as other vascular problems. As vascular disease progresses, closed or open wounds, followed by local or systemic infection, may ultimately result in amputation despite optimal medical-surgical care.

Trauma is the next most common cause for amputation. Motor vehicle accidents and work-related injuries along with higher risk recreational activities account for the majority of these amputations. There is a greater incidence of lower limb loss, although upper limb loss comprises nearly 10% of amputations, particularly in industrial accidents. Among individuals 10 to 20 years of age, tumor is the most common diagnosis leading to amputation.

Congenital limb deficiency occurs in approximately 24 of 100,000 live births and is nearly twice as common in the upper limb than in the lower limb. No classification system has received universal acceptance, so data collection is inconsistent.

■ Assessment/Evaluation

General Considerations

Assessing amputees involves much more than just choosing substitutes for lost body parts. Amputees must first be evaluated for their ability to function without prosthetic replacements. There will always be times when they will need to function without prosthetic devices, including upon waking, when an injury to the residual limb is present, or any time they prefer not to use prostheses.

First, assess the overall health of the patient, including the cardiopulmonary system. If there are general health limitations, they may affect the patient's progress; focus the rehabilitation program on achievable goals. To assess possible functional limitation, observe the patient, without a prosthesis, perform a transfer independently or with an assistive device such as a walker or a cane. If the amputee can perform this activity, he/she should have the necessary balance and coordination to wear a prosthesis functionally.

Energy requirement, measured by oxygen consumption, is the limiting factor in distance of ambulation. A unilateral lower limb amputee using a three-point gait with a walker or crutches consumes approximately 65% more energy than someone with normal gait. Even after prosthetic fitting and training, more energy is required for ambulation. This means that if a patient with a single AKA has the endurance to

Table 3-2. Energy Requirements of Amputees
Using Prostheses

Amputation	Energy Increase (% Above Normal)
Unilateral, below knee	10–20%
Bilateral, below knee	20–40%
Unilateral, above knee	60–70%
Bilateral, above knee	>200%

ambulate with a walker, he should be able to traverse approximately the same distance with an AKA prosthesis. Conversely, if the patient cannot ambulate with a walker due to weakness or fatigue, he/she is unlikely to be able to use a prosthesis to improve function. Levels of energy consumption have been measured for amputees after training with prostheses (Table 3-2).

Assess the patient's mental status. The patient must be able to learn new tasks, including putting on (donning) and removing (doffing) the prosthesis, observing skin for injury inside the prosthetic socket, and caring for the device. Also assess the patient's social support system, since the family and/or caregiver must provide whatever the patient may be lacking physically, cognitively, or environmentally.

Consider the patient's condition with respect to the cause of the amputation. If the amputation was a result of limb ischemia, there may be a similar problem in the other limb. If the amputation was related to cancer, there may be metastatic disease.

Document any other impairments, such as blindness, severe arthritis, stroke, or end-stage renal disease, that may interfere with the patient's functional capacity. Finally, focus your attention on the amputation site itself.

Limb Evaluation

Regardless of the amputation site, there are a number of standard measurements that must be recorded for the residual limb, as follows:

- length of terminal appendage from a fixed proximal land-mark (length of bone and soft tissue may differ);
- appearance and mobility of the scar, and state of healing of the scar;
- soft tissue coverage of the residual limb, particularly of distal bone;
- skin integrity of the residual limb;
- sensation in the residual limb;
- overall shape of the stump;
- range of motion (ROM), both passive and active, in the joints of the residual limb; and
- strength of the remaining musculature of the limb.

Considerations about the residual limb have a different emphasis for the upper extremity amputee, since the function of the arm is to position the hand or terminal device for use, while the function of the leg is to bear weight during ambulation.

▇ Treatment

Ideal rehabilitation management begins before the actual amputation. The potential amputee should be shown a typical prosthesis and what can be accomplished with this device. The exercise program needed after the amputation can be explained and even initiated if the amputation is not imminent.

Preprosthetic Training

Training, if not initiated prior to the surgery, begins as soon as the amputation occurs. It consists of two portions, rehabilitating the person to return to an independent state without a prosthesis, and preparing the residual limb for application of the prosthesis. The amputee should be trained to be independent in all aspects of daily living, including bathing, grooming, toileting, and hygiene. Instructions in transfer activities and mobility at the wheelchair level as well as with an appropriate gait device allow the lower limb amputee to become self-sufficient in these activities.

Prosthetic Fitting

The exact time of fitting depends on many factors. First, the patient must meet the criteria for a suitable candidate using all of the assessment criteria described. The suture line must be healed. The level of stump maturity required at fitting depends on the prosthetic approach to be used. The prosthetist fits most lower limb amputees while the patient is standing; therefore, the patient must have the endurance to stand, sometimes up to 20 minutes. Most prostheses are custom fitted and are made with total contact sockets. Such a socket is created by applying plaster cast material to the limb and making a "negative" mold of the limb. The cast is then filled with a plastic material that forms a "positive" replica of the limb. This serves as the model from which the plastic prosthetic socket is molded.

Prostheses are either preparatory or definitive. A preparatory prosthesis uses exactly the same prosthetic principles for encasement of the residual limb, weight bearing, and suspension of the prosthesis as the definitive model. The sole difference lies in using the preparatory socket to assist in the maturation of the residual limb, usually occurring in 3 to 4 months, while permitting earlier use of the prosthesis. The use of a preparatory socket may allow a better fit in the final prosthesis since the process better accommodates changes in the maturing stump. The socket usually needs modification or replacement when the limb is ready for definitive fitting. The final prosthesis in this system is the definitive prosthesis.

If a definitive prosthesis is ordered as the initial device, it will be the only prosthesis. It is fit after the residual limb has matured completely during the preprosthetic program. Usually the preprosthetic program is longer, because the patient is not casted for the prosthesis until there is complete shrinkage and shaping of the stump. The definitive system has the advantage of being less expensive. Many third-party payors will purchase only one initial prosthesis for policy holders.

Prescription Writing

The prosthetic prescription should in general contain the following items:

* materials used to construct the prosthesis, and how these will perform the weight-bearing or weight-transmitting functions of the prosthesis;
* socket type with any needed additions or modifications;
* suspension system;
* prosthetic components which will replace amputated joints;
* terminal device (hand or foot/ankle) replacement component; and
* stump socks or other supplies.

Prosthetic Training

Regardless of the site of limb loss, the amputee needs to learn to care for the prosthesis and how the component parts work. The patient also needs to learn to don and doff the prosthesis, as well as to inspect the skin over friction points and pressure areas.

▪ Complications

Complications may occur after the prosthesis is in use. Frequent problems include stump skin breakdown, irritation, or pain. An improperly fitting prosthesis may cause irritation, ulceration, or abrasion of the skin at pressure areas in the socket. The stump should be inspected as well as the prosthesis. Bony prominences with overlying skin damage, but without a corresponding area of relief in the socket, may be noticed. Brawny edema, induration, and discoloration of the skin of the distal stump in a circular shape may indicate "choking." This occurs when the residual limb becomes larger, typically from excessive weight gain, and no longer fits in the total contact socket. If a gap exists between the skin of the distal stump and the distal socket wall, pressure causes edema fluid to accumulate. This can lead to extensive skin breakdown, but can be corrected by socket modification or by refabrication of the socket. Local skin problems such as furuncles may also occur and prevent comfortable prosthetic function. The patient should be instructed to keep the skin of the stump clean by washing thoroughly at least twice a day.

Bony spurs and exostoses, bony outgrowths of the distal ends of the bones, are more common in the upper limbs and in electrical injuries, and may impair prosthetic fitting. Lack of coordination of the muscles of the upper extremity residual limb may impair prosthetic success more than in lower extremity loss.

Pain may inhibit successful prosthetic use. Amputees may be particularly prone to "phantom pain," pain that appears to originate in the amputated portion of the limb. This is due to signals arising from the nerves proximal to the amputation site which carried sensation from the amputated portion. The presence of persistent pain generators (such as chronic infection) before the amputation may predispose the amputee to more severe phantom pain. Phantom pain does not respond like acute pain to interventions such as narcotics, but may be controlled by agents used to treat neurogenic pain. Effective agents include tricyclic antidepressants such as doxepin (Sinequan), anti-arrhythmic agents such as mexiletine (Mexitil), or membrane-stabilizing agents such as phenytoin (Dilantin). Physical treatments such as desensitization massage may be taught by a therapist and used by the patient to control pain. Transcutaneous electrical nerve stimulation (TENS), heat, or cold may also be effective.

The stump may contain a painful neuroma, diagnosed by palpation of a tender mass, which creates radiating pain in the distribution of the nerve when the tender area is percussed. All nerves, when severed, develop neuromas to some degree. However, large neuromas, or those in critical locations in the stump, may interfere with prosthetic gait and require surgical revision of the stump. In addition, painful conditions in residual limbs are not limited to factors related to the amputation or prosthesis. A lumbar herniated nucleus pulposus (HNP) in an amputee may cause pain to radiate down the residual limb. Several of the usual clues used to diagnose this condition may be missing, including lower lumbo-sacral dermatomes for assessing sensation, distal muscles for assessing strength, or the patellar or Achilles tendons for assessing reflexes. Compounding the problem is the prosthetic gait, which may predispose to HNP due to increased stress across the lumbar spine.

Follow-Up

The prosthesis itself wears out over time, and may malfunction. The socket, certain joint components, or the entire prosthesis may need to be replaced. The average prosthesis usually lasts at least 2 years, even with very heavy use. A prosthesis may last more than 10 years and still be quite useable for a less vigorous individual.

Outcome

Once the patient has been fitted with a prosthesis, the functional outcome may be quite good. Unless there is an underlying disease process, the residual limb should not deteriorate. The patient should be followed at intervals for the first 12 to 18 months after fitting. The patient then reaches a steady state with the prosthesis and only needs to be seen when complications arise. The prosthetist generally follows the amputee in order to make many of the minor adjustments that are required over the years. Any major change or replacement of the prosthesis requires a prosthetic prescription from the physiatrist, so intermittent follow-up is appropriate for the duration of the patient's life. As with all aspects of rehabilitation, it is important to remember that the patient is the one who ultimately determines the definition of successful prosthetic use. Not all amputees wear their prostheses during all waking hours. Success is achieved if the individual has reached maximal functional potential. However, cost issues should also be considered. An individual should not be prescribed a prosthesis if assessed as having no chance of using it successfully.

■ Rehabilitation by Specific Amputation Sites

Below Knee Amputations

General Considerations

Cardiopulmonary status is not usually a significant issue at this level, since the energy consumption in ambulation is less with a prosthesis than that before prosthetic fitting (ambulation with walker or crutches). However, overall status should still be considered. The general test of ability to ambulate without a prosthesis still gives a general idea of the patient's overall fitness. Mental status is important since the patient will need to learn to don the prosthesis and learn a slightly different pattern of gait.

Residual Limb Assessment

Tibial length ideally should be 5 to 7 inches, or approximately one third of the original tibial length. The fibula should be no longer than the tibia, and ideally should be slightly shorter. Measure tibial length from the medial joint line of the knee rather than the tibial tuberosity, a more diffuse landmark. A bone length of less than 2 inches provides such a short lever arm that prosthetic use may be difficult. Residual tibial length of more than 8 inches makes standard fitting difficult. Extremely long residual limbs in BKAs have poor muscle coverage, because the distal one third of the lower leg is covered mostly by tendon rather than the gastrocnemius/soleus muscle, providing poor padding over the end of the tibia. This predisposes it to skin break-down. In addition, the lever arm of the limb is longer, resulting in greater force on the distal skin during gait, and compounding the breakdown problem.

The scar(s) may be aligned in any direction, but should not adhere to the underlying tissues. Adherent tissue creates more shear force on the skin inside the socket and may lead to more frequent skin breakdown during ambulation. Soft tissue integrity is particularly important at the end of the bone. Usually the gastrocnemius muscle is brought over the end of the tibia and surgically secured. The surgeon often tapers the end of the tibia to remove the sharp edge of the transected bone. The most common site of skin breakdown in the below-knee stump is at the anterior distal end of the stump, where the prosthesis rubs. There must also be good skin integrity over the patellar tendon and anterior flares of the tibia because these are the major weight-bearing areas. The stump should be a slightly tapered cylinder, not tender and pliable distally, rather than firm and unyielding. There should be minimal edema.

Assess knee range of motion; active full extension is necessary for good prosthetic function. There should be at least 70 degrees of active knee flexion. Hip extension should be full. Strength in all muscle groups about the knee and hip should be measured as good (4/5 on manual muscle testing) or as normal (5/5).

Preprosthetic Training

Training consists of shaping and maturing the stump for prosthetic application, as well as addressing joint mobility and strength in the entire residual limb. Upper limbs are strengthened for the use of gait assistive devices.

A specific exercise prescription must be written for active ROM for both the knee and the hip. If there is any contracture of either joint, order static stretching. Order strengthening exercises of the knee extensors and flexors as well as all the major hip muscle groups.

There are several appropriate methods for shaping and

maturing the BKA stump. The method used by the physiatrist depends in part on the surgeon's preference. The most rapid method for getting the limb ready for the prosthesis is the Immediate Fit Rigid Dressing. With this method, the residual limb is placed in a plaster cast to midthigh level in the operating room. This dressing prevents any postoperative edema, thereby speeding stump maturation. The knee is in a few degrees of flexion within the cast, but will not develop a flexion contracture. This dressing is left in place for 10 to 14 days, and then replaced with another rigid dressing, or with a preparatory prosthetic socket with a pylon that allows partial weight bearing on the residual limb. The key element in this method is keeping the stump encased at all times; otherwise, edema and induration of the stump occurs.

When the Immediate Rigid Fit Method is not used, stump wrapping should be used to control edema beginning immediately after surgery. An elastic bandage such as an Ace wrap should be applied to the distal thigh level, in a figure-of-eight method with greater pressure distally than proximally. This method is shown in Figure 3-1. A 4-inch wide wrap is routinely used for BKA stumps. The wrap is initiated proximally (step 1) and then is brought around the distal corner of the stump (step 2). The wrap is then brought proximally again (step 3) and wrapped around the remaining corner of the distal end (step 4).

Avoid circumferential wraps; these may act as tourniquets and trap edema distally, actually exacerbating the problem. The wrap should be as tight as possible without causing pain. It should be reapplied each time it loosens, potentially every 3 to 4 hours. If the knee is at risk for a flexion contracture, a posterior plaster mid-thigh length splint should be used. Progressively firmer wrapping should be performed as the suture line heals, even if sutures are in place. The use of bandaging material over the wound should be discontinued as soon as possible so that better shaping may be accomplished.

Wrapping must continue at all times for the first year, even after the prosthesis is prescribed, whenever the prosthesis is not worn. The patient must be instructed to apply this independently. TuboGrip, a tube-shaped elastic wrap,

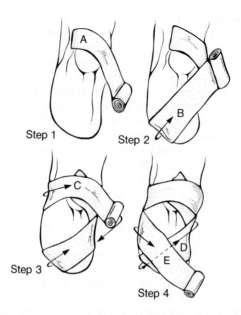

Figure 3-1.   Figure-of-eight method of BKA stump wrapping.

may be substituted for the conventional elastic bandage. If adequate shrinkage is not obtained prior to measuring the patient for the prosthesis, then the prosthesis itself will force the edema out of the limb, rendering the socket too large. This may cause loosening and instability of the prosthesis during gait, potentially requiring major revision or replacement of the prosthetic socket.

Give special care to the suture line. Since there are several layers of tissue that are closed over the cut end of bone, the scar, including both skin and all subcutaneous layers, is likely to adhere to the bone. Write therapy orders for scar mobilization, which involves gentle massage of the skin around the suture line, to reduce adherence to underlying tissue and bone. This should be initiated as soon as tolerated and be performed more aggressively once the sutures are out. The patient should actively perform scar mobilization using skin lotion as a lubricant.

Prosthetic Fitting

The socket used in a below knee prosthesis is called a patellar tendon bearing (PTB) prosthesis. In this socket, the body weight is borne on the patellar tendon, the anterior proximal tibia surface medially and laterally, and the remaining soft tissues of the proximal anterior muscular compartment of the calf. The reason for this is that the distal end of a BKA stump is poorly suited for weight bearing because of pain and propensity for skin breakdown. The socket may be lined with a soft material, called a soft insert, if extra skin protection is needed in addition to stump socks because of fragile skin or an unusually shaped limb. A distal end pad may be prescribed to cushion the bottom of the socket if the hard socket wall is not well tolerated.

Weight is transferred from the socket to the foot via either an exoskeletal or endoskeletal system. In the exoskeletal system, the plastic shell of the socket extends to the terminal device and transmits body weight from the stump to the floor. In the endoskeletal system, a metal pipe joins the socket to the terminal device, transmitting the weight. The pipe is covered with a soft foam cosmetic cover. The exoskeletal prosthesis is more durable; the endoskeletal prosthesis is more cosmetic, but may require more expense for upkeep, as the foam cover is easily torn and requires frequent replacement. The alignment of the endoskeletal prosthesis may be adjusted by the prosthetist, while the exoskeletal prosthesis is a fixed device that cannot be adjusted once fabricated.

The prosthesis is fastened to the limb by a suspension system. The usual PTB suspension system consists of a supracondylar cuff suspension, a small leather cuff attached to the top edge of the socket at the medial and lateral sides. It encircles the distal thigh just above the patella and is secured by a buckle. An alternative suspension system is the PTB-SC or PTS, patellar tendon bearing/supracondylar cuff suspension. This system has a PTB socket which extends laterally above the femoral condyles. The socket has removable pads that, when slid into place, narrow the upper margin of the socket above the condyles and afford suspension, keeping the prosthesis firmly attached to the limb during the swing phase of gait. This system is appropriate for the patient with a short stump or when pistoning (the stump sliding in and out of the socket) is a problem.

The typical terminal device used as the ankle/foot mechanism is a solid-ankle/cushioned-heel (SACH) foot. The cushioned, compressible heel mimics ankle plantar flexion, allowing for a smooth gait. At heel strike, the cushioned heel of the SACH foot compresses, enlarging the surface area of contact with the floor and bringing the forefoot to the floor sooner, stabilizing the patient's balance. If the patient is very active, an energy storing terminal device such as the Seattle Foot or Flex Foot may be used. These devices contain a strong, flexible shank which bends at heel strike, storing energy. The foot recoils at toe-off, generating a force which mimics plantar flexion and gives a push-off which more closely replicates that in normal gait. The typical BKA prosthetic prescription is written as in Table 3-3.

Prosthetic Training

Gait training in physical therapy with the prosthesis should be initiated as soon as the device is fabricated. The average length of training for a BKA patient is 2 weeks. Begin gait training using parallel bars as support until the patient is ready to leave the bars and use a cane or walker. Avoid the use of crutches with the prosthesis as poor gait patterns may develop. The skin should be checked frequently by the therapist and patient for non-blanching that may indicate significant tissue injury and be a prelude to skin breakdown. If present, prosthetic adjustment may be necessary, and the patient should not wear the prosthesis again until any skin lesions are healed.

Above Knee Amputation

General Considerations

Cardiopulmonary status is of more significance in the AKA. The AKA patient needs approximately 65% more energy (as measured by oxygen consumption) during prosthetic gait

Table 3-3. Typical BKA Prosthetic Prescription

> Right BKA prosthesis
>
> PTB socket
>
> Endoskeletal prosthesis
>
> Soft insert
>
> Distal end pad
>
> Cosmetic cover
>
> SACH foot
>
> Cuff suspension
>
> Supplies: stump socks

than that used in normal bipedal gait. Therefore, the patient's general health status is more of a concern than that of a patient with a BKA. Mental status is critical because the prosthesis is more difficult to don than a BKA prosthesis and the patient has to learn a gait pattern that differs significantly from the norm.

Femoral length should ideally be more than 10 inches; as a general rule, the longer the better. This length is measured from the proximal edge of the greater trochanter. Femoral length of less than 8 inches makes it difficult to control the stump in the prosthetic socket. With prosthetic devices available today, any femoral length over 10 inches can be fitted well. The positioning of the scar is not critical for fitting, but the scar should not adhere to any underlying tissue or be deeply invaginated. Bone should be covered with full thickness soft tissue. Carefully inspect the skin in the groin and ischial areas for open areas or lesions. Sensation is usually intact unless areas of skin grafting are present. The stump should be a tapered cylinder. If excess tissue is present over the adductor tendons, the residual limb will be difficult to fit into the prosthesis, causing a painful pinching of the adductor roll between the top edge of the prosthesis and the ischium. The skin in the region of the groin tends to be quite glandular, and excreted material may become impacted in the glands, leading to skin lesions such as furuncles or abscesses. This should first be treated with education about frequent and effective hygiene, and if the problem persists, with an antibiotic solution such as Cleocin-T, a topical antibiotic particularly effective against anaerobic bacteria. Sweating may be a problem inside the socket and may be controlled by Dry-Sol, a potent antiperspirant.

Hip ROM, a critical measurement, is very difficult to assess accurately in AKAs. The shorter and larger the stump, the more difficult hip ROM is to measure. When the leg is amputated through the femur, the only hip muscle groups which maintain their distal insertion sites are those which attach to the greater and lesser trochanters. The effect of the muscles that insert more distally, such as the hamstrings, is lost. The unopposed pull of these residual muscles, specifically the gluteus and iliopsoas muscles, places the femur in a flexed, abducted, and externally rotated position. In addition, the patient who tends to remain in sitting or side-lying positions with the hip flexed can quickly develop a hip flexion contracture. With a short or bulky stump, the femur may be flexed, abducted, or externally rotated inside the stump, even when the stump appears to be in a neutral position. The limb may appear to have full ROM, though the hip joint itself may have significant contractures which will impair prosthetic gait.

Hip extension can be accurately assessed by the Thomas test. The patient is placed in a supine position while the examiner fully flexes the contralateral hip. The patient is instructed to hold the thigh against his chest, thus controlling the rotation of the pelvis to allow accurate measurement of hip extension. Full flexion of the contralateral hip should be confirmed by checking that the lumbar lordosis is completely flattened. This ensures full posterior rotation of the pelvis, securing the angle of the pelvis in relation to the exam table. Then the residual limb is placed in internal rotation and adduction. Only then can the extension of the hip of the residual limb be accurately assessed. A patient may have up to a 60-degree hip flexion contracture and still appear to have full hip extension if the Thomas test is not used, because anterior pelvic rotation, femoral external rotation, and femoral abduction allow the femur to lie flat on the exam table, mimicking full hip extension. However, a hip flexion contracture greater than 10 degrees is enough seriously to impair ability to ambulate with an AKA prosthesis.

Strength in the hip must also be accurately measured. The two hip muscle groups needed by the above-knee amputee during gait are the abductors and the extensors. Half of normal hip extension is provided by the hamstrings, which are severed during the surgical procedure. Therefore the degree of weakness must be carefully measured. The hip abductor muscles can only be measured with the hip in extension and internal rotation. With any degree of hip flexion or external rotation, the examiner will actually be measuring the strength of the hip flexors, as the action of these muscles will substitute for weak abductors.

Preprosthetic Training

Active ROM exercises are ordered for the hip. The hip is at risk for flexion contracture, so static stretch must be ordered. Control the position of the femur within the stump so that it is kept in internal rotation and adduction. Position the pelvis so that the lumbar spine is not forced into lordosis instead of stretching the hip flexors. Lying prone is an ideal method of providing static stretch to the hip flexors, though it may be difficult for older patients or those with moderate contractures to tolerate. Progressive stretching may be accomplished by adding pillows under the residual limb. Order strengthening exercises for the key hip muscle groups, the extensors and abductors.

Residual limb shaping and maturing also start immediately by wrapping with an elastic bandage, usually 6-inch wide Ace wrap. The postoperative wound bandaging should be discarded as rapidly as possible to assure more rapid shaping. For the patient who cannot effectively wrap the residual limb, a stump shrinker may be substituted. A shrinker is a strong elastic presized bandage that covers the distal end of the stump. It has the advantage of being easier to don and the

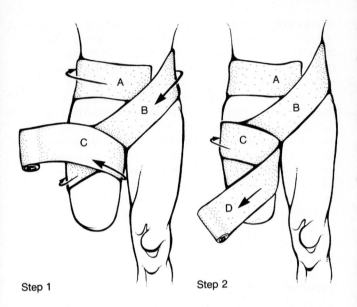

Step 1

Step 2

Figure 3-2. Figure-of-eight method for AKA stump wrapping.

Step 3

disadvantage of being a fixed size. As the stump shrinks, the stump shrinker's compression diminishes, while wrapping provides a custom fit with each application. It is vital that the wrap or the shrinker include the entire residual limb, with special care that the medial stump is wrapped proximally to the adductor tubercle, to avoid an adductor roll. The figure-of-eight wrapping method is used as in Figure 3-2. A six-inch wrap is typically used for AKA stumps. The process is similar to that used on BKA stumps. To adequately secure the compressive dressing high in the groin, especially with short residual limbs, the elastic wrap must go around the waist or a belting device must be used with the stump shrinker.

Prosthetic Fitting

Prosthetic materials used for the socket and weight-transmitting portions of the AKA prosthesis are the same as for the below knee prosthesis. However, since the weight-transmitting portion is longer in the AK prosthesis, the lighter weight of the endoskeletal system is of greater consequence than in a BKA prosthesis.

AKA sockets are of two types, the quadrilateral socket and the CAT-CAM (contoured adducted trochanteric-controlled alignment method) or narrow mediolateral (ML) socket. Currently, the narrow ML socket is more commonly prescribed. Both of these sockets are total contact sockets. In the quadrilateral socket, weight bearing occurs on the ischial tuberosity, with the patient effectively "sitting" on a posterior shelf at the brim of the socket. Stump position within the socket is maintained by pressure from the anterior wall of the socket against the thigh, which keeps the ischial tuberosity in position on the posterior brim. Thus, the empty socket has a rectangular shape when viewed from above, with the narrow dimension in the anterior-posterior plane.

In contrast to the quadrilateral socket, weight bearing on a narrow ML socket is on the lateral aspect of the femur, in the area just below the greater trochanter. This is accomplished by compressing the stump in the socket medially.

From above this socket is oval in appearance, narrower in the mediolateral plane, and is custom-molded to the residual limb along the entire length of the socket.

Suspension in AKA prostheses is provided by the shape of the socket itself or by a belt around the waist. The socket suspension is called a suction socket. The socket is made airtight with a one-way air valve placed distally, and is used without stump socks. When the stump is inserted into the socket, all the air is forced out through the valve. The prosthesis tends to pull away from the stump during the swing phase of gait, but negative pressure between the stump and the socket keeps the prosthesis from sliding off. This socket is difficult to apply and even small volume changes in the stump may create difficulties in donning the prosthesis. If the socket is not applied properly, an air leak may occur and suction is lost, allowing the prosthesis to slide distally and impairing function. The most common suspension belt is a Silesian belt, a webbed strap attached to the lateral brim of the socket. It fits around the opposite iliac crest, thereby holding the socket in place. In the young amputee, a suction socket is the optimal choice. In the older or less vigorous amputee, a semisuction socket, or a looser fitting suction socket with stump socks, in conjunction with a Silesian belt, may be ordered.

The knee joint is chosen in accordance with the patient's needs. An amputee with good balance and an average activity level would best be served by a constant friction knee. If balance is a concern, a safety knee is prescribed. This type of knee joint swings freely as long as a vertical load is not applied. If vertical force is applied, the knee locks in place. If the amputee begins to stumble and fall, the knee locks even when flexed, allowing weight bearing. Thus, the amputee has time to regain balance. In the very active amputee, consider prescribing a hydraulic knee. The fluid in a hydraulic knee allows the knee to move at various speeds depending on the force applied. This allows an individual to walk at varying speeds, an advantage over the constant friction knee.

The foot/ankle device typically used in AKA prostheses is a single axis foot. This terminal device has an ankle joint which moves freely in a plantar- and dorsi-flexion plane.

Table 3-4. Typical AKA Prosthetic Prescription

> Right AKA prosthesis
>
> Narrow ML socket (suction socket)
>
> Endoskeletal prosthesis
>
> Cosmetic cover
>
> Safety knee
>
> Single-axis ankle
>
> Silesian belt (semisuction suspension)

Thus, plantar flexion occurs immediately upon heel strike, placing the prosthetic foot fully on the floor and making the stance phase more stable on the prosthetic limb. A typical AKA prosthetic prescription details each of these components (Table 3-4).

Knee Disarticulation Amputations

Knee disarticulation amputations are not common; patients are fitted with prostheses similar to AKAs. The prosthesis therefore still extends proximally to the ischial tuberosity. This long lever arm provides strong control of the prosthesis during gait. However, the prosthetic knee must be added distally to the socket, which places it more distally than the position of patient's own knee. The center of knee rotation can be preserved by use of a polycentric prosthetic knee joint, which shifts the axis of rotation proximally, approximating normal knee function during gait. However, since total leg length must be the same as that on the contralateral side when the patient stands, the knee joint is located more distally. Therefore, the lower leg segment must be shorter. This causes the prosthetic knee to protrude further than the opposite knee when the patient sits, which may be unacceptable from a cosmetic standpoint. Provide thorough preamputation counseling for such a patient so that an informed decision may be made about the level of amputation.

Upper Extremity Amputations

General Considerations

Cardiopulmonary and overall medical status are of minor importance in the decision to fit the upper extremity amputee with a prosthesis. However, accurate assessment of the patient's mental status is extremely important since new skills of donning the prosthesis and manipulating the terminal device must be learned.

Residual Limb Assessment

In the acute treatment phase, when considering stump length the general rule is to save all that is possible. Soft tissue coverage of bones is necessary whenever possible, especially at the distal aspect. The stump shape should mimic that of the normal limb; it should not be distally edematous or bulbous. The stump soft tissue and skin should move easily, without adhering to underlying structures. Scars should be well-healed and not painful. The presence of exostoses or bone spurs should be determined.

Preprosthetic Training

Order active ROM for each remaining joint immediately after amputation. Give special attention to the shoulder joint in order to preserve full range in the glenohumeral joint, especially external rotation. Order static stretch, if needed. Order strengthening for all remaining major muscle groups. If a myoelectric prosthesis might be considered, order surface electromyographic (EMG) biofeedback training of the muscles to be used to operate the prosthesis.

Begin stump wrapping immediately. Principles described in the lower limb sections also apply here. There may be multiple surgical scars which are likely to adhere to underlying bone. Begin scar mobilization as soon as any adherence is noted, as well as routinely when the scars are fully healed.

The hand of the unaffected limb in a unilateral amputee will almost certainly become the dominant one regardless of prior handedness. The occupational therapy prescription should include orders to instruct the patient in performing activities of daily living (ADLs) one-handed, as well as assisting in changing hand dominance if the previously dominant hand is absent.

Prosthetic Fitting

Prosthetic replacements are either body-powered or myo-electric. In most cases, the body-powered prosthesis is ordered, at least as the initial device. Prosthetic weight should be kept to a minimum. Usually an exoskeletal system with a total contact socket is prescribed. The suspension system in the body-powered prosthesis also serves as the cabling system to transmit body movement into function of the terminal device. Traction on the operating cable opens the terminal device, and strong rubber bands close the device for grasping. The most common type of suspension used is a Northwestern Ring Figure-of-Eight, shown in Figure 3-3.

The wrist joint replacement unit does not usually function as a true wrist, but rather has a "quick disconnect" receptacle which allows a variety of terminal devices to be interchanged. Alternatively, a constant friction wrist unit may be ordered which allows wrist flexion and extension, and which is lighter. The elbow "joint" in a BE prosthesis consists of external hinges which are aligned with the patient's elbow. The elbow joint in an AE prosthesis usually consists of an internally locking elbow with a turntable. The elbow is switched between locked and unlocked positions by placing traction on a second "switching" cable, usually operated by shoulder depression. When the elbow is locked, traction on the operating cable opens the terminal device. When the elbow is unlocked, traction on the operating cable flexes the forearm segment of the prosthesis. The forearm is extended by force of gravity. The turntable allows the forearm to be moved passively toward and away from the body, mimicking internal and external rotation of the humerus. When a shoul-

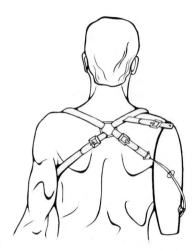

Figure 3-3. Posterior view, Northwestern 0-ring figure-of-eight suspension device for AE prosthesis.

der joint is required following a shoulder disarticulation amputation, a constant friction hinge, which may be passively positioned, is ordered.

The terminal device is the most important part of an upper extremity prosthesis, and may be either a hook or a hand. The hook is a functional device, while the hand, whether designed as a functional unit or solely for cosmetic effect, is not as functional. There are at least fifty different hook terminal devices, the most common being the Dorrance 5X for BE amputees and a Dorrance 5XA for limbs amputated above the elbow. Both types use a cover made of rubber, which is easily torn or marred.

Myoelectric Prostheses

A myoelectric prosthesis uses small electric motors to power movement of the terminal device. The myoelectric prosthetic hand closely resembles a human hand, and is usually positioned in a "three-jaw chuck" grip, in which the stationary thumb opposes the mobile index and middle fingers in a pinching movement. This movement is controlled by the wearer via surface EMG electrodes which sense the activity of the muscles in the residual limb, usually the wrist extensors. Activation of this muscle group triggers activation of the motor, which is incorporated into the prosthetic wall. A battery pack is also incorporated into the prosthesis and requires daily charging. A myoelectric prosthesis may use a harness similar to a body-powered prosthesis, or may simply be slid over the residual forearm and suspended from the epicondyles. As an alternative to the myoelectric hand, a myoelectric hook terminal device may be installed, and may be slightly more functional, though less cosmetic. A myoelectric elbow joint is also available, though the large forearm segment is difficult to move with the small motors available. The major disadvantage of myoelectric devices at this time is their extremely high cost, particularly for AE amputees. Also, the myoelectric hand uses a rubber cosmetic cover which is easily torn and is expensive to replace.

Prosthetic Training

Training in the use of an upper extremity prosthesis is performed by an occupational therapist. The patient should attend daily for the first 2 weeks, tapering to 3 times a week, for a total of 20 to 25 training sessions. The patient should learn how to place the terminal device where desired and how to open and close it. The amputee needs to learn to place the terminal device visually, since it has no proprioceptive component. Independence in ADLs is a primary goal of therapy.

Pediatric Amputees and Limb-Deficient Children

Children with congenital amputations (better termed "limb deficiencies") are prone to an additional complication not usually seen in adults, exostosis, or bony overgrowth. The child's skeletal system retains the ability to grow, leading to the development of new bony prominences at the ends of long bones that outgrow the covering skin and soft tissue. This may lead to skin breakdown and infection, and may require surgical correction.

Prosthetic fitting in the child should follow developmental guidelines. Upper extremity prosthetics may be provided when the child begins to sit, about age 6 months. Lower extremity prostheses may be provided when the child begins to stand and walk, age 9 to 14 months.

▓ Suggested Readings

Atkins DJ, Meier RH, eds. *Comprehensive Management of the Upper-limb Amputee.* New York: Springer-Verlag, 1989.

Esquenazi A, Leonard JA, Meier RM, et al. 3. Prosthetics. *Arch Phys Med Rehabil* 1989;70 (Suppl):207.

Inman VT, Ralston HJ, Todd J. *Human Walking.* Baltimore: Williams & Wilkins, 1981.

Leonard JA, Meier RH. Prosthetics. *In* DeLisa J, ed. *Rehabilitation Medicine.* Philadelphia: J.B. Lippincott, 1993.

Northwestern University Medical School Prosthetic-Orthotic Center. Lower- and upper-limb prosthetics for physicians, surgeons, and therapists (course notebook), 1989.

Sanders GT. *Lower Limb Amputations: A Guide to Rehabilitation.* Philadelphia: F.A. Davis, 1986.

Sherman RA. Published treatments of phantom limb pain. *Am J Phys Med* 1980;59:232–44.

Wu Y, Krick H. Removable rigid dressing for below-knee amputees. *Clinical Prosthetics and Orthotics* 1987;11:33–44.

C. George Kevorkian

4

Arthritis

Introduction

There are many varieties of arthritis. In general, rheumatoid arthritis, osteoarthritis, and the spondyloarthropathies are the main arthritides managed by the physiatrist. However, principal comments here can be applied to most other forms of arthritis.

Rheumatoid Arthritis

Definition

Rheumatoid arthritis (RA) is a common, chronic polyarthritis which may be classified as a diffuse, multi-system, connective tissue disease. The hallmarks of RA are positive testing for immunoglobulin M (IgM) rheumatoid factor; bilateral, usually symmetrical joint disease; erosive changes noted radiographically; and persistent inflammatory synovitis.

After a general discussion of RA, the management of the RA hand and foot will be described in detail.

Epidemiology

The prevalence of RA in the population is approximately 1%, and increases with increasing age. Women are affected about three times more frequently than men, although this

Susan J. Garrison (Ed.): *Handbook of Physical Medicine and Rehabilitation Basics.* First Edition. Copyright © 1995 J. B. Lippincott Company

gender difference is reversed in children. RA has a worldwide distribution. A genetic predisposition does seem to exist, as first-degree relatives of persons with seropositive erosive disease are five to six times more likely to develop severe RA. A strong association with the major histocompatibility complex gene product, HLA-DR4, and a preponderance of whites and Japanese with classic or definite RA have been demonstrated.

Etiology and Pathology

Various theories have been advanced to explain RA, including infective agents, cellular hypersensitivity, genetic predisposition, and immune complex involvement. None has gained unequivocal acceptance. The exact role of rheumatoid factor is still uncertain.

A probable early event in the disease process is an antigen-antibody reaction at the synovial level with activation of complement. Acute pathological findings include microvascular injury; edema of subsynovial tissues; and synovial lining cell proliferation.

In established disease pathological examination of the synovium reveals edema, villous synovial projections, and hypertrophy and hyperplasia of the synovial lining cells (both A and B type cells). Vascular changes such as capillary obstruction, neutrophil infiltration, areas of thrombosis, and perivascular hemorrhage are common. Mononuclear cells predominate in the subsynovial stroma. Mechanisms favoring and/or resulting in a chronic disease process are unknown. As inflammation continues, pannus, an inflammatory synovial mass, is laid down. Pannus may ultimately invade bone and cartilage and lead to joint damage.

Clinical Features

The onset of RA is usually gradual; however, 15 to 20% of patients experience it suddenly. Symptoms such as fatigue, anorexia, malaise, weight loss, weakness, and generalized "aches and pains" usually herald the onset of RA. RA is initially polyarticular in approximately 75% of patients. The small joints of the hands and feet are most affected. Ultimately the hand involvement predominates, with PIP joints affected in 85% of patients, metacarpophalangeal (MCP) joints in 70%, and wrists in 80%. Other joints such as the knees, cervical spine, feet, and temporomandibular are commonly, though less frequently, affected.

Clinical features of involved joints include pain, swelling, limitation of movement, stiffness, and various signs of inflammation, such as erythema and synovitis. Morning stiffness, considered a result of synovial congestion, joint capsule thickening, and an increased volume of synovial fluid, is common.

The clinical course of RA is highly variable. Approximately 10% of patients have a mild, transient polyarthritis followed by a lasting remission; less than 10% have destructive polyarthritis. The remaining 80% exhibit a characteristic waxing and waning of symptoms. The degree of articular severity and the presence of extra-articular manifestations generally do not correlate; however, both of these are more likely to be severe in patients with high titers of rheumatoid factor.

Patients rarely die of RA. Death results typically from associated features such as vasculitis, cervical spine subluxation, complications of drug therapy, and infection. The course of the disease naturally varies with the individual patient, but certain aspects indicate a less favorable outcome. These include insidious onset (patients who perhaps present too late), youthful onset, being female and/or being Caucasian, seropositivity, rheumatoid nodules, and high titers of rheumatoid factor, C-reactive protein and/or haptoglobin.

Numerous authors have proposed functional classifications for RA patients. Steinbrocker's practical, enduring criteria are listed in Table 4-1.

The term "symmetrical," used radiologically, refers to bilateral joint involvement, though not necessarily to the same degree. Bony ankylosis is rarely a feature. See Table 4-2.

Table 4-1. Functional Criteria in RA

Grade	Definition	Remarks
I	Capable of all activities	—
II	Moderate restriction	Physical abilities adequate for normal activities, despite handicaps of discomfort or limited motion of one or more joints
III	Marked restriction	Activity limited to self care and a few duties of a nonstrenuous occupation
IV	Bed and/or chair bound	Capable of little or no self care

Adapted from Steinbrocker O, Traeger CH, Batterman RC. Therapeutic criteria in rheumatoid arthritis. *JAMA* 1949;140:659–662.

Management

A management profile of rheumatoid arthritis can serve as a generic model for physiatric care of the arthritides. Comprehensive management of the arthritis patient involves prescription of appropriate medications as well as utilization of a variety of resources familiar to physiatrists. Aspirin, in doses

Table 4-2. Radiological Features of RA

Early Changes	Late Changes
Soft tissue swelling	Uniform narrowing of joint (cartilage space)
Juxta-articular osteoporosis	Bone destruction
Marginal erosions	Joint malalignment and subluxation

of 3 to 6 grams daily, is the accepted initial drug of choice. Begin at a dosage of 0.9 gram orally QID and increase gradually each 4 to 5 days as tolerated. Obtain serum salicylate levels (22–30 mg/dl) periodically. A level producing tinnitus obviously needs to be reduced. Doses below 3 grams/day are usually only analgesic.

If aspirin is contraindicated, cannot be tolerated, or does not produce the desired therapeutic effect, a trial of nonsteroidal anti-inflammatory agents (NSAIDs) is indicated. If these agents fail to suppress the disease process, a variety of drugs such as gold, steroids, penicillamine, and antimalarials are available, in addition to a variety of experimental drugs and procedures. Consultation with a rheumatologist is recommended at this level of disease management.

Physiatric Management

The physiatrist is familiar with the wide array of resources available for optimal treatment of arthritis patients. He/she is ideally suited to lead the arthritis rehabilitation team (see Table 4-3), prescribing, coordinating, and teaching the patient's treatment regimen.

The goals of arthritis rehabilitation are to:

- maintain or improve range of motion;
- prevent deformities;
- limit disability;
- protect susceptible joints;
- decrease pain and stiffness;
- use joints and muscles efficiently and safely;
- improve strength in selected muscles;
- improve endurance; and
- control weight and maintain appropriate nutrition.

Efficient arthritis rehabilitation is characterized by a motivated, well-informed patient, following a regimen prescribed and coordinated by a knowledgeable physician, administered by a registered, well-trained therapist, and coordinated with other medical/surgical treatments. The reg-

Table 4-3. The Arthritis Rehabilitation Team

Physiatrist

Patient and family

Patient educator

Occupational therapist

Physical therapist

Pharmacist

Nurse

Psychologist/Psychiatrist

Dietician

Social worker

Vocational counselor

imen should include sufficient instructional treatments, an ongoing basic home program, and modification of the program as disease state changes. Poor rehabilitation outcome can result from the omission of these elements. Formal treatments that do not provide functional improvement or relief after several weeks should either be modified or discontinued. The patient and family should be aware that physical medicine and rehabilitation (PM&R) treatments do not cure arthritis, substitute for adequate rest, replace prescribed medications, or usually result in rapid improvement.

Agents used for arthritis rehabilitation include heat, cold, hydrotherapy, exercise, rest, mechanical agents, education, and/or other agents.

Heat

A variety of reasons have been advanced to explain the mechanisms of analgesia production by heat, such as local axon reflex, endorphin production stimulation, gating theories, and others. Any or all may be significant. See Table 4-4. Use

Table 4-4. Heat Apparati

Rationale	Agents	Deep Heat
• Analgesic	• Infrared lamp	• Shortwave
• Sedative	• Baker	• Microwave
• Antispasmodic	• Contrast baths	• Ultrasound
• Metabolic	• Hydrocolator packs	
• Remote effects	• Fluidotherapy	
	• Whirlpool	
	• Hot tub bath	
	• Paraffin baths	
	• Electric blankets and heating pads	

any as desired. There is no first-line superficial heating apparatus of choice. Deep heating apparti includes shortwave, microwave, and ultrasound. Avoid the use of these over acutely or subacutely inflamed rheumatoid joints.

Cold

Heat and cold have similar analgesic and antispasmodic effects. Their metabolic and remote effects are essentially opposite. Application of cold typically aggravates joint stiffness; therefore, use cryotherapy with caution, even though this modality is effective in treating acutely inflamed soft tissue. See Table 4-5.

Hydrotherapy

The mechanical buoyancy effect of water immersion helps to decrease stress in weight-bearing joints and allows for easier ambulation. Such therapy can occur in a wading tank. See Table 4-6.

Table 4-5. Cryotherapy

Rationale	Agents
• Analgesic	• Cold water
• Metabolic	• Ice packs
• Antispasmodic	• Ice massage
• Antispastic	• Slush
• Remote effects	• Evaporants

Table 4-6. Hydrotherapy

Rationale	Agents
• Sedative	• Whirlpool
• Mechanical	• Hubbard tank
• Sensory	• Wading tank
	• Therapeutic pool
	• Showers
	• Douches
	• Peloids
	• Contrast baths

Other Therapeutic Agents

Any or all may be used as appropriate. See Table 4-7. Use of pressure gradient gloves may reduce finger swelling; however, their use is controversial.

Exercises

Most arthritic patients cannot tolerate total body muscle strengthening. Judicious selection of muscles to be strengthened is essential. Remember the cervical spine and temporo-

Table 4-7. Other Therapeutic Agents

Local Injections

TENS

Biofeedback

Acupuncture

Operant conditioning

Pressure gloves

mandibular joint (TMJ). See Table 4-8 for exercise goals, and Table 4-9 for types of exercises. Any or all may be suitable. Isometric exercises are preferred, of ten repetitions or less, usually in selected muscles such as the hip extensors and quadriceps.

Modify or temporarily discontinue any exercise or activity that apparently increases pain, stiffness, or swelling persisting for 24 hours or more. Though isometric exercises are preferred, low-resistance isotonic exercises are safer for the elderly and for those patients for whom isometric exercises are contraindicated, such as severe hypertensives. See Figure 4-1.

Table 4-8. Goals of Exercises

Preserve or improve ROM

Increase strength in selected muscles

Improve endurance

Prevent deconditioning

Improve coordination

Improve function

Relax tense muscles

Improve posture

Table 4-9. Classification of Exercises

Passive (maintains ROM)

Active assistive (increases ROM)

Active (maintains ROM, improves endurance)

Resistive (increases strength)

Stretching

Re-education

Coordination

Relaxation

Postural

Deep breathing

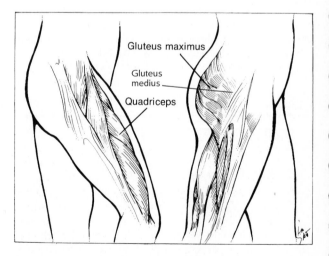

Figure 4-1. Important muscles to strengthen and keep strong for sit to stand and stair-climbing activities.

Table 4-10. Effects of Rest

Beneficial	Harmful
Decreases pain	Psychological Effects
Decreases joint metabolism	Depression
	Anxiety
Decreases joint inflammation	Dependency
	Muscle Atrophy
Useful adjuvant to antiinflammatory medication	Deconditioning
	Postural deconditioning
May minimize cartilage and collagen destruction (unproven)	Deep vein thrombosis
	Negative calcium and nitrogen balances
	Increased tendency to contracture formation

Rest

Instruct the patient to get 10 hours of bed rest daily, but not to become inactive. See Table 4-10 for the effects of rest.

Assistive Devices

Prescribe activities of daily living (ADL) devices liberally as needed for common activities. Such devices include utensils with built-up handles, modified pens and grip pencils, reachers, and so forth. Also, teach joint-sparing techniques.

About one-third of RA patients have some significant mobility difficulty. Mobility devices include canes with handle modification, or platforms; crutches; walkers, with platforms (volar armrests); and shoes. Other transportation aids include stair gliders (elevators); wheelchairs, including electric models; and adapted vans and automobiles.

Education

Patient education should be ongoing, especially education about scientific, efficacious medical treatment opposed to unproved "quick-fix" miracle cures.

Information about home, employment, and recreational adaptations to physical disabilities must be repeated over time as the patient ages and the disease progresses. Family members also benefit from continued exposure to this information.

The local Arthritis Foundation is a source of educational materials as well as peer support groups and trained counselors. Medical social workers, home health services, and vocational rehabilitation also educate patients through evaluation and training.

The Rheumatoid Hand

An understanding of the pathophysiology and kinesiology of the rheumatoid hand is essential for adequate treatment. See Figure 4-2 for major hand-deforming forces.

The wrist is affected early in most patients, often resulting in a flexion contracture. Radial deviation of the metacarpals commonly precedes and contributes to the more noticeable ulnar deviation at the MCP joints. A zigzag then results, mainly because of the direction of pull of the extrinsic finger flexors and extensors.

However, normal anatomical factors exist which enhance ulnar deviation, including the following:

* the long finger flexors pull ulnarly during power grip;
* the shape of the metacarpal heads (heads of IV and V are normally ulnarly directed; the radial condyle has a more prominent shoulder);
* the radial collateral ligament is longer and thinner than the ulnar and therefore more easily stretched;
* intrinsic muscle factors, particularly the ulnar insertions of the intrinsics which are more efficient than the radial; also, the abductor digiti minimi pulls ulnarly; and finally,

Ulnar Deviation of Fingers

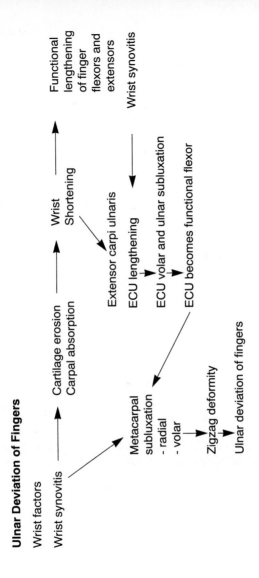

Figure 4-2. Hand Deforming Forces in RA

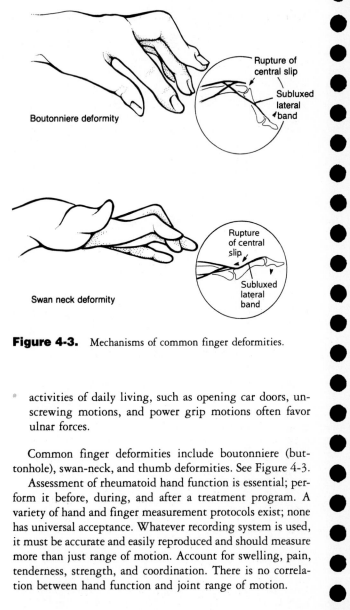

Figure 4-3. Mechanisms of common finger deformities.

activities of daily living, such as opening car doors, un-
screwing motions, and power grip motions often favor
ulnar forces.

Common finger deformities include boutonniere (but-
tonhole), swan-neck, and thumb deformities. See Figure 4-3.
Assessment of rheumatoid hand function is essential; perform it before, during, and after a treatment program. A
variety of hand and finger measurement protocols exist; none
has universal acceptance. Whatever recording system is used,
it must be accurate and easily reproduced and should measure
more than just range of motion. Account for swelling, pain,
tenderness, strength, and coordination. There is no correlation between hand function and joint range of motion.

Treatment of the Rheumatoid Hand

A treatment protocol for the RA hand should include the use of splints, modalities, and exercises.

Splints

Theoretically, splinting should enforce the beneficial effects of rest and result in symptomatic improvement, especially in the acute disease stages. The major goals are to:

- relieve pain;
- maintain position of function;
- discourage abuse of affected joints; and
- assist function, both pre- and post-surgically.

Splint immobilization should assist in reducing synovitis and resulting pain. Evidence is inconclusive as to whether splints prevent deformities from occurring, or correct deformities already present. Pre- and post-surgical splints are highly individualized, often intricate, and not utilized by the typical RA patient. Splints employed for achieving the goals above include resting splints, active or functional splints, and dynamic splints.

Resting splints are the most practical and useful. These should almost always be prescribed to patients in the acute stage. If both hands are involved, the patient should alternate usage daily. In the acute stage, resting splints should provide a 10 to 20 degree wrist cock-up, in order to keep the wrist aligned properly, supply some radially directed force to the fingers to offset ulnar deviation, and provide support under the heads of the proximal phalanges to prevent volar subluxation and keep the MCP joints extended. Subluxation and deformity of the long finger flexors and extensors as a result of RA make the hand intrinsics usually tight and dominant. The resting splint should keep the hand in a predominantly neutral position.

Functional splints provide some support to an isolated joint while allowing use of the hand. Dynamic splints utilize

springs or rubber bands in an attempt to improve alignment
or range of motion.

Therapeutic Modalities

The major indications for the use of these modalities include
analgesia, decrease of joint stiffness, and skin softening in
selected cases. Selection of a specific modality usually depends upon patient preference and ease of use in the home.
They include paraffin baths (portable models available), contrast baths, hand whirlpools, fluidotherapy, and microwave
mittens.

Application of cold can relieve pain and reduce swelling,
spasticity, and spasms. However, because its use increases
joint stiffness, it is contraindicated in both the acute and
chronic stages of RA.

Exercises

The purpose of exercises for the RA hand is to preserve
function and prevent deformities. The basic hand exercise
prescription includes:

*   stretching of interossei (flexing distal interphalangeal
    (DIP) and proximal interphalangeal (PIP) while extend-
    ing MCP joint);
*   active range of motion exercises for wrist, thumb, and
    fingers; and
*   re-education and gentle manual resistance exercises for
    the weakened finger extensor muscles.

Exercises such as squeezing a rubber ball or sponge are
contraindicated. Since they primarily involve the lumbricales
and finger flexors, already mechanically dominant forces in
RA, these exercises increase the development of muscle imbalance and hand deformities. Use only active or gentle active assistive range of motion exercises (AROM or AAROM);
avoid passive range of motion (PROM).

Table 4-11. Shoe Design Elements

Extra-depth shoe

High, wide toe box

Crepe sole

Rocker bottom

Steel shank (from heel to MTP joint)

Firm heel counter

Tie lacing with multiple lace holes (for wide pressure distribution)

Velcro tongue closures

Rheumatoid Foot

The majority of RA patients have foot deformities. Gait analysis of such patients commonly reveals a slower gait velocity, decreased step length, and foot pronation. A prolonged double support phase is common; initial ground contact is with the medial border of the pronated foot. Treatment consists of footwear modifications, use of modalities, and exercises. Specific shoe design is shown in Table 4-11. Common problems and interventions are presented in Table 4-12.

A variety of custom molded shoes are now available and may be necessary in treating a severely deformed foot. If pain and disability become intractable, a final solution may be the use of a tendon patellar weightbearing brace to unload the ankle.

Use caution in making modifications to a shoe; it often becomes heavier and therefore may not be practical for the patient. See Table 4-13.

Exercises/Modalities

No single exercise protocol meets the needs of all RA patients with foot involvement. Generally, the essentials of any

Table 4-12. Common RA Foot Problems and Interventions

Problem	Intervention
Forefoot	
Metatarsalgia (including involvement of first metatarsal phalangeal joint)	Metatarsal bar
	Rocker bottom to shoe
	Metatarsal pad insert
	Plastazote insert
	Inner sole wedge
Hallux valgus	Extra-depth shoe with wide toe box
Hammertoes	
Midfoot	
Midtarsal joint pain	Use of tennis shoes
	Adhesive arch strapping
	Steel shank
Hind foot	
Painful subtalar joints and painful heel	Crepe sole
	Padded heel insert
	UCBL orthosis
	Plastic heel cup
	Arch supports
	Steroid injections
	PTB weightbearing brace

Table 4-13. Shoe Modifications

Heel pads, cups

UCBL insert (especially for plantar fascitis)

Plastozote insert

Metatarsal bars and/or inserts

Medial heel wedge/Thomas heel (for pronation)

Lateral shoe wedge

exercise program include heel cord stretching, AROM of
the ankle and subtalar joints, and flexion and extension of
the toes. Instruct the patient to perform these daily. Foot
whirlpools may provide analgesia and can be used at home.

▓ Osteoarthritis

Definition

Osteoarthritis (OA), also known as degenerative joint disease,
is the most common joint disease of human beings and is
considered to be the leading cause of disability in the elderly.
OA is characterized pathologically by the progressive deterioration and ultimate loss of articular cartilage with reactive
changes at the joint margins and in the subchondral bone.

Epidemiology

The prevalence of OA markedly increases with increasing
age. This condition is rare in children and young adults. A
simple scheme classifies OA as either idiopathic (primary), or
secondary (attributable to an obvious underlying cause); the
idiopathic group is the most common.

Age, gender, vocation and avocation, race, and heredity all
may play a role in the clinical manifestations of OA. In
elderly populations, OA is more common in the thumb and
other finger joints in women; hip OA is more common in
men. The clinical patterns of joint involvement often relate
to prior vocation or avocation. For example, OA is common
in the ankles of ballet dancers, although this is an uncommon
site in the overall population. Native Americans are more
likely to develop OA than Caucasians; Chinese in Hong
Kong have a lower incidence than Caucasians. Female relatives of a woman whose distal interphalangeal joints are involved (Heberden's nodes) are more likely to develop OA of
these joints. The exact role of obesity as a primary etiological
factor is still uncertain.

Clinical Features

Clinical manifestations of OA usually include gradual development of joint pain, stiffness, joint enlargement, and associated limitation of movement. Typically, only one or a few joints are involved. Early in the disease, pain results from, or is aggravated by, joint use and is relieved by rest. With progression of the disease, pain at rest may become common, as well as pain brought on by minimal movement. Joint enlargement may result from synovitis, increased synovial fluid, or cartilage and bone proliferation. Joints commonly involved include interphalangeal joints, thumb base, hip, knee, and spine.

Treatment

The conservative treatment of OA involves drug therapy, reduction of joint load, and rehabilitative therapy. Drug therapy is essentially symptomatic, and simple analgesics such as aspirin should be used initially. NSAIDs should be prescribed if severe joint inflammation is present or a trial of analgesics has failed. Systemic glucocorticoids are usually not indicated, but intra- or periarticular injections of a depo-glucocorticoid may, if necessary, provide symptomatic relief.

Methods to relieve joint loading include:

- correction of postural abnormalities;
- orthotics;
- well-padded shoes, such as running shoes;
- use of a cane or walker;
- judicious rest, though not prolonged immobilization; and
- weight loss.

The principles of rehabilitative therapy are similar to those previously described for RA.

▪ Ankylosing Spondylitis and Other Spondyloarthropathies

Ankylosing spondylitis (AS) is the prototype disease of a group of interrelated seronegative spondyloarthropathies. Disorders also included in this classification are Reiter's disease, certain forms of psoriatic arthritis, juvenile chronic polyarthropathy, acute anterior uveitis, reactive arthritis, and the enteropathic arthritides. These disorders are not considered rheumatoid variants. Common features of the spondyloarthropathies include:

- seronegativity for IgM rheumatoid factor;
- association with sacroiliitis/ankylosing spondylitis;
- presence of enthesopathy (inflammation/ossification at the site of ligamentous insertion into bone);
- association with the histocompatibility antigen, HLA-B27;
- tendency to familial clustering as well as overlap (two or more spondyloarthropathies in the same family); and
- association with certain "co-diseases" such as psoriasis, chronic inflammatory bowel diseases, urethritis, and acute anterior uveitis.

Ankylosing spondylitis will be reviewed as a typical representative of this group.

Definition

The term ankylosing spondylitis (AS) is not necessarily ideal for this disease, as only a small minority of patients progress to a bent, fused spine. Moll has defined ankylosing spondylitis as a chronic disorder of the spine and sacroiliac joints, in which inflammatory lesions are associated with progressive stiffening of the spine and radiological calcification of spinal ligaments.

Among the most widely accepted criteria for diagnosis of AS are those developed in Rome (1961) and New York (1966). The most common way to satisfy the criteria is radio-

logical evidence of grade III or IV bilateral sacroiliitis together
with a history of pain and/or limitation of motion. The
presence or absence of the HLA-B27 antigen does not alone
confirm the diagnosis. This disease is almost always diagnosed
by means of a radiological examination confirming sacroiliitis.
Therefore, a patient with symptomatic sacroiliitis, though
lacking the HLA-B27 antigen, may still have AS.

Epidemiology

The prevalence in Caucasians is approximately 1%. The sex
ratio for sacroiliitis is almost identical, but males are much
more likely to have progressive spinal disease. Thus, a male:fe-
male ratio of 3:1 to 5:1 is suggested. The geographical distribution of AS is similar to that of the HLA-B27 antigen, and is
therefore rare in African and American blacks and Japanese.
The disease usually presents between 15 to 35 years of age.

Clinical Features

Common symptoms include a gradual onset of low back pain,
usually worse in the evening. Morning stiffness is common;
activity usually decreases the discomfort. Typical musculoskeletal clinical features are shown in Figure 4-4. In
established cases, spinal mobility and chest expansion are
reduced. Various sacroiliac "stress tests" are not reliable clinical indicators. Progressive postural changes, such as forward
stoop, are associated with tightness of heel cords, hamstrings,
flexors, and pectorals. Some conditions associated with AS
include ulcerative colitis, psoriasis, urethritis, iritis, aortic
incompetence, and cardiac conduction defects. See Figure 4-5.

Radiology

Radiological features include:

* sacroiliitis—changes vary from blurring of the joint margin to sclerosis and eventual SI joint fusion

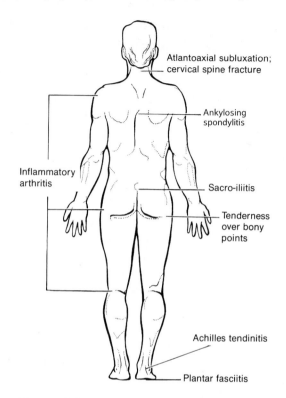

Figure 4-4. Musculoskeletal clinical features of AS.

- spinal changes—syndesmophyte formation; in severe cases, the classical fused-bamboo spine; ossifying diskitis; intervertebral fusion; and fractures.
- other abnormalities—erosion and ankylosing of peripheral joints (particularly hip), ischial tuberosity whiskering, and periosteal elevations. For severe hip conditions, total hip arthroplasty is usually preferred to other forms of hip surgery (re-ankylosis).

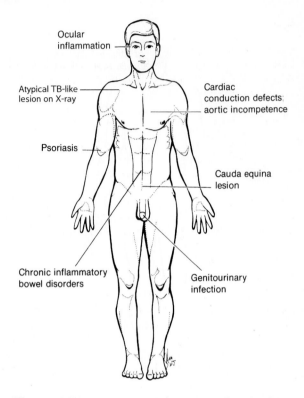

Figure 4-5.   Non-musculoskeletal clinical features of AS.

Laboratory

Rheumatoid factor is almost always negative; the HLA-B27 antigen is positive in at least 98% of cases. Erythrocyte sedimentation rate, alkaline phosphatase and creatine phosphokinase are usually abnormal at some stage of the disease.

Management

Comprehensive physiatric management includes use of medication, physical therapy, and patient education.

Medication

Indomethacin (Indocin) (up to 200 mg/daily) and phenyl-butazone (up to 400 mg/daily) are currently recommended drugs of choice. Try other NSAIDs if these are not tolerated.

Physical Therapy

The objectives of physical therapy in treatment of AS are to maintain normal spinal column position, strengthen spinal muscles, increase breathing capacity, maintain joint mobility, and relieve symptoms. Exercises include deep breathing, back extension and strengthening, stretching of pectorals, hip flex-ors, hamstrings, and heel cords; trunk mobility; and neck and shoulder mobility. Modalities may be employed as needed.

Patient Education

An education program includes a description of the disease and its course, with a rationale of needed exercises and devel-opment of posture consciousness. The need for adequate rest should be stressed, and the use of proper sleeping surfaces, including a hard mattress with few, if any, pillows. Advise the patient to avoid undesirable physical activities such as body contact sports.

Outcome

The prognosis of AS is usually better than that of rheumatoid arthritis, in that only a minority of patients ultimately devel-op a significant disabling spinal deformity. Progressive dis-ease is less common in women.

Suggested Readings

Bellamy N. *Prognosis in the Rheumatic Diseases.* Dordrecht: Kluwer Academic Publishers, 1991.

Convery FR, Minteer MA, Amiel D, Connett KL. Polyarticular disability: a functional assessment. *Arch Phys Med Rehabil.* 1977;58:494–499.

Ehrlich GE. *Rehabilitation Management of Rheumatic Conditions.* Baltimore, MD: Williams & Wilkins, 1980.

Feibel A, Fast A. Deep heating of joints: a reconsideration. *Arch Phys Med Rehabil.* 1977;58:69–71.

Hicks JE, Gerber LH. Rehabilitation of the Patient with Arthritis and Connective Tissue Disease. *In:* DeLisa JA, Gans B, eds. *Principles and Practice of Rehabilitation Medicine.* 2nd ed. Philadelphia, PA: J.B. Lippincott, 1993, pp. 1047–1081.

Kelley WN, Harris ED, Ruddy S, Sledge CB. *Textbook of Rheumatology.* 4th ed. Philadelphia, PA: W.B. Saunders, 1993.

McCarty DJ. *Arthritis and Allied Conditions.* 11th ed. Philadelphia, PA: Lea and Febiger, 1989.

McGuire T, Kumar VN. Rehabilitation management of the rheumatoid foot. *Orthopaedic Review* 1987;16:83–88.

Moll JMH. *Rheumatology in Clinical Practice.* Oxford, England: Blackwell Scientific Publications, 1987.

Pincus T, Callahan LF, Bradley LA, Vaughn WK, Wolfe F. Elevated MMPI scores for hypochondriasis, depressions and hysteria in patients with rheumatoid arthritis reflect disease rather than psychological status. *Arthritis and Rheumatism* 1986;29:1456–1466.

Rodnan GB, Schumacher HR. *Primer on the Rheumatic Diseases.* 8th ed. Atlanta, GA: Arthritis Foundation, 1983.

Schutt AH. Physical medicine and rehabilitation in the elderly arthritic patient. *Journal of the American Geriatrics Society.* 1977;25:76–82.

Smith RD, Polley HF. Rest therapy for rheumatoid arthritis. *Mayo Clinic Proceedings* 1978;53:141–145.

Spiegel JS, Spiegel TM, Ward NB, Paulus HE, et al. Rehabilitation for rheumatoid arthritis patients. *Arthritis and Rheumatism* 1986;29:628–636.

Steinbrocker O, Traeger CH, Batterman RC. Therapeutic criteria in rheumatoid arthritis. *JAMA* 1949;140:659–662.

Swanson AB, Swanson GD. Pathogenesis and pathomechanics of rheumatoid deformities in the hand and wrist. *Orthopedic Clinics of N.A.* 1973;4:1039–1056.

Swezey RL. *Arthritis: Rational Therapy and Rehabilitation.* Philadelphia, PA: W.B. Saunders, 1978.

5

Katie Irani

Burns

■ Definition

Burns represent a major health problem throughout the world. The United States has the highest incidence of burns among industrialized countries. In 1982, more than 2 million people required medical attention for burns and about 10,000 deaths were burn related. Only motor vehicle accidents cause more accidental deaths than burns. Structural fires account for less than 5% of hospital admissions for burns, but they are responsible for more than 45% of burn-related deaths, which are largely due to smoke inhalation. The decline in fire-related deaths over the last 25 years is attributed to better fire-fighting techniques, improved emergency medical systems and increased use of smoke detectors.

Advances in medical care of burned patients have improved the survival rate. An expansion of specialized centers for burns has resulted not only in improved care, but also in major advances in multidisciplinary research for burn management. Post-burn disability has increased, due to the increased survival rate. The number of annual disability days secondary to burn injuries is estimated at 9 million. Physical Medicine and Rehabilitation should be involved in the care of burn patients from the onset, through the acute stage, and during long-term follow-up.

Susan J. Garrison (Ed.): *Handbook of Physical Medicine and Rehabilitation Basics*. First Edition. Copyright © 1995 J. B. Lippincott Company

■ Epidemiology

A peak incidence of burns occurs in children 1 to 5 years of age; most of these are scalds from hot liquids. Accidents due to flammable liquids are the major cause of burns in teenagers and adults, most commonly males from 17 to 30 years old. Burns are more prevalent in nonwhite, male, and lower socioeconomic groups. See Table 5-1.

■ Classification by Depth of Burn

Burns are customarily classified into superficial (first), partial thickness (second), and full thickness (third) degree burns. See Table 5-2.

Determination of burn depth is difficult in the first few hours or days, particularly differentiating between deep partial and full thickness burns. Appearance remains the most reliable indicator. Burn depth is best determined by the rate and the completeness of healing after 3 weeks.

■ Classification by Severity of the Burn

The American Burn Association has classified thermal injuries as major and minor. See Table 5-3.

The surface area of the body burned is often estimated by using the "Rule of Nines" as developed by Pulaski and Tennison. A rough method of calculation, it is unreliable in

Table 5-1. Burn Classification by Etiology

Percentage	Etiology
95	Thermal
5	Chemical and Electrical
Rare	Radiation

Table 5-2. Burn Classification by Depth

Type	Cause	Part of Skin Involved	Clinical Findings	Healing Characteristics
Superficial (first-degree)	Sunburn, ultraviolet, short flash fire	Superficial, epidermis	Erythema, edema, painful	Within 3–7 days, no scar, no pigment changes
Partial thickness (second-degree—superficial)	Scalds, spills, flashes of flame	Epidermis; most of basal layer remains	Pink or mottled red, blisters, weeping, painful	Less than 3 weeks, minimal scar pigment changes ±
Partial thickness (second-degree deep)	Immersion, scalds, flame	Epidermis and dermis; only the basal layer lining the appendages remains	Cherry red or pale; pain ±; skin pliable	Greater than 3 weeks, severe hypertrophic scar formation may occur; may need grafting
Full thickness (third-degree)	Flame, electrical, chemical	Total skin destruction; may also involve deeper structures like fat, muscles, and bone	Tan or pearly white, leathery odor of burned flesh, non-pliable, wrinkled, especially over joints and bones, parchment-like, thrombosed vessels, anesthetic	Requires grafting

Modified from *Comprehensive Rehabilitation of Burns*. Fisher SV, Helm PA, eds. Baltimore: Williams & Wilkins, 1984. p. 13.

Table 5-3. Classification of Burn Severity

Minor burn
15% TBSA*, 1st and 2nd degree burn in an adult

10% TBSA, 1st and 2nd degree burn in a child

2% TBSA, 3rd degree burn in child or adult, not involving eyes, ears, face, or genitalia

Moderate burn
15–25% TBSA, 2nd degree burn in an adult

10–20% TBSA, 2nd degree burn in a child

2–10% TBSA, 3rd degree in child or adult, not involving eyes, ears, face, or genitalia

Major burn
25% TBSA, 2nd degree burn in an adult

20% TBSA, 2nd degree burn in a child

All 3rd degree burns greater than 10% TBSA

All burns involving hands, face, eyes, ears, feet, or genitalia

All inhalation injuries

Electrical burns

Complicated burn injuries involving fractures or other major trauma

All poor risk patients—pre-existing conditions such as head injury, closed head injury, cerebrovascular accident, psychiatric disability, emphysema or lung disease, cancer, diabetes, etc.

*TBSA designates total body surface area.
From Helm PA, Kevorkian GC, Lushbaugh MS, et al. Burn injury: rehabilitation management in 1982. *Arch Phys Med Rehabil* 1982;63: 6–16.

children under 15 years of age. The body is represented by 9 and its multiples and the perineum makes up the last 1%. See Figure 5-1.

A more accurate estimation of the total body surface area burn was developed by Lund and Browder. See Figure 5-2.

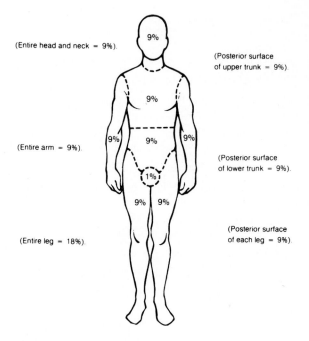

(Entire head and neck = 9%).

9%

(Posterior surface of upper trunk = 9%).

9%

(Entire arm = 9%).

9% 9% 9%

(Posterior surface of lower trunk = 9%).

1%

9% 9%

(Posterior surface of each leg = 9%).

(Entire leg = 18%).

Figure 5-1. Rule of Nines according to Pulaski and Tennison. A rapid, easily remembered method of calculation, but relatively inaccurate. (From Solem LD. Classification. *In:* Fisher SV, Helm PA. *Comprehensive Rehabilitation of Burns,* Baltimore: Williams & Wilkins, 1984, p. 14.)

In moderate and major burns, first degree burns are not considered in calculating total body burned surface. A patient's palm print is about 1% of the total body surface; use it to estimate the size of a small burn.

■ Assessment/Evaluation

Perform a thorough evaluation including depth of the burn; percentage of body burn; area of the body affected, with special attention to the hands and areas over joint surfaces;

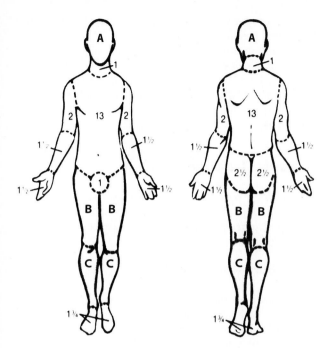

Relative percentages of areas affected by growth

Age in years	Half of head (A)	Half of one thigh (B)	Half of one leg (C)
Infant	9½	2¾	2½
1	8½	3¼	2½
5	6½	4	2¾
10	5½	4¼	3
15	4½	4½	3¼
Adult	3½	4¾	3½

Total percent burned _____ 2° + _____ 3° = _____

Figure 5-2. Lund and Browder Chart: A more accurate method of burn calculation commonly used by burn physicians. (Reproduced with permission from Lund and Browder: *Surg Gynecol Obstet* 79:352, 1944(3).)

presence of edema, exposed tendons, and associated fractures. Document presence of pain and/or infection.

Minor burns are the majority of burn injuries requiring treatment, usually on an outpatient basis. For the moderate/major burned patient admitted to the hospital, describe the general condition, associated injuries, and mental and respiratory conditions. Consider these additional factors in formulating the rehabilitation program.

▨ Acute Treatment

The goals in burn care are to manage pain, allow rapid wound healing, preserve function, prevent or minimize hypertrophic scarring, and achieve good cosmetic outcome.

Minor Burn—Outpatient Care

These burns are the majority of burn injuries, usually not associated with life-threatening complications. Second degree burns may cause intense pain even though the area of burn may be small. Apply cool saline soaked gauze compresses to achieve immediate temporary pain relief. Avoid ice; the decrease in cutaneous blood flow may increase tissue necrosis. A benefit of effective topical care is long-term pain relief; use of narcotic analgesia is unnecessary.

Cleanse the burn wound thoroughly; debride if necessary, and apply a topical antimicrobial ointment or cream in order to prevent rapid proliferation of bacteria and minimize infection. Sulfadiazine cream 1% is commonly applied; any broad spectrum antibiotic can be used. Cleanse the wound once or twice daily with soap and water and reapply the topical antibiotic and dressing. Cover the wound with thick mesh gauze to absorb exudate and protect it with a loosely wrapped elastic gauze bandage. An oral antibiotic is usually unnecessary with a small burn. Administer tetanus toxoid if the patient has not received tetanus immunization in the last 10 years.

In an outpatient setting, biologic and synthetic dressings

may be used on second degree burns. Follow the patient daily until the graft adheres.

Patients with pain due to burns across joints assume flexed positions that may lead to contractures. Prevent contractures by early active range of motion (AROM) exercises. Use sustained stretch to maintain range. Splints are usually not necessary. After healing, use pressure bandages until the skin is soft and supple.

Moderate/Major Burns

Moderate/major burns are routinely treated on an inpatient basis, with a physiatrist as a member of the burn team. The main issues to address are positioning, splinting, and range of motion exercises.

Positioning

An anticontracture positioning program is essential. Use therapeutic positioning techniques to decrease edema, preserve function, and prevent contractures as well as localized neuropathies.

Total body positioning and positioning of specific injury sites are combined to control edema, facilitate wound care and maintain range of motion. See Figure 5-3. Simple elevation of burned extremities, while maintaining full extension, helps in edema control. If elevation of legs and upper body is required, scrotal swelling may develop in males. Use a scrotal support and a change in position, if possible. Individualize positioning; compromise if necessary to achieve patient tolerance, which varies greatly from one patient to another. Gaining patient cooperation may be a problem. Adults may voluntarily maintain proper positioning except during sleep; only night splinting may be needed. Children may require splinting both day and night. If a patient is active during the day, use only night splinting to maintain the ROM gained during the day.

The position of comfort is the position of contracture.

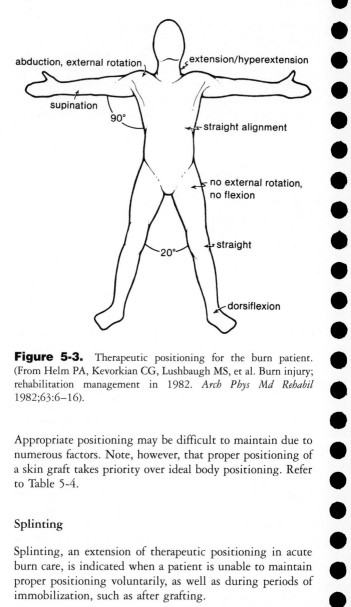

Figure 5-3. Therapeutic positioning for the burn patient. (From Helm PA, Kevorkian CG, Lushbaugh MS, et al. Burn injury; rehabilitation management in 1982. *Arch Phys Md Rehabil* 1982;63:6–16).

Appropriate positioning may be difficult to maintain due to numerous factors. Note, however, that proper positioning of a skin graft takes priority over ideal body positioning. Refer to Table 5-4.

Splinting

Splinting, an extension of therapeutic positioning in acute burn care, is indicated when a patient is unable to maintain proper positioning voluntarily, as well as during periods of immobilization, such as after grafting.

Table 5-4. Factors Affecting Positioning

Associated injuries
  Airway problems
  Fractures

Tracheostomy

Ventilator dependency

Intravenous/arterial lines

Urinary catheters

Pre-existing conditions
  Arthritis
  Neuromuscular diseases

Skin grafts

Surgery

Hands require special attention. Splint immediately to prevent edema and maintain range of motion. Use a volar splint with the wrist in about 10 to 15 degrees of extension, the metacarpal phalangeal joints (MCPs) in 60 to 70 degrees of flexion, and the proximal interphalangeal (PIPs) and distal interphalangeal joints (DIPs) in full extension with the thumb in an abducted, opposed position. Keep exposed tendons moist with moist wraps and biological dressing. These tendons can quickly become dry and denatured, and then snap or rupture. For exposed tendons use continuous splinting, keeping them in a slack position to prevent tension until they are healed or covered.

Use continuous splinting in unresponsive patients, uncooperative patients, hand burns, exposed tendon injuries, and peripheral nerve injuries.

Assess splints frequently for proper fit and alignment. If pain, tingling, numbness, inflammation, or tissue maceration are present, immediately adjust the splint to prevent further damage. Continuously applied splints should be assessed at least 3 times a day.

Commonly used splints are listed in Table 5-5.

Table 5-5. Commonly Used Splints

Area of Burn	Optimal Position	Splint
Hands	Wrist—10 to 15° of extension	Volar splint
	MCP—60 to 65° of flexion	
	PIP, DIP—full extension	
Elbow-cubital (volar aspect)	Full extension and supination	Anterior volar conforming splint
		Three-point conforming splint
		Posterior elbow extension splint after grafting
Shoulder and axilla	90° of abduction, external rotation	A firm density foam wedge
		Conforming axillary splint
		Airplane splint
Hip	Full extension— 20° of abduction, no external rotation	Triangular foam wedge and
		Hip abduction, extension splint (primarily used in children)
Knee	Full extension	Posterior knee extension splint
		Three-point extension splint
Ankle and foot	90° dorsiflexion, no inversion	Posterior dorsiflexion splint
		Anterior conforming splint

Exercise

The goals of exercise are to reduce edema, maintain range of motion and prevent skin contractures. When the patient is medically ill in the early post-burn period, emphasize proper positioning and splinting. Initiate PROM exercises to maintain joint mobility. Encourage the patient to participate actively in positioning. Perform gentle passive, active assistive, and AROM exercises 2 to 3 times a day, even in cases of circumferential burns necessitating escharotomies. Exercises are best tolerated after the application of topical cream and biological dressing. After isolated joint motion exercises, perform patterned movements involving multiple joints. Use a gentle sustained stretch over the burned area. This is more effective in preventing skin contractures than multiple, fast, individual joint motions.

Begin activities of daily living (ADLs) and ambulation as soon as possible. This helps the patient psychologically by fostering ego development and a sense of independence. ADLs demonstrate motor skills and coordination; early ambulation reduces problems from immobility and maintains strength and endurance. If there are lower limb burns, use short, frequent ambulation sessions. Avoid prolonged periods of standing or walking. Elevate the legs when sitting or resting to minimize dependent edema. Wrap the legs with elastic bandages before standing and walking to decrease swelling of the lower limbs. If the soles of the feet are affected, use an extra padding of dressing and/or foam-soled slippers. Ambulation is contraindicated with exposed tendon or joint capsule, or severe burns of the feet with swelling or infection.

As healing progresses, add functional strengthening activities to the exercise program. Observe carefully for complaints of muscle soreness, fatigue, or joint pain.

Immediately after grafting, discontinue exercises to the grafted areas but continue ROM to the surrounding ungrafted areas. Expect full ROM in 7 to 10 days after grafting in most cases. Treat donor sites as open wounds, with ROM exercises to prevent limitation of movement.

Hydrotherapy

Three types of cleansing techniques for open wounds are as follows:

Local wound care involves small areas as well as areas of the body, such as the face and ears, which are difficult to treat with hydrotherapy.

Immersion hydrotherapy with the water temperature about 96–98°F usually lasts for 15 to 20 minutes. Avoid extended submersion; there is potential for loss of electrolytes. Cross contamination between different wound sites as well as contamination from normal body flora can occur. Use heating elements to prevent excessive cooling in patients with large wounds and inadequate thermoregulation. Use water agitation to remove debris and creams, irrigate wounds, soften eschars, and increase patient comfort.

Nonsubmersion hydrotherapy (spray technique) occurs with the patient on a stretcher, and uses a hose or shower head suspended at an angle over a Hubbard tank. Use a water temperature of 100°F to allow for loss of warmth as the water is sprayed. This method allows easier protection of IV catheters and tracheostomies, as well as easier access to and cleaning of the perineal area. The spray loosens eschar and removes dead tissues and extraneous material from wounds, thereby decreasing the pain of scrubbing and debridement. More extensive manual debridement is possible using nonsubmersion hydrotherapy than during the 20-minute time limit of submersion.

Generally, discontinue hydrotherapy for 3 to 5 days following autograft or homograft. Hydrotherapy can be continued after heterograft.

Post-Excisional Therapy and Grafting Procedures

Early incision and grafting significantly reduces the period of acute burn rehabilitation. Early tangential and full thickness excision obviates the need for painful, protracted manual debridement. In consultation with the surgical staff prior to grafting procedures, decide positioning alternatives to be used during the post-graft immobilization phase. Discontinue hydrotherapy for about 3 to 5 days after grafting. Continue ROM exercises following excisional therapy and/or application of heterograft. Reinstate ambulation after 8 to 10 days of lower limb grafting. Apply elastic wraps from toes to groin before ambulation to prevent dependent edema, vascular stasis and bleeding under the grafts.

Convalescent Phase of Burn Rehabilitation

The convalescent phase begins as wounds are covered, grafts have taken, and the patient is medically stabilized. Evaluate the patient's home environment and family support. Instruct in appropriate assistance. Address any necessary home environmental changes. Treat any related physical problems such as contractures and weakness. There are multiple common problems seen in the convalescent phase, as listed below.

SKIN PROBLEMS AND CARE

Healing skin is fragile. There are often small open areas and blisters. The skin is nonsupple and dry. Avoid hydrotherapy and use of strong astringent or antiseptic soaps due to the drying effect; nearly healed areas will crack and break down. Avoid tub soaking; simple washing and showering is adequate. Use dry mesh dressing over open areas. Apply it wet; allow it to dry; change it 2 to 4 times a day after soaking to prevent removing new epithelium. If the open area is fairly large, use a topical agent such as silver sulfadiazine or bacitracin.

Blistering of the newly healed skin is common and may be a recurring problem. Keep the skin clean and lubricated; avoid any kind of friction or trauma. Drain small blisters with a sterile needle, flatten with a dressing, and allow to crust and heal. Open large blisters, treat conservatively, and allow to heal. Cauterize small overgranulated areas with silver nitrate sticks.

Healed skin is dry and breaks down easily since it lacks normal lubrication and pliability. Keep healed areas lubricated with a mild, non-irritating agent such as mineral oil, aloe vera cream or cocoa butter. Apply lightly and rub gently, as often as necessary, avoiding a greasy residue.

As healing occurs, massage with a gentle stroking motion, using a lubricant. Avoid friction and blistering. Begin deep massage as the skin becomes less fragile. This increases skin pliability and decreases sensitivity of the healed areas.

Alleviate hypersensitivity by the use of graduated pressure gradient materials. Initially, use elastic bandage, progress to elastic stockinette, then double layers of stockinette, and finally, commercially made pressure garments.

HYPERTROPHIC SCAR FORMATION AND MANAGEMENT

If allowed to heal spontaneously, deep second degree burns develop hypertrophic scarring. Hypertrophic scars usually manifest at 3 months after a burn. If a scar is red, raised, and firm, it will form hypertrophic tissue.

Children develop hypertrophic scarring more often than adults; blacks and Asians are more susceptible to hypertrophic scar formation than other races.

Control scar hypertrophy with external pressure. Continuous pressure approximating capillary pressure of 25 to 30 mm Hg changes the collagen configuration from whorls to more organized layers.

Use commercially available pressure garments that are worn continuously, except for bathing and possibly exercise. These garments cause shearing on wearing. Prepare the skin for commercial garments by using graduated gradient pressure to increase skin tolerance. Small blisters and breakdowns do not preclude the use of these garments. These garments must be worn until the scar is completely matured, which is usually around 12 to 18 months.

Noncompliance is a difficult problem. It can result from difficulty in donning the garment, pain on wearing, inability to understand fully the scar healing process, poor emotional support, and/or from psychological problems.

If tissue contracture occurs, use slow sustained stretch of a contracted area. Put the scar on a maximum stretch and apply a thick coating of paraffin at a temperature of about

118°F to prevent burning of the newly-healed, sensitive skin. Cover and leave in place for 20 to 30 minutes. Use splints, elastic wraps and weights to maintain the stretched position. Immediately after treatment, perform massage and stretching exercises to increase range of motion.

SPLINTING

Total contact or conforming splints are commonly used to provide static, total contact, continuous firm pressure which produces suppleness and flattening of the scar tissue, thus allowing more excursion. These splints are used for the following problems: (1) When scarring and band formation occurs over the posterior knee or dorsum of the foot and ankle. Often these are used at night only, and the patient is encouraged to use the part actively during the day. (2) When the burns are over contoured areas like the face and neck. Transparent, rigid face masks and neck conformers are custom-made and are worn continuously until the scar is matured and soft. (3) When hard pressure is needed under the axilla or in the web spaces between the fingers to prevent webbing.

Dynamic splinting, commonly used in the hand and with nerve damage, is used to stretch out a contracture. This works best when the patient is relaxed. Use serial splinting to stretch out an existing contracture.

GENERAL RECONDITIONING

As the skin heals, incorporate general conditioning and strengthening exercises. Use coordination exercises for gross and fine motor re-education.

Psychosocial Aspects of Moderate to Major Burns

Adjustment to severe burn injury is influenced by numerous factors. Refer to Table 5-6.

Table 5-6. Influences on Adjustment
Premorbid personality
Family stability
Extent of the burn
Location of the burn
In-hospital and outpatient environment
Attitudes of the burn team members and the family
Community support systems

Acute Stage

The patient may be disoriented, fearful and in pain. Survival issues may be the patient's central focus, especially while in the intensive care setting. Repeat information and give reassurance. Involve family and friends early in patient support and comfort. Provide consistent and accurate information to the patient and family; discuss every aspect of the recovery progress. In addition to medication, use techniques to involve the patient actively in the control of pain such as relaxation techniques, breathing exercises, hypnosis, and guided imagery.

Subacute Phase

Survival is no longer an issue. The patient has anxieties and fears about the future, including appearance, work, family, and social acceptance. Depression, withdrawal, and emotional lability may be seen. Provide emotional support from the team and family, as well as psychotherapy and counseling as needed.

Convalescent Phase

Adjustments to psychological problems usually continue during the first year. Long-term problems are not usually present. If face or hands are involved and/or a premorbid psychological problem existed, expect long-term adjustment problems.

■ Complications of Burns

Neuromuscular Complications

Common problems include localized compression or stretch neuropathies, generalized peripheral neuropathy, intramuscular injection injuries, and electrically induced neurological sequelae.

Localized nerve injury or stretch injury is often preventable. The ulnar and peroneal nerves and the brachial plexus are most frequently affected. Avoid poor positioning, including lengthy static positioning. A frog-lying position, with the hip flexed, abducted and externally rotated, the knee flexed and the foot plantar flexed, stretches the peroneal nerve at the fibular head. Direct pressure at the fibular head, as in prolonged side-lying, may result in peroneal neuropathy. The ulnar nerve may be compressed externally or internally in the cubital tunnel when the elbows are flexed and arms pronated for prolonged periods of time. Massive edema can cause carpal tunnel syndrome; this may require surgical decompression. Tight bulky dressing after grafting may cause direct pressure neuropathy, which is most commonly seen in the peroneal nerve at the knee.

Tourniquet injury involving compression of the nerve may occur during surgery. The tourniquet can cause direct pressure injury to the underlying tissues and ischemic injury to the distal parts.

The brachial plexus may be affected when the patient lies prone with the arms fully abducted, externally rotated and with elbows flexed for a number of days following grafting. Upper plexus stretch results from lying on the side with the arm hanging across the chest and off the bed. Another possible mechanism of brachial plexus injury is compression between the clavicle and the first rib (when the upper extremity is suspended), with the arm fully abducted and externally rotated in the supine lying position. Avoid this stretch and pressure by forward flexing the arm about 30 degrees at the shoulder.

Avoid repeated intramuscular injections in the same muscle; this causes muscle injury. These are seen frequently in the deltoid on the unburned side. The patient complains of shoulder pain with limited range of motion and deltoid weakness. Prevent this complication by use of a rotating injection schedule; educate the patient, as well as nursing personnel, about its importance.

A diffuse peripheral neuropathy is reported in 15% to 29% of burned patients, excluding electrical burns, with more than 20% of the body burned. The etiology is undetermined. The patients complain of generalized weakness which is mistakenly attributed to disuse. The neuropathy tends to improve with time, though some patients complain of fatigue and poor endurance for months or even years.

Neurological consequences of electrical burns include paraparesis, quadriparesis, radiculopathies, plexopathies, and peripheral nerve injuries at entrance and exit wounds. Signs and symptoms of spinal cord damage may not be apparent for a latency period of up to 1 year.

Musculoskeletal Complications

Hetertopic Ossification

Heterotopic ossification is new bone formation in tissues that normally do not ossify. Sometimes ossification is seen in the soft tissues surrounding a joint.

The elbow is most commonly involved. The usual signs and symptoms of pain, redness, and swelling may not be apparent. A sudden loss of ROM in a previously mobile joint is usually the first sign. Spontaneous resolution of bony mass can occur, especially in children.

Calcific Tendinitis

This is seen most commonly in the shoulder joint following burn injury. It can cause severe pain and limitation of movement. Use deep heat with ultrasound, active assistive to

AROM exercises and anti-inflammatory agents; consider steroid injections.

Joint Dislocation/Ankylosis

Joint dislocation is rarely seen as a result of faulty positioning during acute stage and/or following scar tissue contracture, particularly in hand burns. Joint ankylosis in small joints is seen following hand burns.

Scoliosis/Kyphosis

In children, asymmetrical trunk burns can lead to scoliosis. Scarring and contracture produces scoliosis with concavity toward the scar. Hip and knee contractures cause leg length discrepancy which may later contribute to scoliosis. This can be prevented with early trunk mobilization.

Kyphosis may develop with burns of the anterior chest, neck, and shoulders. Use proper positioning, postural exercises, pressure garments and/or total contact body jackets as early as necessary to prevent this deformity. Surgical excision of the scar may be required.

Amputation

Tissue destruction in severe thermal injuries, especially of the hand and foot, can result in amputation of digits. Severe electrical injury often necessitates limb amputation, sometimes multiple.

Outcome

The outcome after a burn injury depends on the combined efforts of the patient and a well-organized multidisciplinary burn team. If left to spontaneous recovery without intervention, severe scarring and contractures can occur. In the acute stage, the patient has to be followed very closely and intensive therapy initiated. Associated injuries like fractures, dislocations, inhalation burns, and extensive body burns prolong the rehabilitation course.

Follow-Up

After discharge, the patient is followed less intensively in therapies. Depending upon the extent of the body burn, the patient will need 2 to 3 sessions per week of supervised therapies.

Check pressure garments for excessive pressure and skin breakdown. These garments usually last for 3 to 4 months. Issue two pairs of garments for washing and wearing alternately.

Some patients develop temporary or permanent intolerance to heat and cold. Avoid prolonged exposure to heat or cold. Warn patients against vigorous outdoor activities until tolerance develops.

Sunburn occurs easily as long as skin discoloration is present; avoid direct sunlight exposure. Advise the patient to use sunscreens, cover the healed area with clothing, and plan outdoor activities in the early morning and late evening. Sunlight exposure after application of sunscreen can begin gradually, with caution, after about 6 months.

Follow a severely burned patient for at least 18 to 24 months, until the scar is completely matured and all rehabilitation complications have been resolved.

■ Suggested Readings

Deitch EA. The management of burns. *N Engl J Med.* 1990;18:1249–1253.

Fisher SV, Helm PA. *Comprehensive Rehabilitation of Burns.* Baltimore: Williams & Wilkins, 1988.

Helm PA, Kevorkian CG, Lushbaugh MS, et al. Burn injury: rehabilitation management in 1982. *Arch Phys Med Rehabil* 1982;63:6–16.

David X. Cifu

6

Cancer Rehabilitation

▪ Overview

Currently one million people in the United States are under active treatment for cancer; 1.5 million are considered cured. The lifetime probability for developing cancer is one in three. Over 600,000 people per year are diagnosed with cancer. Fifty percent of all cancers occur in persons over 65 years of age. A variety of factors, including type of cancer, therapeutic interventions, variable periods of bed rest, and the co-morbidity often seen in the elderly, combine to produce significant long-term or permanent functional loss as a result of cancer. Timely cancer rehabilitation can return the individual to functional independence, thereby improving quality of life.

▪ Functional Assessment

The functional status of a cancer patient can be correlated with the outcome of the underlying disease. The Karnofsky Performance Status Scale, the most widely used measure of the functional status of cancer patients, allows a consistent means of categorization. Match rehabilitation goals to the patient's functional level. See Table 6-1.

Susan J. Garrison (Ed.): *Handbook of Physical Medicine and Rehabilitation Basics*. First Edition. Copyright © 1995 J. B. Lippincott Company

Table 6-1. Karnofsky Performance Status Scale

General Category	Index	Specific Criteria
Able to carry on normal activity, no special care needed	100	Normal, no complaints, no evidence of disease
	90	Able to carry on normal activity, minor signs or symptoms of disease
	80	Normal activity with effort, some signs or symptoms of disease
Unable to work, able to live at home and care for most personal needs, varying amount of assistance needed	70	Cares for self, unable to carry on normal activity or to do work
	60	Requires occasional assistance from others, but able to care for most needs
	50	Requires considerable assistance from others and frequent medical care
Unable to care for self, requires institutional hospital care or equivalent, disease may be rapidly progressing	40	Disabled, requires special care and assistance
	30	Severely disabled, hospitalization indicated; death not imminent
	20	Very sick, hospitalization necessary; active supportive treatment necessary
	10	Moribund
	0	Dead

Mor V, Laliberle L, Morris JN, Wiemann M: The Karnofsky Performance Status Scale: an examination of its reliability and validity in a research setting. Cancer 53:2002–2007, 1984.

▐ Treatment

The regimen utilized to maintain function includes mobilization, activity, nutrition, social support systems, and pain
control. This overall program is used in combination with
specific interventions based on the organ systems affected.
Cancer rehabilitation concentrates initially on early discharge
from the acute care setting. Continued rehabilitation occurs
in the home environment. The intensity of the rehabilitation
effort and the clinical setting depend on the type, site and
extent of involvement of the cancer.

Mobilization

Use daily bedside physical therapy to teach independence in
bed mobility, through such activities as rolling from side to
side and moving from a supine to a sitting position, as well as
transfer skills, such as bed to chair. Nurses reinforce these
learned activities.

Progressively increase the patient's time out of bed. Use a
sitting program for patients who have difficulty with sitting
secondary to orthostatic disturbances or skin breakdown. Assess skin integrity prior to and after sitting to prevent breakdown. Patients are to be out of bed, in a chair, throughout
the day, as much as tolerated.

Activity

Encourage patients to do as much for themselves as possible,
such as dressing, grooming, and feeding, as well as to use
their own strength for mobility, either ambulating or pro-
pelling a wheelchair. Provide reachers, gait devices, and other
aids to allow independent function. Physical appearance is
important; encourage the use of wigs, make-up, and other
aspects of cosmesis such as prosthetic facial features and
limbs and modified clothing.

Formulate an individualized program for stretching, positioning, self range of motion, strengthening, and condition-

ing, in addition to regular physical and occupational therapy. Educate family and friends in ways to encourage and support independent activities.

When the patient achieves enough functional independence to be discharged, teach a specific home program of exercises to promote continued improvement. Consider a home safety evaluation. Schedule periodic evaluations and home or outpatient physical and occupational therapies, if needed. Consider the patient's expected functional outcome when ordering expensive equipment; devices may not be useful if the patient soon experiences a physical decline.

Social Support

The use of a multidisciplinary team approach (including an oncologist, a physiatrist, appropriate therapist(s), a social worker, a psychologist, an oncology nurse, a dietician, and, of course, the patient) is necessary in order to attempt to address all concerns. Select facilities such as the acute care hospital, the hospice, and the home with supportive care, through awareness of availability and the patient's care needs and wishes. Involve family members and friends, as appropriate, to achieve a smooth transition from one environment to another and to maintain adequate patient care.

Nutrition

Encourage good nutrition. Offer foods pleasant in appearance, smell, and taste. Anorexia, changes in ability to smell and taste, oropharyngeal and esophageal lesions and infections, and problems with digestion and absorption are common.

Maintain independent feeding and, if possible, independent preparation of food, by promoting mobilization and activity. Preserve the patient's autonomy as much as possible. Supplement the diet liberally as soon as possible with foods high in calories and protein to maintain strength and endurance. Obtain assistance from dieticians and nutritionists.

Use enteral feeding or intravenous hyperalimentation only as a last resort to support nutritional needs. The oral route is the most physiological approach.

Pain Management

Pain is present in 40% of intermediate-stage cancer, and 60 to 80% of advanced-stage cancer. Cancer pain as categorized by Foley allows for a systematic treatment regimen (See Table 6-2).

First, ascertain the type of cancer pain present. Categorize the patient using this pain classification. Treatment of the underlying cancer is the first line of therapy. Surgery, radiotherapy, and chemotherapy directed at the tumor may all result in decreased pain.

Next, use non-narcotic pain relievers such as aspirin, acetaminophen, and nonsteroidal anti-inflammatory drugs in combination with physical modalities such as vibration, transcutaneous electrical nerve stimulation (TENS), massage, and heat or cold. Encourage continued mobilization and activity. Avoid physical modalities utilizing heat over an area of known tumor involvement.

As the next line of treatment, prescribe an oral opioid, in

Table 6-2. Foley's Cancer Pain Classification

I. Patients with acute cancer-related pain associated with diagnosis of cancer or associated with therapy

II. Patients with chronic cancer-related pain associated with cancer progression or therapy

III. Patients with pre-existing chronic pain and cancer pain

IV. Patients with a history of drug addiction and cancer-related pain

V. Patients dying with cancer-related pain

Foley KM: Cancer Pain Syndromes. *J Pain Symptom Manag* 2(2):S13–S17, 1987.

combination with a non-narcotic pain reliever depending on the degree of pain and the clinical situation. In cases of acute pain syndromes, as well as in terminal patients, utilize narcotic medications more rapidly and liberally.

When appropriate opioid preparations are ineffective, consider invasive neurosurgical and anesthetic procedures performed by experienced personnel as useful adjuvants for pain control.

In addition to pharmacological intervention, use behavioral approaches such as relaxation training, distraction, guided imagery, hypnosis, and behavioral training.

▩ Complications

Bony Metastases

Obtain bone scans and X-rays when there is evidence of bony involvement such as fracture, bone pain, or specific tumor type, in order to define the extent of the problem. While local immobilization using, for example, a sling or a halo-vest, or radiation therapy may forestall fractures, surgical correction, specifically intramedullary rodding, is necessary to promote weight bearing and continued activity. Additionally, surgical intervention is indicated prophylactically in all cases where greater than 50% of the bone cortex is destroyed, or in lesions greater than 3 centimeters in diameter.

Orthopedically repair pathologic fractures by pinning, rodding, or replacing rather than casting or otherwise immobilizing, in order to allow early mobilization and weight-bearing.

Treat pain from metastases with local immobilization, medications, physical modalities, radiation therapy, and/or chemotherapy (hormonal manipulation). If the pain is intractable, surgical intervention is indicated.

Amputation

With the advent of limb salvage procedures, amputation secondary to cancer has become less frequent, particularly in children. Rehabilitation following limb salvage is similar to that of joint replacement patients; however, expect a longer period of immobilization and/or non-weightbearing. In addition, more extensive bracing and assistive devices may be required.

Fit the patient with a conventional prosthesis as soon as possible, following basic principles of amputee rehabilitation. (See Chapter 3, Amputations.)

Observe for common problems, including poor skin healing, as a result of radiation and chemotherapy, weight fluctuations, and generalized deconditioning.

Neurologic Involvement

Rehabilitate the patient with primary or metastatic spinal cord cancer using principles of spinal cord injury rehabilitation. (See Chapter 17, Spinal Cord Injury.)

Primary and metastatic brain tumors may present with headache, focal neurologic deficit, seizures, or diffuse encephalopathy. Following acute treatment such as surgery, radiation therapy, and corticosteroid administration, employ stroke rehabilitation techniques. (See Chapter 19, Stroke.)

Abnormalities of the neuromuscular system, both focal, such as Pancoast tumor and compression neuropathy, and systemic, such as peripheral neuropathy, may be the result of cancer or may be treatment-related. Diagnose and treat these problems, using rehabilitative strategies for neuromuscular diseases. (See Chapter 14, Peripheral Neuropathy and Chapter 11, Neuromuscular Diseases.)

Breast Cancer

Advances in breast surgery have eliminated many of the complications associated with radical mastectomy such as edema, pain, immobility, and poor cosmesis. Educate the patient about appropriate positioning, range of motion, pain control, and activities.

The patient will be immobilized at the shoulder at the time of surgery. On the fourth postoperative day, begin active motion of the affected elbow, wrist, and hand, as well as the unaffected upper limb. Initiate motion of the affected shoulder in the supine position at day 5 to 7. Progress to upright activities when the sutures are removed at 2 weeks. At that time, add activities of daily living (ADLs) and strengthening for the patient's home program. Most patients require compression with an elastic bandage, followed by use of a custom-fitting gradient pressure garment for management of edema. In the rare patient who develops lymphedema despite appropriate interventions, use pneumatic intermittent compression and/or compression garments, such as a custom glove and sleeve.

Suggested Readings

Dietz JH. Rehabilitation of the cancer patient. *Med Clin N Amer.* 1969;53(3):607–624.

Foley KM. Cancer pain syndromes. *J Pain Symptom Manag* 1987;2(2):S13–S17.

Hirsh D, Grabois M, Decker N. Rehabilitation of the cancer patient. *In:* DeLisa JA, ed. *Rehabilitation Medicine: Principles and Practice.* Philadelphia, PA: J.B. Lippincott, 1988 pp. 660–670.

Laban M. Rehabilitation of patients with cancer. *In:* Kottke FJ, Stillwell GK, Lehmann JF, eds.: *Krusen's Handbook of Physical Medicine and Rehabilitation.* 4th ed. Philadelphia, PA: W.B. Saunders, 1990 pp. 1102–1111.

Portnoy RK. Practical aspects of pain control in the patient with cancer. *Cancer J Clin* 1988;38(6):327–351.

Recommendations for Cancer Prevention. *Department of Cancer Prevention and Control Manual.* Houston, TX: The University of Texas M.D. Anderson Cancer Center, 1989.

Donna Schramm
Anjali Jain

7

Cardiovascular Conditioning Exercise and Cardiac Rehabilitation

Cardiovascular Fitness, Exercise Testing and Prescription

Consider the human organism to be a cardio-pulmonary-muscular system designed to do work, that is to move mass over distance. The maximal ability of the individual to do work reflects his or her cardiovascular fitness: the gold standard of measurement of cardiovascular fitness is maximal oxygen consumption, or VO_2 max. Maximal oxygen consumption is defined as the level of exercise achieved by an individual at the point when fatigue or symptoms prevent further exercise. Oxygen consumption is not a convenient method of determining fitness because of the specialized equipment required to measure oxygen use. Therefore, more practical and clinically useful means of evaluating cardiovascular fitness is necessary.

Oxygen consumption (VO_2) consists of heart rate (HR), stroke volume of the heart (SV), arterial oxygen content of the blood (CaO_2) and the ability of the end-organ, or muscle, to extract oxygen from the blood before it is dumped into the venous system ($CaO_2 - CvO_2$). The mathematical relationship of these variables is the Fick Equation: $VO_2 = HR \times SV (CaO_2)$; or at maximal oxygen consumption: VO_2 max $= HR_{max} \times SV_{max} \times (CaO_{2max} - CvO_{2min})$. Clinically, the

Susan J. Garrison (Ed.): *Handbook of Physical Medicine and Rehabilitation Basics.* First Edition. Copyright © 1995 J. B. Lippincott Company

HR and HR max, or maximal heart rate, are used to evaluate how hard a person is working (in terms of that person's maximal cardiovascular ability). The maximal heart rate an individual can obtain decreases physiologically with aging; maximal heart rate can be approximated by subtracting age from 220: 220 − age in years = maximal obtainable heart rate. This estimation is only a rough guideline, however; the only way in which an individual's maximum heart rate can be determined is by exercise treadmill testing.

Exercise testing on a treadmill, or with an arm ergometer for persons unable to walk, assists in determining the maximal heart rate an individual can achieve. Because heart rate is proportionally related to oxygen consumption by the Fick Equation, the maximal heart rate provides some indication of cardiovascular fitness or the maximal amount of internal work that can be done.

A second type of work to consider is the external work that is being accomplished. Some individuals will have more efficient cardio-pulmonary-muscular systems than others and therefore will accomplish more external work at the same heart rate or oxygen consumption than the inefficient individual. However, an inefficient cardio-pulmonary-muscular work system can become more efficient. This is the goal of cardiovascular exercise; when efficiency improves as a result of cardiovascular conditioning exercise, a training effect is said to have occurred. The Fick Equation, $VO_2 = HR \times SV \times (CaO_2 - CvO_2)$, suggests the possible variables that might be made more efficient by a cardiac conditioning exercise program. Studies suggest that in normal subjects at maximal work levels, conditioning exercise increases VO_{2max} by increasing SV and by increasing end-organ extraction, meaning increasing $(CaO_2 - CvO_2)$.

Maximal heart rate is physiologically set and age dependent. The practical and clinical corollary to this increased efficiency is that at submaximal external work levels, after training effect has occurred, a lower HR, lower SV, and lower myocardial oxygen demand will be required to do the same amount of external work as compared to pretraining HR, SV, and myocardial oxygen demand. Other factors in addition to exercise affect variables in the Fick Equation (Table 7-1).

Table 7-1. The Effects of Exercise and Other Factors on Maximal Oxygen Consumption (Maximal Cardiovascular Fitness)*

	Determinants of Max Values	Effects of Exercise in Normal Persons	Effects of Exercise in Cardiac Patients
HR_{max}	Age, sinus node medications	—	Potential HR_{max} may be lower due to medications or disturbed chronotropic response post MI
SV_{max}	Heart size, conditioning effects (contractility, preload, afterload), disease effects on wall motion and valves	Increases (increased LV mass and ED diameter)	Disease effects may decrease
CaO_2max	Pulmonary diffusion, ventilation and perfusion and adverse disease processes, inspired F_iO_2 (altitude) anemia, smoking decrease	—	Co-morbid pulmonary disease may decrease
CvO_2max	Skeletal aerobic enzymes, fiber types, genetics, muscle disease, capillary bed		The greatest training effect occurs peripherally
CaO_2-CvO_2	O_2 extraction by muscle, sympathetic redistribution of blood to active tissues	Increases	The greatest training effect occurs peripherally

*Adapted from Yanowitz FG, ed. Coronary Artery Disease Prevention. New York: Marcel Dekker, 1992.

The amount of exercise necessary to induce a cardiovascular conditioning effect in a normal person is 30 to 60 minutes of aerobic exercise three to five times per week at an intensity of 70% of maximal heart rate. Aerobic exercise is defined as a rhythmic, repetitive exercise using large muscle groups that adequately induces a heart rate response; activities may include brisk walking, jogging, biking, or swimming. The 30 minutes of aerobic activity is always preceded by stretching warm-up and cool-down periods of 10 to 15 minutes each. In persons younger than 35 to 45 years starting an exercise program, use maximal heart rate (220 − age); however, perform a maximal exercise treadmill test in persons older than 45 years or over 35 years with any risk factors for coronary artery disease (CAD). A submaximal or symptom-limited stress test is necessary if a cardiac event has occurred.

Persons who have sustained a cardiac event are prescribed a different intensity of exercise. They also participate in 30 minutes of aerobic activity, preceded and followed by 15 minutes of stretching, but intensity is 60% of maximal heart rate obtained on a symptom-limited exercise treadmill test.

Some patients with chronic stable angina will predictably have onset of pain at certain levels of exercise-induced heart rate and systolic blood pressure, called the double product (HR × SBP), or the rate-pressure product. These patients should exercise 10 beats per minute below their symptomatic heart rate to develop a training effect. As they become more conditioned, meaning fit, they will be able to do more external work, even though they never exceed their symptomatic heart rate.

Exercise Stress Testing

There are many published protocols of exercise treadmill testing. In general, exercise treadmill protocols increase the external workload, in regular increments of 1 to 3 METS depending on the protocol, in regular time intervals, or every 2 to 3 minutes. MET, or work load, is increased by speeding up and/or elevating the treadmill. For example, a person undergoing a diagnostic maximal treadmill test may use a

Bruce protocol that rapidly progresses to 3 METS activity and increases 2 to 2.5 METS in intensity every 2 minutes. On the other hand, a cardiac patient during a predischarge low-level symptom-limited test would probably undergo a modified Bruce, or a Naughton protocol that starts at a level of 1.5 METS and even after 12 minutes only reaches an intensity of 4 METS.

The term METS is often used in exercise physiology. One MET, equal to 3.5 ml O_2/kg/min, describes energy required for the average person to sit quietly at rest, arms and trunk supported. Activities of increased workload are described in terms of this average metabolic rate. For example, self-care activities, on average, are at 3 MET workload and cause average people to require three times the O_2 consumption that they would resting quietly; slowly climbing stairs is a 5 to 7 MET activity and the average person will increase O_2 consumption 5 to 7 times.

There are at least three strategies for exercising a patient during an exercise treadmill test (ETT). These strategies differ in intensity, rate of increase of intensity, and type of patient studied. The strategies include: maximal ETT, submaximal ETT, and symptom-limited low-level ETT. It is probably safest for the resident physician and patient to clarify with the cardiologist or ETT lab physician which protocol and strategy will be used. It should be noted that all ETTs (maximal, submaximal, and low-level symptom-limited) should end if symptoms occur. This requirement necessitates that the attendant of an ETT is aware of and can recognize the criteria for ending an ETT. Table 7-2 compares features of maximal, submaximal, and symptom-limited, low-level stress tests; however, use of these terms is not universally accepted.

In the evaluation of patients who have sustained cardiac events, submaximal or symptom-limited, low-level tests might be used; each institution has its own protocol for testing. Be aware that there are different protocols and strategies of testing; clarify the test to be used and criteria for ending the test with the attending physician. Throughout any treadmill test, monitor EKG, patient appearance, blood pressure, heart rate, and symptomatology. Stop the test at

Table 7-2. Submaximal and Symptom-limited Exercise Tolerance Test (ETT)

	Maximal ETT	Sub-maximal ETT	Symptom-limited ETT
Endpoint	Symptoms of cardiovascular insufficiency or disease	Symptoms of cardiovascular insufficiency or disease	Symptoms of cardiovascular insufficiency or disease
	Maximal obtained HR (some labs)	Predetermined % of age-predicted maximal HR (often 60%)	Maximal HR obtained
			Completely free of symptoms or signs of CAD
	Age-predicted maximal HR (some labs)	Predetermined MET level (often 5 METS)	
		Predetermined Borg PRE (perceived exertion level)	
Protocol	Fast increase in intensity (e.g. Bruce protocol)	Variable: check your lab's protocol; often low-level	Low level: low MET initiation point and small increments of increase MET intensity (e.g. Naughton, Modified Bruce)
Special Uses	(Check your lab's protocol)	Tracking patient fitness in conditioning exercise program, patient after cardiac event (some labs)	Patient post cardiac event (some labs)

patient request, if equipment fails, or for increasing angina, 2-mm horizontal or down-sloping ST depression or elevation, supraventricular or ventricular tachycardia, exercise-induced intraventricular conduction delays, exercise-induced hypotension, severe hypertension, bradycardia or significant heart block, or progressive ventricular ectopy.

Contraindications to ETT are essentially the same as those to Phase 1 of a cardiac rehabilitation program (described on p. 133), and also include digitalis or other drug effect and presence of a fixed-rate pacemaker.

For cardiac patients performing a low-level stress test, poor prognosis is associated with inability to achieve 5 METS activity, malignant ventricular arrhythmias, exercise-induced hypotension, and significant ST segment elevation or depression.

▣ Cardiac Rehabilitation

Successful cardiac rehabilitation restores the cardiac-impaired patient to optimal physiologic, psychosocial, and vocational function by involving the patient, as soon as is medically safe after a cardiac event, in a multidisciplinary program of exercise and education. The medical goals of cardiac rehabilitation are to recondition the cardiac patient so that he or she may tolerate daily activities, and to educate the patient so that he or she may make lifestyle choices that modify risk factors for heart disease and reduce the risk of recurrent disease. Another goal is to provide the patient with adequate confidence, stamina, and knowledge to resume safely vocational, recreational, and sexual activities.

The typical patient involved in a cardiac rehabilitation program has a diagnosis of CAD and has just experienced a myocardial infarction or coronary artery bypass graft procedure (CABG). However, patients with other cardiac diseases or surgical interventions may benefit from cardiac rehabilitation programs (Table 7-3). People who have not yet had a cardiac event but who have significant risk factors for CAD should be included in exercise conditioning and given instructions about risk factor modification after medical evaluation.

Table 7-3. Diagnoses of Patients Who May Benefit from
Cardiac Rehabilitation

Myocardial infarction	Status post surgical-correction of congenital cardiac defects
Status post CABG	
Status post coronary-angioplasty	Status post cardiac-transplantation
Status post valve-replacement	Compensated congestive heart failure
Status post valvuloplasty	Chronic stable angina
Persons with increased risk for CAD, after medical clearance	

A standard cardiac rehabilitation program has three
phases. Each of the three phases has activity and education
components as well as goals, but differs with respect to location and duration of the phase, amount of supervision, and
intensity of activity (Table 7-4). Phase 1 activities include
low metabolic demand activities that are performed up to 30
minutes several times per day. The goals of Phase 1 are to
avoid the sequelae of immobility (refer to Chapter 10, Immobilization), to tolerate self-care activity and household ambulation by the time of discharge from acute care, and to intro-
duce the concepts of low-fat diet, the benefits of exercise, and
independence in administering medication.

Phase 2 activities begin with light aerobic activities 1
hour each day (including warm-up and cool down periods),
three days a week. Patient and family education sessions
regarding diet, prevention of disease progression, symptom
recognition, sensible exercise, stress management, and other
pertinent issues continue. By the end of Phase 2, the cardiac
patient should have adequate information and training to
sustain healthy habits. These include lifestyle adjustment to
minimize further cardiac risk and to resume premorbid activities safely.

text continues on page 128

Table 7-4. Three Phases of a Cardiac Rehabilitation Program

	Location	Initiation	Duration	Monitored	Activity/Intensity
Phase 1	Inpatient	2–4 days	Hospitalization	Yes	Progress to independent self-care and short distance ambulation
Phase 2	Outpatient	3 weeks from onset	8–12 weeks	Yes	Progressive cardiac conditioning 1 hour 3 times per week (target heart rate based on submax ETT)
Phase 3	Community	After Phase 2	Lifetime	No	Maintenance of cardiac conditioning 1 hour 3 times per week

Table 7-5. Members of a Multidisciplinary Cardiac Rehabilitation Team

Team Member	Possible Duties
Physician	Prescribe medications
	Prescribe activity with appropriate precautions
	Prescribe appropriate diet
	Consult and supervise other health care personnel
Nurse	Review medications and their identification, adverse effects, purposes, and administration
	Review disease process and symptom identification
Physical Therapist	Demonstrate and teach proper exercise techniques as prescribed by M.D.
	Assist in symptom identification during activity

Occupational Therapist	Instruct in energy conservation techniques, relaxation techniques, work simplification techniques
	Instruct in proper execution of ADLs
Nutritionist	Diet instruction and grocery planning to achieve the recommended low-fat, low-cholesterol, low-sodium, or diabetic diet
Psychologist	Address symptoms of anxiety or depression
	Instruct in stress management techniques
	Address stressors related to psychosocial situation
Social Worker	Obtain educational and employment history and make referrals to intervene where financial or vocational difficulties can be anticipated
	Address family questions and concerns
Vocational Rehabilitation Counselor	Vocational retraining and relocation

text continued from page 124

Typically, physicians are involved in prescribing exercise, medications, and dietary modifications; however, the roles of other health care professionals and the issues they address are also important. Team members may include nurses, physical and occupational therapists, a psychologist or psychiatrist, nutritionist, social worker, and vocational rehabilitation counselor (Table 7-5).

Seventy to 80% of cardiac patients return to work; however, only 30% of cardiac patients in lower socioeconomic levels or with lower educational achievement are able to return to work. Take a complete social history; prioritize the social worker's efforts to anticipate financial and vocational needs. The vocational counselor will initiate vocational assessment. The occupational therapist performs a worksite evaluation and may recommend job modifications or identify excessive isometric work. The most common psychological reaction to a cardiac event is anxiety and depression, which is usually self-limiting, but may last beyond 6 months in up to 30% of patients. A psychologist or psychiatrist should be involved or at least available to the cardiac rehabilitation team; many patients will need to learn stress management techniques. The occupational therapist may instruct in relaxation techniques.

Coronary Artery Disease: Risk Factors and Modification

Most patients in cardiac rehabilitation programs are recovering from the sequelae of CAD, as opposed to other cardiac pathology such as congenital, myopathic, or valvular disease. In the United States CAD remains the number one cause of death, killing over 500,000 Americans annually. Thrombus formation in an atherosclerotic artery is found in the majority of persons who die of transmural myocardial infarction.

The United States' age-adjusted mortality rate for myocardial infarction (MI), however, is declining; in the 1950s this rate was 226 per 100,000, but by 1987, age-adjusted mortality for CAD had declined almost 50% to 124 per 100,000. Decline in mortality rate is attributed to advances in medical treatment and technology, including pre-hospital care, the wide availability of coronary care units, the use of thrombolytic agents, and improved diagnostic techniques and surgical interventions. However, a significant decline in the age-adjusted mortality rate of CAD has been attributed to patient-implemented lifestyle changes to reduce risk of cardiac disease.

Risk factors for atherosclerotic CAD include elevated serum cholesterol, cigarette smoking, hypertension, diabetes mellitus, advanced age, male gender, history of previous cardiac event or abnormal EKG, and a family history of CAD before the age of 50 years. The control of hypertension has not been shown to decrease cardiac risk, possibly because the medications used increase serum lipids. However, dietary and medical control of hyperlipidemia, smoking cessation, increased exercise, and modification of "Type A" behavior may also slow atherosclerotic disease progression or reduce disease recurrence or mortality (Table 7-6).

Instruction in the prevention of the progression or recurrence of CAD through risk factor modification is a significant portion of the cardiac rehabilitation program.

Cardiac Rehabilitation: Phase 1

Cardiac rehabilitation usually has three distinct, successive phases. The phases of cardiac rehabilitation, when successful, lead to a cardiac patient's functioning safely at maximal physiological, psychosocial, and vocational ability through an independent, self-monitored program of aerobic exercise, stress management, sensible diet, and recommended medical follow-up. Phase 1, the inpatient acute phase of cardiac rehabilitation, is the initiation point and cornerstone for all other phases. Activity resumption and prescription, dietary changes and education, stress management techniques, and planning for vocational, family, and sexual needs begin in this stage.

Table 7-6. CAD Risk Factor (RF), Effects on CAD with Modification

Risk Factor	Modifiable	Decreased CAD, progression if RF improved	Decreased CAD even if RF improved	Decreased CAD death if RF improved
Advanced age	No			
Male gender	No			
Family History CAD	No			
Sedentary lifestyle	Yes	Questionable	Moderate aerobic activity in the general population leads to fewer CAD events	Possibly
Elevated lipids	Yes	Yes (demonstrated with vegetarian diet, with low-fat diet, and lipid lowering medication)	Control of lipids reduces risk of first cardiac event; effect on recurrence not ascertained	Yes
Smoking	Yes		Yes	Yes
Hypertension risk	Yes	Control does not reduce CAD risk, but is desirable to reduce cerebrovascular accidents		
Diabetes Mellitus	Yes	No effect shown	Possible	
Type A Personality				

Physicians should prescribe activity with appropriate precautions and monitor the patient's response to prescribed activity. The initial management of patients with acute ischemia is bed rest, with appropriate medical evaluation and treatment (Table 7-7). Patients ordered bed rest longer than 3 to 4 days are at risk for complications of immobility (refer to Chapter 10, Immobilization). In order to prescribe activity with appropriate precautions, examine the patient and review the chart for signs and symptoms that might contraindicate or limit activity (Table 7-8). Record these findings.

Begin activity when the patient is free of chest pain and early complications have been ruled out, usually at 36 hours to 4 days after admission. Approach activity cautiously if there are findings of moderate hypertension, moderate aortic stenosis, co-existent chronic medical disease, incisional drainage, sinus tachycardia, or ventricular aneurysm. Patients with uncomplicated cardiac events or first degree heart block, sinus bradycardia, and infrequent premature ventricular contractions (PVCs) may generally proceed with Phase 1 activity. Appropriately prescribed and monitored early activity and ambulation is safe and does not increase risk of complications. The patient must be monitored during and after activity for signs and symptoms of activity-induced cardiovascular dysfunction (Table 7-9). Always stop activity if adverse symptoms occur.

Precautions written as part of the exercise prescription should reflect the physician's concern for activity-induced adverse cardiovascular effects. While in Phase 1, the patient should not participate in activity that raises the heart rate above 20 beats per minute over the resting heart rate. In Phase 1, activities are performed for 5 to 30 minutes, 2 to 3 times each day; CABG patients progress slightly faster than MI patients. A sample program of a multistep, graded-activity program for Phase 1 cardiac rehabilitation is in Table 7-10.

Goals the patient should achieve by the time of discharge, meaning the end of Phase 1, include self-care and activities of daily living (ADLs) and household ambulation, except stair

text continues on page 135

Table 7-7. History and Exam Findings of Significance in the CAD Patient

Historical Features	Physical Findings	Diagnostic Studies
Continued angina	Resting hypertension	CPK values
		CPK-MB values
		LDH values
Peri-operative or extended infarct	Orthostatic or symptomatic hypotension	EKG
		Chest x-ray (pneumonia, edema)
Post or concurrent history of CVA, COPD, renal and/or hepatic disease, systemic ASVD, arthritis, electrolyte imbalance, diabetes	Uncompensated heart failure: rales, edema, jugular distension, hypoxia, tachypnea, S3 gallop, fever; sinus tachycardia over 120, incisional drainage (CABG)	Telemetry strips for atrial fib and flutter, degrees of heart block, PVC triplets, more than 6 PVCs/min
Fixed-rate pacemaker	Focal neurologic signs	Ventricular fib and tachycardia
Medications which reduce heart rate response	Signs of PVD, arthritis, skin pressure	Echocardiogram for pericarditis or critical aortic stenosis
Febrile illness, PE, DVT	Tubes and drains that limit mobility (central, chest, surgical, etc.)	

Table 7-8. Complications Contraindicating Activity

Continued angina

Severe resting hypertension

Symptomatic, orthostatic or exercise-induced hypotension

Second or third degree heart block

Severe atrial or ventricular arrhythmias

Acute febrile or medical illness or instability such as
pneumonia, GI bleed

Cardiogenic shock or uncompensated heart failure

Pericarditis

Critical aortic stenosis

Table 7-9. Signs and Symptoms of Activity-Induced
Cardiovascular Dysfunction

Angina

Nausea

Dyspnea

Altered mental status

Activity-induced hypotension

Fatigue

Pallor

Cyanosis

Hypoxia

Activity-induced dysrhythmia

Table 7-10. Sample Phase 1 Cardiac Rehabilitation Activity Outline

Step	MET Workload	Location	Activities
1	1.5	Patient room	Ankle pumps, deep breathing and cough; P-AAROM all limbs; feed self
(initiated in ICU prior to PM&R consult)			
2	1.5	Patient room	Above; plus, transfer to bedside commode and chair; light grooming
(Initiated in ICU prior to PM&R consult)			
3	1.5	Patient room	AROM, stretching, up in chair, bathing, slow paced ambulation
4	1.5 to 2.0	Nursing station	Supervised ambulation for 75 feet, dressing activity
5	1.5 to 3.0	Nursing station or gym	Ad lib ambulation on nursing station, 2 to 3 stairs, ADLs at sink; ambulation 100 to 300 feet, stationary bike (no resistance) for 3 minutes, warm-up activity
6	1.5 to 3.0	Gym	Ambulate 500 feet, 2 sets of steps or 8 stairs, 5 minutes stationary bike; teach to take pulse rate

text continued from page 131

climbing. The patient should also understand and be able to take medications independently, adhere to prescribed diet, check pulse rate, and identify symptoms of recurrent disease. Occasionally, before discharge or at 3 weeks after the CAD event, the patient undergoes a submaximal, or in some cases, a symptom-limited exercise treadmill test to determine the level of cardiovascular fitness, work capacity, or symptomatic heart rate for the purposes of Phase 2 exercise prescription.

Almost all ADLs can be performed at an energy cost of 4 METS or less. Stair climbing requires 5 to 6 METS. Patients unable to achieve normal ADLs without symptoms have severe impairment of the cardiovascular system by the New York Functional Classification System (Table 7-11).

If a cardiac patient only tolerated 4 METS of activity intensity on a Naughton ETT protocol, he or she would not be ready to perform the 5 to 7 MET activity of stair climbing.

Cardiac Rehabilitation: Phase 2

Once the patient is discharged from the hospital, the comprehensive cardiac rehabilitation program moves into higher gear. The goal of Phase 2 is to provide the patient with the information and experience that will permit him or her to pursue an independent cardiac conditioning and wellness program after graduating from the structured program. This phase usually begins within 2 weeks of discharge from the hospital, and sessions last 1 hour per day, 3 times per week for 8 to 12 weeks. Phase 2 usually takes place in a hospital or clinic. Requiring close physician supervision, this phase places emphasis on exercise and physical reconditioning; frequently, patients are monitored by telemetry during exercise.

As already discussed, initial exercise intensity is determined by results of a submaximal or symptom-limited, low-level ETT. Intensity is increased on a weekly basis as symp-

text continues on page 139

Table 7-11. New York Heart Association Functional Classification System

Class	Limitation of Activity	METS	O_2 Consumption
I	No limits, no symptoms with ordinary activity	7 or more	24 cc/kg/min or more
II	Symptoms with ordinary activity; comfort at rest	5–6	17–21 cc/kg/min
III	Comfort at rest; symptoms with less than normal activity	3–4	10–14 cc/kg/min
IV	Discomfort with any activity; may have symptoms at rest	1–2	3.5–7 cc/kg/min

Table 7-12. Suggested Activity Levels for Phase 2 Cardiac Rehabilitation

Level	Timing	Activities
1	3–4 weeks p/MI	8 minutes × 2 on stationary bike at 35% MET obtained on ETT (MET-ETT)
	monitored	8 minutes × 2 on arm ergometer at 30% MET obtained on ETT
		12 minutes at 50% MET-ETT on treadmill
2	4 weeks	8 minutes on bike at 45% MET-ETT × 2
		8 minutes on arm ergometer at 35% MET-ETT × 2
		12 minutes at 60% MET-ETT on treadmill
3	4–5 weeks	Same, except increase treadmill intensity to 70% of MET-ETT
4	5 weeks	Bike: 12 min at 45% MET-ETT
		Arm ergometer: 8 min × 2 at 45% MET-ETT
		Treadmill: 12 min at 75% MET-ETT
5	5–6 weeks	Bike: 15 min at 45% MET-ETT; otherwise, the same
6	6 weeks discontinue monitor if stable	Arm ergometer: 8 min × 2 at 45% MET-ETT
		Treadmill: 15 min at 75% MET-ETT

(continued)

Table 7-12. (*Continued*)

Level	Timing	Activities
7	6–7 weeks after MI	Bike: 15 minutes at 3.7 METS
		Arm ergometer: 8 min × 2 at 4.5 METS
		Treadmill: 14 min at 3.9 METS
		Rowing machine: low resistance for 3–5 min
8	7 weeks	Bike: 15 min at 4.9 METS
		Arm ergometer: 8 min × 2 at 5.5 METS
		Treadmill: 20 min at 3.9 METS
9	9 weeks	Bike: same
		Arm ergometer: 8 min × 2 at 6.4 METS
		Treadmill: 22 min at 6 METS
10	11 weeks	Bike: 15 min at 6.1 METS
		Arm ergometer: same; Treadmill 25 min at 6 METS
11	12 weeks	Bike: same; Arm ergometer: 25 min at 6 METS
11	12 weeks	Bike: same; Arm ergometer: same; Treadmill 27.5 min at 6 METS
12	13 weeks	Bike: same; Arm ergometer: same; Treadmill 30 min at 6 METS

text continued from page 135

toms and conditioning permit. There are many published protocols of activity, but a suggested activity outline is provided (Table 7-12). Contraindications to Phase 2 are essentially the same as those to ETT or Phase 1.

In general, the patient begins Phase 2 at an external intensity level of 5 METS and through aerobic conditioning progresses to 8 METS activity before discharge to Phase 3, after 8 to 12 weeks.

Education about diet, stress, medication, exercise, and symptomatology continue in Phase 2. Preparations to return to work, including job site evaluation, or duty modification, are completed in this phase.

By discharge, the patient should be ready for the responsibilities of Phase 3, including a daily self-administered exercise program, carryover of lifestyle associated with low cardiac risk, and compliance with medications and medical follow-up. The patient should also have adequate knowledge of his or her disease and symptoms to pursue vocational, recreational, and sexual activities safely.

Cardiac Rehabilitation: Phase 3

Phase 3 of cardiac rehabilitation should be considered a permanent change in lifestyle, and should continue throughout the person's life to minimize cardiac disease morbidity and mortality.

■ Suggested Readings

American College of Sports Medicine. *Guidelines for Exercise Testing and Prescription.* Philadelphia: Lea and Febiger, 1986.

Brammel HL. Rehabilitation of the cardiac patient. *In* DeLisa JA, Gans B, eds. *Rehabilitation Medicine: Principles and Practice.* Philadelphia: J.B. Lippincott, 1988, pp. 671–688.

Chaitman B. Exercise stress testing. *In* Braunwald E, ed. *Heart Disease: A Textbook of Cardiovascular Medicine.* Philadelphia: W.B. Saunders, 1992, pp. 161–179.

Dennis CA. Rehabilitation of the patient with coronary artery disease. *In* Braunwald E, ed. *Heart Disease: A Textbook of Cardiovascular Medicine.* Philadelphia: W.B. Saunders, 1992.

Flores AM, Moldover JR, Garrison SJ. Cardiovascular, pulmonary, and cancer rehabilitation. *Arch Phys Med Rehabil* 1990;71:S230–254.

Pollock ML, Pels AE, Foster C, Ward A. Exercise prescription for rehabilitation of the cardiac patient. *In* Pollock ML, Schmidt DH, eds. *Heart Disease and Rehabilitation,* 2nd ed. New York: John Wiley and Sons, 1986, pp. 477–513.

Yanowitz FG, ed. *Coronary Artery Disease Prevention.* New York: Marcel Dekker, 1992.

Martin Grabois
Jon VanDeventer

8

Chronic Pain

▓ Introduction

Chronic pain is difficult and frustrating to control. Patients
who experience it are often viewed as management problems,
and therefore, as undesirable. Most physicians, including
medical students, house officers, and practitioners, often lack
understanding, have little training and even less interest in
management of chronic pain. The aim of this chapter is to
provide an understanding of chronic pain syndromes, a thorough summary of evaluation techniques available, and treatment techniques utilized in its management. Hopefully, this
increased knowledge will result in improved management of
chronic pain patients.

▓ Chronic Pain Characteristics

Pain, in general, is an unpleasant sensory and emotional response to a stimulus associated with acute or potential tissue
damage lasting less than 3 months. Acute pain is a normal
symptom resulting from a noxious stimulus. It serves a useful
biological purpose by warning the organism of injury, and
causing it to seek help and guard the affected body part. It is
usually time-limited and its intensity gradually decreases as

Susan J. Garrison (Ed.): *Handbook of Physical Medicine and Rehabilitation
Basics*. First Edition. Copyright © 1995 J. B. Lippincott Company

Table 8-1. Characteristics of Chronic Pain

Persists long after healing should have occurred.

Alteration of behavior and mood: depression, "pain behaviors," anger, moodiness, and anxiety.

Limitation of activity: deconditioning, loss of strength, and flexibility.

Vocational dysfunction and financial distress.

Altered marital, family, and social relationship: stress, conflict, withdrawal, and dependency.

Not always clear relationship to organic pathology.

Litigation, disputes with insurance carriers or worker's compensation.

Multiple nonproductive tests, surgeries, medical treatments, and therapies.

Inappropriate or excessive use of medication and medical services.

the noxious stimulus is removed. Chronic pain, in contrast, is not a symptom, but is itself a disease with specific characteristics (Table 8-1). It may be associated with chronic pathology such as degenerative joint disease (DJD), or simply with persistent symptoms long after recovery from a disease or injury should have occurred. When it lasts longer than 6 months, chronic pain represents an interaction of organic and physical factors with environmental and psychological factors.

■ Epidemiology

Accurate statistics on the incidence and cost of chronic pain are difficult to locate and substantiate. However, the incidence continues to grow and accelerate; the economic loss is staggering.

■ Etiology and Pathophysiology

The study of chronic pain is relatively new. It is not certain whether it is one condition or whether multiple subtypes exist, and there is no universally accepted model of its etiology and pathology. Some postulate disorders of the central nervous system (CNS) such as dysfunction of pain modulation systems, and disorders of neuroactive peptides and neurotransmitters. Others propose the involvement of peripheral mechanisms, such as persistent local tissue pathology, peripheral nerve dysfunction, and biomechanical abnormalities, while some emphasize psychosocial factors such as operant learning of pain behaviors, family/marital network dysfunction, and economic/legal disincentives to recovery. In any case, chronic pain results when acute pain is not adequately evaluated and/or treated, when curative treatment or control is not available, or when pain-reinforcing complications such as secondary gains, social, economic, or psychosocial factors are prominent. Thus, in a small but significant number of acute pain patients, the pain continues and even intensifies in nature. The physical sensation of pain is complicated by physical factors such as inactivity, psychological factors such as depression, and environmental factors such as compensation (Figure 8-1).

■ Concepts of Treatment

The best treatment for chronic pain is prevention. This involves identifying contributing factors and addressing them in the early stages of the pain syndrome. As acute pain changes to subacute pain, these contributing factors usually become apparent. At this point a comprehensive interdisciplinary team approach is indicated, with appropriate use of medication, modalities, and gradual introduction of physical reconditioning activities. Identifiable psychosocial and environmental issues, although not usually prominent at this stage, must be recognized and managed. However, once these factors become prominent and last longer than 6 months the treatment strategy must be altered.

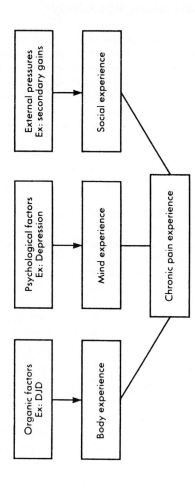

Figure 8-1. Chronic pain: interaction of organic, psychologic and social factors. (From Grabois M. Chronic pain. *In* Goodgold, *Rehabilitation Medicine*. St. Louis: C.V. Mosby, 1988, p. 664.)

When pain becomes chronic it increases in complexity, and the patient becomes more resistant to treatment. Concepts used in the treatment of acute pain such as inactivity, surgical intervention, narcotic medications, and physical modalities will not usually result in success. It is at this point that the concept of pain clinics or programs which involve multidisciplinary and comprehensive evaluation and treatment becomes appropriate and essential. Treatment goals address improving the quality of life and functional capabilities of the individual with alleviation or modification of pain if possible, and the remedy of factors which contribute to the perpetuation of the chronic pain syndrome.

Pain Team and Patient Selection

Members of the multidisciplinary team are listed in Table 8-2. The physician usually provides overall leadership and is the patient manager. Nonclinical administrative management

Table 8-2. The Pain Rehabilitation Team

Clinical	Administrative	Consultants
Physiatrist/patient manager	Program Coordinator	Pharmacologist
Psychologist and/or psychiatrist	Secretarial/clerical staff	Dietician
Physical Therapist		Recreational Therapist
Occupational Therapist		Chaplain
Vocational Counselor		Other physician specialists
Social Worker		
Rehabilitation Nurse		

Table 8-3. Guidelines for Candidate Selection for the Pain Management Program

The candidate:

has had chronic pain of more than 6 months' duration;

can comprehend the abstract principles of the pain management program;

is independently mobile (for attendance of appointments);

is cooperative and willing to follow the principles of the pain management program;

has had appropriate evaluation techniques performed and/or reviewed;

has had appropriate surgical and conservative treatment for pain; and

accepts concept of program.

may be in the hands of a coordinator. In smaller programs, however, these positions may be combined.

The physician is responsible for the initial evaluation and referral to the team. All members of the team subsequently evaluate and assist in the selection of appropriate patients. Evaluations are on a one-to-one basis. The team makes the decision to accept or reject a potential patient during a team conference. Appropriate patients are those who demonstrate chronic pain, are motivated to participate, do not have complicating factors such as secondary gains, and accept the concepts and goals of the pain program (Table 8-3).

■ Assessment and Evaluation

The etiology of the pain syndrome is evaluated and the treatment plan formulated through a comprehensive pain evaluation, including a complete history, physical examination, and functional evaluation from the medical and psychosocial point of view. Obtain appropriate diagnostic tests and pain measurements. Make the evaluation as objective and quantitative as possible. Obtain and review the patient's pertinent medical records. Review a pain questionnaire completed by the patient prior to your examination. (Figure 8-2).

History

Emphasize the following components in the clinical history:

- Pain description: location, radiation characteristics, time sequence, what makes it worse or better, and patient's activity level;
- Prior pain evaluations: physicians, hospitalizations, and diagnostic tests performed;
- Psychosocial/vocational evaluation: behavioral responses to pain, adjustments to impairment and disability, family and working history and dynamics; and
- Past treatment: medical, surgical, and rehabilitative.

Physical Examination

Perform the initial comprehensive physical examination in a traditional manner. Concentrate on the musculoskeletal and neuromuscular systems, as well as body mechanics. Evaluate other systems more thoroughly depending on the location of the pain (e.g.: chest pain suggests cardiac evaluation).

Measurement of Pain and Its Effects

While the measurement of induced acute pain is relatively easy and reproducible, the measurement of chronic pain is not. Pain is a subjective phenomenon; it is not directly measurable. Hence, it is the effects of chronic pain that are measured. A combination of techniques is needed to evaluate appropriately the chronic pain patient, including measures of

text continues on page 152

Figure 8-2. The following four pages show a sample pain management program questionnaire.

Complete the entire form by checking or circling answers.
Fill in blanks. Use ink only.

NAME: _____   DATE: _____

ADDRESS: _____   AGE: _____

PHONE: _____   BIRTH DATE: _____

OCCUPATION: _____   MARITAL STATUS: _____

REFERRING PHYSICIAN: _____   LEVEL OF EDUCATION: _

1. Onset of pain (Give specific date; if accident, describe.) _____

2. Surgery for pain (list below/none)

Procedure	Date	Surgeon
_____	____	_____
_____	____	_____
_____	____	_____

3. Location of pain:
   Indicate on the diagram the following:
   a. Entire painful area (xxxxx)
   b. Single most painful spot (*)
   c. Numbness (ooooo)
   d. Tingling area(s) (-----)

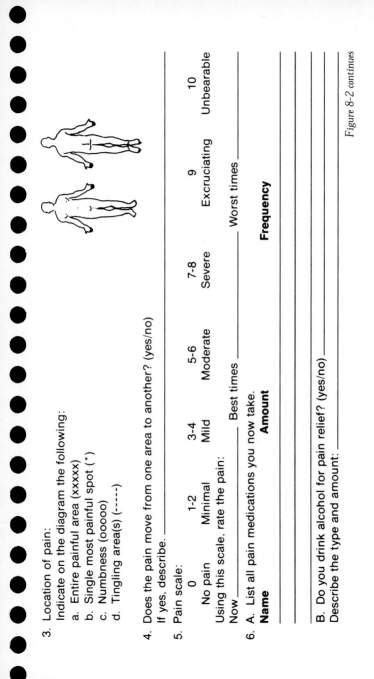

4. Does the pain move from one area to another? (yes/no)
   If yes, describe. _____

5. Pain scale:

0	1-2	3-4	5-6	7-8	9	10
No pain	Minimal	Mild	Moderate	Severe	Excruciating	Unbearable

   Using this scale, rate the pain:
   Now _____ Best times _____ Worst times _____

6. A. List all pain medications you now take.

Name	Amount	Frequency

   B. Do you drink alcohol for pain relief? (yes/no) _____
      Describe the type and amount: _____

Figure 8-2 continues

Figure 8-2. (*Continued*)

7. A. Circle all physical and/or occupational therapies you have experienced for pain treatment:

Hot packs   Cold packs   Paraffin   Laser

Exercises   Massage   Fluidotherapy   TENS

Ultrasound   Whirlpool   Neuroprobe   Biofeedback

Other _____

B. Place a check mark by those that gave the most relief.

8. Using (X) for decreases, (O) for increases, indicate the effect of the following:

___ walking   ___ sleeping   ___ sexual activities   ___ alcohol

___ sitting   ___ fatigue   ___ bending   ___ medications

___ standing   ___ tension   ___ working   ___ bowel movements

___ reclining   ___ exercise   ___ house cleaning   ___ lifting

9. In a 24-hour period, indicate the hours you spend

in pain _____; reclining because of pain _____;

reclining for other reasons _____; sleeping _____.

10. Circle the numbers indicating pain limitations.

Activity	Normal	Mildly limited	Moderately limited	Severely limited
Walking	1	2	3	4
Running	1	2	3	4
Bending	1	2	3	4
Lifting	1	2	3	4
Sitting	1	2	3	4
Stair climbing	1	2	3	4
Resting	1	2	3	4
Sexual Activities	1	2	3	4
Working	1	2	3	4
Hobbies	1	2	3	4

11. Were pain not a problem, what would you like to do that you cannot do now? _____

12. When did you last work your regular job? _____ (date)

13. Is your case Workman's Compensation? _____ (yes/no)

14. Are you involved in a lawsuit because of the pain?   yes/no

    Describe: _____

text continued from page 147

self-reported pain, biomechanical, physiological, psychological/behavioral, functional, familial/social, and medical parameters. Some of these parameters are provided in Table 8-4, while Table 8-5 lists several accepted, published scales in use. In both tables, items utilized at Baylor College of Medicine are noted with an asterisk.

A few key points are as follows: (1) The measurement of chronic pain and its effect is in its infancy; there has been a proliferation of assessment instruments and methods which await further study, but none is universally accepted. (2) Rehabilitative pain management programs emphasize improving patient functioning, rather than focusing primarily on the relief of pain. Functional evaluation, especially in the area of activities of daily living (ADLs), household activities, vocational activities, and mobilization (sitting, standing, transferring and ambulation), must be included in the comprehensive measurement of pain patients. Often the key question is how much a patient can do, rather than how much it hurts. (3) Assessment characteristics should be multiple and broad since patients may improve on some parameters and not others; for instance, "up time" or vocational status may improve, while subjective pain ratings remain the same.

Diagnostic Tests

Consider diagnostic studies an extension of the clinical examination. Findings of diagnostic studies vary little from those of the primary disease process. Do not repeat diagnostic studies previously performed satisfactorily, especially if there has been no significant change in the clinical examination. Order studies only if the diagnosis has not yet been established or if the results will change your treatment approach.

Classification of Patients

At the conclusion of the evaluation process it may be helpful to classify patients into categories based on their symptoms, objective findings, and psychosocial findings. This then has

Table 8-4. Assessment Methods of the Effects of Chronic Pain

Subjective Pain	Whole body diagram*
	Pain intensity rating scales*
	Visual analogue scales*
	General pain measurement (McGill Questionnaire)*
Biomechanical	Flexibility* (ROM measurements)
	Endurance* (activity duration, such as walking; treadmill or ergometer testing)
	Strength* (number of repetitions lifting a given weight; performance on Cybex or KinCom machine; static and dynamic body mechanics
Physiological	EMG muscle tension* (biofeedback)
	Critical evoked potential
	Autonomic responses
	Oxygen consumption (VO_2) with exercise
Psychological/Behavioral	Personality factors* (Minnesota Multiphasic Personality Inventory [MMPI])
	Mood (Beck Depression Inventory)
	Frequency of "pain behaviors"
	Stress management and coping skills*
	"Meaning" of pain to patient/family*

(continued)

Table 8-4. (*Continued*)

Functional	Basic ADL skills*
	Housework
	Yard work
	"Up time" (activity diary)*: sitting, standing, walking, reclining, lying
	Hobbies
	Prevocational and/or vocational status
Familial/Social	Marital distress
	Family distress
	Social withdrawal
	Contribution of family, social, and economic systems to maintaining pain behavior
Medical	Patterns of medication usage*
	Use of healthcare system
	Effectiveness of therapies
	Sleep patterns
	Effects of other health problems

*Measures used at Baylor College of Medicine

implications for the treatment approaches to be utilized. The Brena and Chapman Emory Pain Estimate Model attempts to achieve this concept. It has been modified with examples as shown in Table 8-6.

▣ Pain Management Program

The present structure of the Baylor College of Medicine Pain Management Program at The Methodist Hospital is outlined in Figure 8-3. The program is available on an inpatient or

Table 8-5. Accepted Published Tests

Pain
McGill Pain Questionnaire*

Functional Status
Sickness Impact Profile

Pain and Impairment Relationship Scale

Functional Assessment Screening Questionnaire

Psychological Status
Minnesota Multiphasic Personality Inventory (MMPI)

Back Depression Inventory

Several Factors in Single Scale
Picaza Scale*

Hendler Screening Test for Chronic Back Pain Patients

Emory Pain Estimate Model

*Used at Baylor College of Medicine

outpatient/day hospital basis. Weekly team conferences are held to monitor progress, identify new problems, and modify the treatment plan as needed. Patients may be discharged from the program with 24 hours notice at any time if they are not benefiting from the program.

Treatment Approaches

By the time the patient with chronic pain is seen in a pain clinic, most traditional medical and surgical interventions have been attempted and have been unsuccessful. It is important not to repeat these techniques unless it is felt they have not been utilized properly or unless they may be used in combination with other forms of treatment which could yield

text continues on page 158

Table 8-6. Classification of the Patient with Chronic Nonmalignant Pain with Examples and Treatment Strategies

Class	Symptoms	Objective Findings	Psychosocial Components	Example	Treatment Strategies
IA	High	High correlation	High	Rheumatoid arthritis	Behavior modification approach with emphasis on medication and physical modalities
IB	High	High correlation	Low	Rheumatoid arthritis	Medication and modalities approach
IIA	High	Low correlation	High	Musculoskeletal/low back pain	Behavioral modification approach
IIB	High	Low correlation	Low	Musculoskeletal/low back pain	Physical modalities and exercise

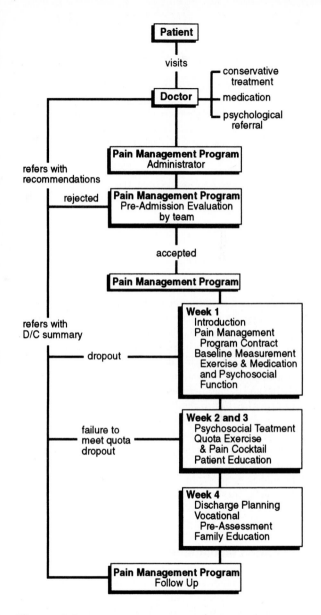

Figure 8-3. Structure of the Baylor College of Medicine Pain Management Program at the Methodist Hospital.

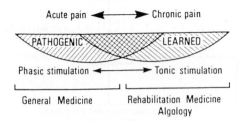

Figure 8-4. Nociceptive spectrum. (From Brena SF, Chapman SL. Management of Patients with Chronic Pain. New York: S.P. Medical & Scientific Books, 1983.)

text continued from page 155

a better result. The goals in treating the patient with chronic pain are to modify and/or reduce medication, modulate the pain response, increase activity, restore physical functioning, and alleviate psychosocial and vocational dysfunction. Basically the techniques utilized should restore patient function to the highest level within the limits of the remaining pain or other physical limitations. This is basically the Physical Medicine and Rehabilitation (PM&R) approach to the treatment of patients with disabilities (Figure 8-4).

Treatment methods are usually employed in combination to achieve treatment goals. For example, remediation of sleep disturbance may require medication adjustment, psychological techniques such as relaxation training or stress management, and an activity/physical restoration program. Integrate treatment techniques into a comprehensive program. Do not use them in isolation.

Medication Management

Avoid narcotic medication in the chronic pain patient; its use tends to enhance chronic pain behavior. Sedatives, hypnotics, and tranquilizers are likewise contraindicated.

The reduction and elimination of contraindicated medications are best accomplished in an inpatient or day-hospital setting utilizing a behavior modification approach. The basic steps in the program are as follows:

1. Switch injectable to oral medications.
2. Continue current medication on an as-needed (prn) basis with strict record-keeping to obtain the typical 24-hour baseline requirement.
3. Allow no new or additional narcotic, tranquilizer, or hypnotic medications.
4. Initiate pain cocktail with active ingredients of methadone or similar medication in an equivalent dose to the currently used narcotic (Table 8-7) in a masking vehicle around the clock, in a pattern of dosage and time interval currently utilized by the patient.
5. Slowly reduce active ingredients of the pain cocktail, with equal increases in the masking vehicle over 3 to 6 weeks to avoid withdrawal (Table 8-8).
6. Discontinue the pain cocktail when the patient is receiving masking vehicle only.
7. Share all information with the patient except the times and amount of reduction of the active ingredients.

This program can be utilized similarly for tranquilizers or hypnotic medications.

Correction of sleep disturbance and alleviation of depression may be accomplished with antidepressants in a single dose given at bedtime. Doxepin or amitriptyline (50–150 mg) is often used in dosages smaller than those utilized to treat depression. Antidepressants, in addition, have analgesic properties, may act synergistically with some non-narcotic analgesics, and may enhance the effectiveness of physical modalities such as transcutaneous electrical nerve stimulation (TENS).

Safe analgesia may be provided by nonsteroidal anti-inflammatory drugs, acetaminophen, and occasionally muscle relaxants.

text continues on page 164

Table 8-7. Narcotic Agonist Analgesics

Drug	Equianalgesic Doses* Intramuscular (mg)	Oral (mg)	Onset (minutes)	Peak (hours)	Duration† (hours)	$T \frac{1}{2}$ (hours)
Alfentanil	nd	na	immediate	nd	nd	1–2‡‡
Codeine	120	200	10–30	0.5–1	4–6	3
Fentanyl	0.1	na	7–8	nd	1–2	1.5–6
Hydrocodone	nd	nd	nd	nd	4–8	3.3–4.5
Hydromorphone	1.5	7.5	15–30	0.5–1	4–5	2–3
Levorphanol	2	4	30–90	0.5–1	6–8	12–16
Meperidine	75	300	10–45	0.5–1	2–4	3–4
Methadone	10	20	30–60	0.5–1	4–6ᵝ	15–30

Morphine	10	60	15–60‖	0.5–1	3–7	1.5–2
Oxycodone (po)	na	30	15–30	1	4–6	nd
Oxymorphone	1	10‡	5–10	0.5–1	3–6	nd
Propoxyphene (po)	nd	130**/200††	30–60	2–2.5	4–6	6–12
Sufentanil	0.02	na	1.3–3‡‡	nd	nd	2.5

nd = no data available; na = not applicable.

*Based on acute, short-term use. Chronic Administration may alter pharmacokinetics and decrease the oral:parenteral dose ratio. The morphine oral—parenteral ratio decreases to 1.5–2.5:1 upon chronic dosing.

†After IV administration, peak effects may be more pronounced but duration is shorter. Duration of action may be longer with the oral route

‡Rectal

ßDuration and half-life increase with repeated use due to cumulative effects.

‖Data based on intrathecal or epidural administration.

**HCl salt

††Napsylate salt

‡‡Data based on IV administration.

From *Drug Facts and Comparisons*. St. Louis: Facts and Comparisons, Inc., 1993, p. 242a.

Table 8-8. Sample Pain Cocktail Regimen

Inpatient days		Pain cocktail format
1–6	Baseline	Patient reports preadmission pattern of "one or two of the 50 mg tablets of Demerol two or three times a day, as needed, at home."
		Physician orders to nurse: "May have Demerol, *prn* pain, not to exceed three 50 mg tablets every 3 hours. Carefully record amount taken."
		Analysis of baseline data: Patient averaged 600 mg of Demerol per 24-hour period, averaging of 3- to 4-hour intervals between requests.
7–9 First cocktail	Prescription to pharmacists:	Demerol, 1920 mg Bevisol, Plebex, or other liquid B complex, 12 ml; cherry syrup qs 240 ml
	Directions:	Pain cocktail, 10 ml po q3h, day and night, *not prn*
	Nursing order:	Pain cocktail, 10 ml po q3h, day and night, *not prn*
		Since contents of the pain cocktail are not on the label, a copy of the prescription must be kept in a separate pain cocktail book.
10–12		Decrease each daily total by 64 mg, $\frac{1}{10}$ of original amount. A 3-day prescription is decreased by 64×3 or 192 mg.
	Prescription to pharmacists:	Demerol, 1728 mg Bevisol, Plebex, or other liquid B complex, 12 ml; cherry syrup qs 240 ml
	Directions:	Pain cocktail, 10 ml po q3h, day and night, *not prn*
	Nursing order:	Pain cocktail, 10 ml po q3h, day and night, *not prn*
13–15	Prescription to pharmacists:	Demerol, 1536 mg Bevisol, Plebex, or other liquid B complex, 12 ml; cherry syrup qs 240 ml

Table 8-8. (*Continued*)

Inpatient days		Pain cocktail format
16–18	Sig:	Pain cocktail, 10 ml po q3h, day and night, *not prn*
	Nursing order:	Pain cocktail, 10 ml po q3h, day and night, *not prn*
	Prescription to pharmacists:	Demerol, 1344 mg
		Bevisol, Plebex, or other liquid B complex, 12 ml; cherry syrup qs 240 ml
	Sig:	Pain cocktail, 10 ml po q3h, day and night, *not prn*
	Nursing order:	Pain cocktail, 10 ml po q3h, day and night, *not prn*
19–21		Demerol, 1152 mg
	Prescription to pharmacists:	Bevisol, Plebex, or other liquid B complex, 12 ml; cherry syrup qs 240 ml
	Sig:	Pain cocktail, 10 ml po q3h, day and night, *not prn*
	Nursing order:	Pain cocktail, 10 ml po q3h, day and night, *not prn*
22–24		Demerol 960 mg
	Prescription to pharmacists:	Bevisol, Plebex, or other liquid B complex, 12 ml; cherry syrup qs 240 ml
	Sig:	Pain cocktail, 10 ml po q3h, day and night, *not prn*
	Nursing order:	Pain cocktail, 10 ml po q3h, day and night, *not prn*
37–39		Demerol 0 mg
	Prescription to pharmacists:	Bevisol, Plebex, or other liquid B complex, 12 ml; cherry syrup qs 240 ml
	Sig:	Pain cocktail, 10 ml po q3h, day and night, *not prn*
	Nursing order:	Pain cocktail, 10 ml po q3h, day and night, *not prn*

(Maintain patient on vehicle for 2 to 10 days, if all is going well, inform patient and ask if continuation of vehicle is desired.)

From Fordyce WE: Behavioral methods for chronic pain and illness. St. Louis: C. V. Mosby; 1979.

text continued from page 159

■ Pain Control

Pain control by techniques other than medication usually involves modulation, perhaps reduction, but rarely elimination of the chronic pain symptoms. The techniques used should be active rather than passive, and have the ability to be utilized by the patient at home. Techniques requiring a therapist or special equipment are usually not appropriate for the chronic pain patient. Like medication, they should be utilized for the shortest time possible with gradual decreases in usage as indicated.

Of the physical modalities, only heat, cold, and transcutaneous electrical nerve stimulation are commonly used in chronic pain management. Others are used sparingly, and most have greater usefulness in acute and subacute pain conditions (Table 8-9). Occasionally they are utilized to treat acute pain superimposed upon a chronic pain syndrome, particularly during the first week to help mobilize the chronic pain patient beginning the treatment program.

Heat in the form of packs, pads, and whirlpool, as well as cold in the form of ice packs are the most common modalities used to treat pain. In the chronic pain patient, they may be employed prior to and after exercise, achieving their effects through their ability to reduce pain and promote muscle relaxation and sedation.

Table 8-9. Modalities Used in Chronic Pain

Nerve blocks

Trigger point injections

Spray and stretch techniques

Acupuncture

Hypnotherapy

Mobilization and manipulation

Surgical treatment

A trial of TENS is indicated in many neurogenic and musculoskeletal pain syndromes. Generally, it is found to be more effective in chronic pain patients without a history of significant surgical intervention and/or high narcotic usage levels. The exact mechanism of TENS is not certain, but possibilities include the direct effects of stimulation of afferent nerves, modification of pain transmission at the level of the dorsal horn in the spinal cord, or the activation of supraspinal pain modulation centers mediated by endorphins. Prior to the rental or purchase of a TENS unit, a trial of therapy with appropriate positioning of electrodes and education in its utilization is indicated. Like most intervention techniques it has a significant placebo effect, and its effectiveness decreases significantly over time.

Biofeedback can be used to provide instantaneous feedback to the patient regarding such parameters as muscle tension and skin temperature. Patients can then be taught to exert control over these and other functions mediated by both the somatic and autonomic nervous systems. In chronic pain patients it can be employed to facilitate relaxation, alleviate muscle tension and anxiety, demonstrate the role of the mind in modifying physical responses, and promote improved sleeping patterns. While results of treatment vary among individuals, the most successful responders seem to be patients with tension headaches, torticollis, musculoskeletal neck pain, and Raynaud's Disease.

Finally, patients must be educated in the management of the many controllable factors which can affect their pain level. These include, for example, the adverse effects of inactivity and deconditioning, poor body mechanics, the use of narcotics, sedatives and tranquilizers, social withdrawal, inappropriate pacing of activities, and a host of others. Of particular importance is education regarding the nature of pain, and the important differences between the approach to acute versus chronic pain.

Treatment of Biomechanical Factors

One of the components of the chronic pain syndrome is activity restriction. This results in deconditioning and the loss of strength and flexibility. There also may be significant abnormalities of static and dynamic posture, as well as impaired biomechanics in sitting, standing, bending, and lifting.

Education, video feedback, and an "obstacle course" may be used to correct biomechanical problems, with a program of flexibility exercises also prescribed if necessary. Exercises to strengthen and restore flexibility of specific muscle groups (e.g., Williams flexion exercises for the low back) and general conditioning exercises (e.g., cycling, walking, swimming) should be started at a low level and systematically increased to recondition the patient. As with the program of medication control, a behavior modification program is utilized. The patient's level of activity and exercise is first determined over a few days. Then a goal is set within the patient's ability and he/she is encouraged to achieve that level regardless of pain complaints. Every few days the goal is reset appropriately at a higher level (Figure 8-5). Reinforcement is through daily positive feedback for accomplishing goals established. Patients are instructed in pacing themselves appropriately.

Psychosocial Intervention

Psychosocial issues relevant to the chronic pain patient are identified through patient and family interviews, behavioral observation, and psychological testing. Treatment may entail group sessions, individual treatment, or behavioral interventions supported by the entire treatment team. Problems requiring treatment commonly include the following: (1) Pain behavior: chronic pain patients often are highly focused on their pain. Conversation may be dominated by references to pain sensations, treatments, and pain-related physical limitations. Similarly, nonverbal behavior may be marked by grimaces, groans, limping, etc. (2) Depression: this is nearly always present and may be reflected in mood, decreased libido, sleep disturbance, and social withdrawal. Grief about losses of physical abilities, social/family role, and previously enjoyed activities must be resolved. Antidepressants may be

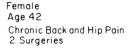

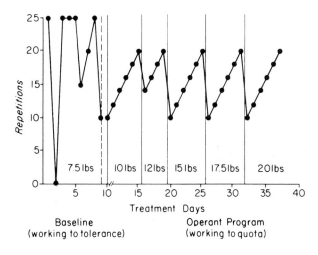

Figure 8-5. Behavioral modification approach to exercise. (From Fordyce WE. *Behavioral Methods for Chronic Pain and Illness.* St. Louis: C.V. Mosby, 1976, p. 173.)

required in addition to psychological therapies. (3) Stress: pain patients face multiple stressors, including pending litigation, uncertainty regarding the future of their economic and health status, and family or marital distress. Treatment may include training in stress management (e.g., relaxation techniques, problem solving) as well as marital, family, or vocational counseling. (4) Marital/family dysfunction: as time passes family members will alter their behavior in adapting to the chronic pain patient. Some of these adaptations may unwittingly contribute to the patient's pain behavior (e.g., giving attention to the patient's complaints, or taking over the patient's household duties when the pain is particularly bad). Enlistment of family cooperation in eliminating dysfunctional behavior patterns is essential in many cases.

Restoration of Functional Activity

Assessment of chronic pain patients' daily activities usually reveals multiple areas of deficits (Table 8-10). Remediation efforts involve the application of several key principles.

* Activities to be worked on must be agreed upon in advance; patients will work best at activities that are important to them.
* Careful task analysis may reveal ways to simplify the activity.
* Principles of energy conservation and pacing must be observed.

Table 8-10. Typical Areas of Functional Activity Deficits in Chronic Pain Patients

"Up time": excessive time spent in bed or reclining in chair or on sofa

Upright sitting and standing tolerance

Self-care: dressing, bathing, grooming

Performance of household chores

Performance of yard work

Participation in avocational pursuits

Task-oriented activities away from home: e.g., grocery shopping

Activities away from home: social, family, community

Vocational activities

Driving

- Physical activities need to be treated as exercise, starting slowly and increasing the activity gradually (e.g., vacuuming initially may need to be done in 3-minute blocks).
- Activity diaries or other forms of monitoring progress must be utilized.

▒ Results

If the goals of pain medication reduction, pain modification, and increased activity are accepted, patients who enter and successfully complete a pain management program can achieve significant success in a cost effective manner. Progress should be measured in objective and quantifiable ways, such as level of medication utilized, strength, sitting tolerance, walking distance, and continued utilization of health resources. The cost effective component of these programs is measured through models developed by Steig and coworkers.

▒ Suggested Readings

Aronoff GM. *Evaluation and Treatment of Chronic Pain.* Baltimore: Urban & Schwarzenberg, 1985.

Brena SF, Chapman SL. *Management of Patients with Chronic Pain.* New York: Spectrum Publications, Inc., 1983.

Fordyce WE. *Behavioral Methods for Chronic Pain and Illness.* St. Louis: C.V. Mosby, 1976.

Grabois M. Chronic pain: evaluation and treatment. *In* Goodgold J, ed. *Rehabilitation Medicine.* St. Louis: C.V. Mosby, 1988, pp. 663–674.

Ng LKY. *New Approaches to Treatment of Chronic Pain: A Review of Multidisciplinary Pain Clinics and Pain Centers.* Rockville, MD: National Institute on Drug Abuse Research, 1981. Monograph 36.

Raj PP. *Practical Management of Pain.* Chicago: Year Book Medical Publishers, 1986.

Reuler JB, Girard DE, Nardone DA. The chronic pain syndrome: misconceptions and management. *Annals of Internal Medicine* 1980;93:588–596.

Steig RL, Williams RC, Gallaher LA. Multidisciplinary pain treatment centers. *Journal of Occupational Medicine* 1981; 23:94.

Wall PD, Melzack R. *Textbook of Pain.* Edinburgh: Churchill Livingstone, 1984.

Walsh NE, Dumitru D, Ramamurthy S, Schoenfeld LS. Treatment of the patient with chronic pain. *In* DeLisa JA, ed. *Rehabilitation Medicine: Principles and Practice,* 2nd ed. Philadelphia: J.B. Lippincott, 1993, pp. 973–995.

Fae H. Garden

9

Limb Fractures

▉ Definition

A fracture is a structural break in a bone, an epiphyseal plate, or a cartilaginous joint surface. While damage to bone is often immediately obvious, damage to the surrounding soft tissues may escape early clinical detection. Damaged soft tissue associated with a fracture is of great clinical significance and may ultimately affect clinical outcome. This chapter will focus on adult limb fractures, their aftercare, and rehabilitation.

▉ Terminology

Refer to Figure 9-1.

Transverse fracture: the long axis of bone and fracture plane are perpendicular. Usually caused by low velocity, bending injuries.

Oblique fracture: the long axis of bone and fracture plane form an angle.

Spiral fracture: produced by a twisting force that causes bone to fracture along shear lines.

Comminuted fracture: more than two fracture fragments present.

Susan J. Garrison (Ed.): *Handbook of Physical Medicine and Rehabilitation Basics.* First Edition. Copyright © 1995 J. B. Lippincott Company

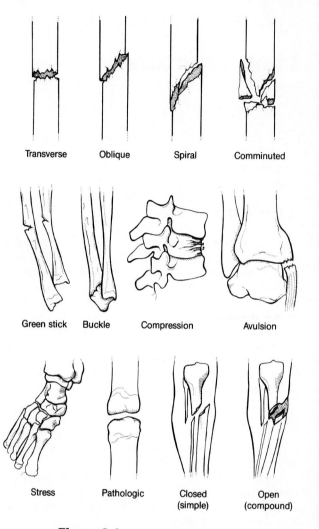

| Transverse | Oblique | Spiral | Comminuted |

| Green stick | Buckle | Compression | Avulsion |

| Stress | Pathologic | Closed (simple) | Open (compound) |

Figure 9-1. Types of limb fractures.

Greenstick fracture: an incomplete fracture produced by angulatory forces. The opposite cortex is intact. Occurs in children.

Buckling (Torus) fracture: a fracture in which one cortex is compacted while the opposite cortex is intact. Occurs in children.

Compression fracture: decreased length or width of bone segments caused by impaction of trabecular bone.

Avulsion fracture: fracture produced by traction forces on bone through the enthesis.

Stress fracture: small cracks in bone that develop as a result of repeated fatigue. Discontinuity of bone can usually be avoided by stopping the repeated stress.

Pathological fracture: interruption of bone at an area that has been weakened by a pathologic process.

Closed (Simple) fracture: fracture surface is not in contact with the skin or mucous membranes.

Open (Compound) fracture: fracture surface communicates with skin or mucous membranes.

▓ Anatomy

The load-bearing capacity of bone can reach up to 10 to 20 times body weight. This is made possible by the elastic properties of bone that allow it to bend slightly when load is applied.

Bone is composed of a compact cortical layer that forms the outer shell and a spongy, interior trabecular meshwork. While both cortical and trabecular components contribute to overall bone strength, cortical bone is able to resist compression or shearing forces better than tension forces.

The ratio of cortical to trabecular components in the adult skeleton is about 4:1. Vertebrae are mostly composed of trabecular bone while long bones such as the radius and ulna are approximately 90% cortical. See Figure 9-2.

The periosteum becomes weaker and less osteogenic with age. Periosteal tearing at the time of a fracture may interfere with surgical reduction procedures. Decreased periosteal osteogenesis in adults results in slower fracture healing and may contribute to delayed union and non-union.

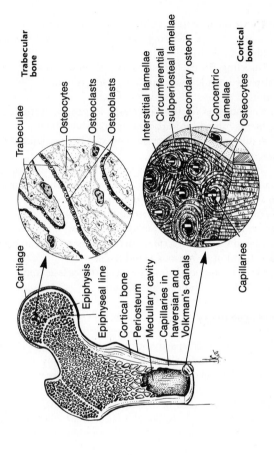

Figure 9-2. Composition of bone.

Cartilage

Epiphysis

Epiphyseal line

Cortical bone

Periosteum

Medullary cavity

Capillaries in haversian and Volkman's canals

Trabeculae

Osteocytes

Osteoclasts

Osteoblasts

Trabecular bone

Interstitial lamellae

Circumferential subperiosteal lamellae

Secondary osteon

Concentric lamellae

Osteocytes

Capillaries

Cortical bone

▌ Epidemiology

In the United States, fractures represent nearly 10% of all reported injuries. A 1976 National Health Survey estimated that for every 10 persons in the United States, fractures account for more than 6 days of restricted activity each year. In addition to huge economic costs, fractures can result in permanent disability and premature death.

Limb fractures occur most often in young males and older females. In the United States, the most common fracture among Caucasian females up until age 75 are Colles' fractures (fracture of the distal radius with posterior displacement of the fracture fragment). After age 75, hip fractures become more frequent. Nearly half of all hip fractures occur in persons over the age of 80. Over 75% of all hip fractures occur in women. The etiology and pathophysiology of hip fractures due to osteoporosis is discussed in Chapter 12, Osteoporosis.

Patients with Colles' fractures rarely require hospitalization or rehabilitation services. Hip fractures, especially in the geriatric population, are associated with high rates of morbidity and mortality. The ability of a person to regain ambulation after hip fracture has been associated with survival.

▌ Etiology/Pathophysiology

Bone is strongest when subjected to symmetrical compression forces. Excessive bending or torsional loads leads to tension failure and fracture. The most common direct cause of limb fractures is a fall. These falls usually occur at home and frequently involve heights of less than six feet. See Table 9-1.

Bone pathology, especially as a result of osteoporosis, may predispose an individual to sustaining a limb fracture. See Table 9-2.

▌ Assessment of Fracture Healing

There is a great deal of variation in fracture healing time from one individual to the next. See Table 9-3.

Motion at the fracture site can delay bone union. Frac-

Table 9-1. Causes of Limb Fractures

Falls

Crush injuries

Motor vehicle accidents

Bicycle accidents

Auto/bicycle/pedestrian accidents

Sports injuries

Fights

Repetitive stress or fatigue

Spontaneous/idiopathic

Table 9-2. Factors Contributing to Limb Fractures

General
   Osteoporosis
   Osteogenesis imperfecta
   Osteitis Deformans (Paget's disease)

Metabolic
   Vitamin C deficiency (scurvy)
   Vitamin D deficiency (rickets)
   Hyperparathyroidism
   Osteomalacia

Inflammatory
   Osteomyelitis
   Rheumatoid arthritis

Ischemic
   Avascular necrosis

Neoplastic
   Primary tumors of bone
   Metastatic carcinoma

Neuromuscular
   Spinal cord injuries
   Anterior horn cell disease
   Myopathies

Table 9-3. Factors Affecting Fracture Healing

Patient age

Amount of fracture displacement

Type of fracture

Location of fracture

Blood supply to fracture

Coexisting medical conditions

tured bones are typically immobilized one joint above and one joint below the fracture site.

In an uncomplicated fracture, microscopic evidence of healing can usually be seen at the fracture site within 15 hours of injury. Radiographic evidence of callus formation is apparent at about 4 weeks following injury. Callus is made up of a mixture of cartilage and woven (fibrous) bone. Callus formation and its progressive replacement by stronger, re-modeled osteomal bone may continue for several years.

The state of fracture healing is determined by clinical examination and radiographic assessment. Even when the patient and the examiner fail to detect movement or pain at the fracture site, the fracture line will still be visible on X-ray. Although immobilization may no longer be required, the bone should not be exposed to excessive stress. Clinical and radiographic assessment should continue on a periodic basis until the fracture line is no longer visible.

■ Rehabilitation Evaluation

The physiatrist must communicate effectively with the patient as well as with the referring surgeon. Elicit a detailed history, including pre-fracture functional status and support systems. Review radiographs and pertinent laboratory values before commencing therapies.

Inspect the affected limb carefully. Document presence

or absence of edema, trophic changes, muscular atrophy, pressure ulcers and/or clinical evidence of DVT. Palpate peripheral pulses above and below the fracture site. Perform a careful neurologic examination to rule out sensory or motor deficits as a result of peripheral nerve injuries. Note any pain elicited by palpation, movement, or weight-bearing of the affected limb. A manual muscle test to determine strength will not be accurate in the early phase of postfracture rehabilitation because of pain and swelling, and may even result in fracture displacement. Document initial passive and active range of motion in joints proximal and distal to the fracture site, as well as the patient's ability to contract muscles voluntarily in the affected limb.

■ Treatment

Descriptions of splinting and fracture reduction techniques may be found in most orthopedic surgery textbooks.

The major goal of rehabilitation management in fracture aftercare is restoration of the patient's normal activity level. See Table 9-4. Patients with lower limb fractures, particularly fractures of the femoral head and neck and traumatic musculoskeletal injuries are those most commonly referred for rehabilitation services. Rapid mobilization lessens the deleterious effects of immobility on the cardiopulmonary and musculoskeletal systems. After the initial immobilization period, consider using a fracture orthosis to facilitate ambulation and to allow progressive weight-bearing. Fracture orthoses are most commonly prescribed for fractures of the tibia and distal femur. See Figure 9-3.

The decision to resume normal activity levels should be made jointly by the physiatrist, orthopedic surgeon, therapist, and patient. Weight-bearing status and length of immobilization will vary according to the type of fracture, its location, and treatment. The following general guidelines pertain to hip fractures. Surgeons often differ in their choice of postoperative rehabilitation protocols.

Femoral neck fractures, either subcapital, intercapsular, or transcervical, are frequently associated with mild groin pain

Table 9-4. General Rehabilitative Measures for Limb Fractures

Goal	Measures
Reduce pain	Oral, non-narcotic analgesics
	Modalities: heat, massage, TENS, fluidotherapy (heat should not be applied until hemostasis is assured)
Reduce edema	Active, assisted exercises
	Elevation of distal and proximal aspects of the limb
	Hydrocollator packs
	Whirlpool bath
	Gentle massage
	Compression garments
Restore range of motion and strength	Active, assisted exercises
	Neuromuscular reeducation
	Resistive exercises (when appropriate)
	Modalities: heat followed by stretching of connective tissue
Return to independence in self-care and ADLs	Adaptive equipment prescription: raised toilet seat, reacher, chair cushion, bathtub bench, long-handled bath sponge, hand-held shower nozzle.
	Ambulatory aids: walker, cane, crutches

that may refer to the knee. Endoprosthetic replacement is often necessary due to the risk of avascular necrosis.

A patient with an intertrochanteric fracture may experience more severe pain and present with apparent shortening and external rotation of the affected extremity. Surgical intervention (open reduction and internal fixation [ORIF]) using pins and plates or a compression screw is often necessary.

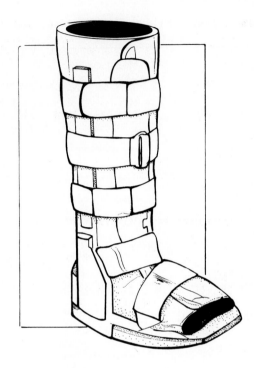

Figure 9-3. Orthotic cast.

Preoperative Care Guidelines

* Examine unaffected joints, opposite leg, and upper limbs.
* Exercise to strengthen hip abductors (if appropriate).
* Discuss postoperative therapy and goals with patient.

Postoperative Care Guidelines (Day 2–3)

* Determine whether cemented or non-cemented prosthesis was used.
* Examine for postoperative complications: sciatic or peroneal nerve paresis, hematoma, or DVT.

- Patients with total hip arthroplasty should avoid hip adduction, internal rotation, and flexion past 90 degrees in the affected limb. An abduction pillow will help maintain proper position while in bed and sitting.
- Partial weight-bearing in parallel bars may begin in patients with cemented hip prosthesis.
- Patients with porous coated and noncemented prostheses should be restricted to touch-down or non-weight-bearing for the first six weeks. The same applies to fractures treated by ORIF.
- Active assisted exercises may begin in the normal anatomic planes of motion.

Postoperative Care Guidelines (Day 4)

- Progress to three-point gait with standard walker crutches (cemented prosthesis) and advance to weight-bearing as tolerated.
- Non-weight-bearing or touch-down weight-bearing with standard walker or crutches if noncemented/porous prosthesis or ORIF.
- Isometric exercises for the quadriceps should be taught prior to discharge.

Outpatient Care Guidelines (6–12 Weeks PostOp)

- Obtain radiographic evaluation of the surgical site.
- Advance to a cane if cemented prosthesis was used.
- Advance to partial weight-bearing with standard walker or crutches if noncemented prosthesis was used.
- Begin low-weight, isotonic exercises to strengthen thigh and hip muscles.

Complications

Non-union at Fracture Site

Failure of a fracture to unite after 5 months may be due to factors such as age, overall health, and motion at the fracture site. Electrical stimulation to enhance osteogenesis and bone grafting are accepted treatment techniques.

Peripheral Nerve Injuries

Minor stretch injuries and swelling can result in neuropraxia. Nerve conduction studies will be abnormal. Recovery typically occurs within 10 weeks after the injury if pressures are removed. More severe stretch injuries and direct nerve trauma may result in axonal degeneration. Surgical repair of lacerated peripheral nerves may be necessary.

Compartment Syndromes

Unrelieved swelling in the tight osteofascial compartments of the limb leads to ischemia of the enclosed muscles and nerves. A patient who experiences severe pain with passive stretch and loss of muscle strength should be suspected of having developed compartment syndrome. Persistent use of analgesics for pain control can mask these symptoms and delay necessary surgical decompression. Displaced supracondylar fractures of the humerus can be complicated by a compartment syndrome and lead to development of Volkmann's contracture, in which the muscles of the flexor forearm are shortened and the fingers contract. Forearm pronation and elbow flexion are also frequently present.

Skin Complications

Immobilization without appropriate pressure relief can and incorrect application of a fracture cast can result in development of a pressure ulcer. Both of these complications are iatrogenic and preventable.

Reflex Sympathetic Dystrophy (RSD)

RSD is a syndrome of pain, hyperesthesia, vasomotor disturbance, and dystrophic changes in the skin and bone of an affected extremity. RSD that occurs after soft tissue trauma

with predominant findings of bony atrophy is referred to as
Sudek's atrophy of bone. The diagnosis of RSD is primarily
clinical and the disorder typically progresses in stages. Paravertebral sympathetic ganglion block is a widely used treatment. Reports of successful treatment of symptoms using
physical therapy. TENS, corticosteroids and phenoxybenz-
amine have appeared in the literature.

▌Suggested Readings

Cummings SR, Kelsey JL, Nevitt MC, O'Dowd KJ. Epidemiology of osteoporosis and osteoporotic fractures. *Epidemiol
Rev* 1985;7:178.

Demopoulous JT. Rehabilitation in fractures of the limbs. *In*
Ruskin A, ed. *Current Therapy in Physiatry,* Philadelphia:
W.B. Saunders, 1984.

Garraway WM, Stauffer RN, Kurland LT, O'Fallon WM.
Limb fractures in a defined population. Part I. Frequency and
distribution. *Mayo Clin Proc* 1979;54:701. Part II. Orthopedic treatment and utilization of health care. *Mayo Clin Proc*
1979;54:708.

Gradisar IA. Fracture stabilization and healing. *In* Gould JA,
Davies GJ, eds. *Orthopedic and Sports Physical Therapy,* 2nd ed.
St. Louis: C.V. Mosby, 1990.

Hoaglund FT, Duthie RB. Fracture and joint injuries. *In*
Schwartz SI, ed. *Principles of Surgery,* 6th ed. New York:
McGraw-Hill Book Company, 1994.

Knapp M. Aftercare of fractures. *In* Kottke FJ, Stillwell GK.
Lehmann JF, eds. *Krusen's Handbook of Physical Medicine and
Rehabilitation.* Philadelphia: W.B. Saunders, 1982.

Miller CW. Survival and ambulation following hip fracture.
J Bone Joint Surg 1978;60A:930.

Opitz JL. Total joint arthroplasty: principles and guidelines for postoperative physiatric management. *Mayo Clin Proc* 1979;54:602–612.

Salter RB. *Textbook of Disorders and Injuries of the Musculoskeletal System,* 2nd ed. Baltimore: Williams & Wilkins, 1983.

Schwartzman RJ, McLellan MD. Reflex sympathetic dystrophy, a review. *Arch Neurol* 1987;44:555.

Waugh T. Arthroplasty rehabilitation. *In* Goodgold J, ed. *Rehabilitation Medicine.* St. Louis: C.V. Mosby, 1988.

Wild D, Nayak U, Isaacs B. Description, classification and prevention of falls in old people at home. *Rheumatol Rehabil* 1981;20:153.

Zuckerman JD, Newport ML. Rehabilitation of fractures in adults. *In* Goodgold J, ed. *Rehabilitation Medicine.* St. Louis: C.V. Mosby, 1988.

Shahzadi Saleem
Carlos Vallbona

10

Immobilization

Immobilization is defined as physical restriction or limitation of body members and of the body in turning, sitting and ambulation. This may result from any of the following:

* neuromusculoskeletal disorders and injuries, such as paralysis;
* orthopedic casts, body jackets, and splints;
* critical illness requiring bed rest;
* prolonged stay in reduced gravity position, such as sitting or recumbency; or
* weightlessness in space, where movements are not restricted, but occur without counteracting forces of gravity.

Prolonged bed rest and inactivity reduce general metabolic activity. This results in decreased functional capacity of multiple body systems, with clinical manifestations of immobilization syndrome. The metabolic consequences are independent of the cause for which immobilization might be prescribed, and are seen both in healthy volunteers and patients with neuromusculoskeletal problems. The outcome however, depends on the degree and duration of immobilization. In a patient who has a neurological or musculoskeletal deficit, the effects of immobilization result in further reduc-

Susan J. Garrison (Ed.): *Handbook of Physical Medicine and Rehabilitation Basics.* First Edition. Copyright © 1995 J. B. Lippincott Company

tion of functional capacity. This causes severe disability; it takes longer to restore these patients to their maximal functional potential.

Awareness of the deleterious effects of prolonged bed rest allows for judicious planning of physical activities, exercise, and rest, thereby preventing immobilization syndrome.

The clinical manifestations of immobilization are summarized in Table 10-1. Some are self-explanatory. Others are described later as they influence patient management. Rehabilitation measures to counteract or prevent disability resulting from immobilization are described at the end of this chapter.

■ Deleterious Effects of Prolonged Immobilization

Musculoskeletal System

Strength

With immobilization, different muscle groups show a variable decrease in strength. The antigravity muscles, particularly those in the lower limbs, are predominantly affected. The scientific literature suggests a 50% decrease in strength with total inactivity. After space flights, astronauts also demonstrate a decrease in muscle strength, with individual variations. Recovery of strength occurs much more slowly than loss of strength. It may take 4 weeks to regain strength that is lost in 1 week, even when the person participates in a maximal strengthening program.

Endurance

A decrease in strength and concomitant effects of immobilization on the cardiovascular system result in decreased endurance.

Table 10-1. The Immobilization Syndrome: Clinical
Manifestations

Central nervous system
Altered sensation

Decreased motor activity

Autonomic lability

Emotional and behavioral disturbances

Intellectual deficit

Muscular system
Decreased muscle strength

Decreased endurance

Muscle atrophy

Poor coordination

Skeletal system
Osteoporosis

Fibrosis and ankylosis of joints

Cardiovascular system
Increased heart rate (adrenergic state)

Decreased cardiac reserve

Orthostatic hypotension

Phlebothrombosis

Respiratory system
Decreased vital capacity (restrictive impairment)

Decreased maximal voluntary ventilation (restrictive impairment)

Regional changes in ventilation/perfusion

Impairment of cougning mechanism

Digestive system
Anorexia

Constipation

(continued)

Table 10-1. (*Continued*)

Endocrine and renal effects
Increased diuresis and extracellular fluid shifts

Increased natriuresis

Hypercalciuria

Renal lithiasis

Integumentary system
Atrophy of the skin

Pressure ulcers

Muscle Atrophy

Muscle atrophy is dependent on the degree, as well as the
cause, of inactivity and disuse. In upper motor neuron disease, spastic paralysis, and immobilization, muscle bulk decreases by 30% to 35%, because increased muscle tone actually prevents complete atrophy. The atrophy involves both
Type I and II fibers, but Type II fibers are predominantly
involved in immobilization atrophy. In the case of lower motor neuron dysfunction and chronic irreversible flaccid paralysis, muscle bulk is reduced by 90% to 95%. If recovery does
not occur, muscle fibers are replaced by connective tissue.

Contracture

Contracture is a loss of range of motion in a joint. It may
result from several causes, such as tightness of connective
tissue, muscle, and joint capsule, as well as a joint disorder.
However, in an immobilized person, mechanical factors are
most important. If a muscle is chronically maintained in a
shortened position, the muscle fibers and connective tissue
adapt to the shortened length, causing contracture on the
relaxed side of the joint. A muscle held in shortened position
for only 5 to 7 days will demonstrate shortening of the

muscle belly due to contraction of collagen fibers and decrease in muscle fiber sacromeres. If this position continues for 3 weeks or more, the loose connective tissue in muscles and around joints will gradually change into dense connective tissue, causing contracture. Contributing factors such as edema, hemorrhage, spasticity, paralysis, pain, muscle imbalance, soft tissue injury, and advanced age compound and enhance formation of contractures. Muscle imbalance is the most important contributing factor. In the immobile patient, lower limb contractures are most common, usually involving the hips, knees, and ankles (two-joint muscles). In the upper limbs, the wrists, shoulders, and elbows are at risk. Similar pathophysiologic changes may occur in the joints of the spine, especially in the cervical and lumbar regions. Development of contractures is one of the most severe, yet in most cases preventable, disabilities that result from immobilization and have a major influence on the functional outcome of rehabilitation. Be aware; anticipate and take measures to prevent contractures. Prevention is preferable to treatment, and is much more cost-effective.

Coordination

A combination of the above factors and disuse results in decreased coordination. In a patient who has a central nervous system (CNS) lesion causing incoordination, the effects of immobilization can make it appear worse.

Osteoporosis

The stimulus of weight bearing, gravity, and muscle activity on bone mass maintains the balance between bone formation and resorption. Several enzymatic factors also play a part. Prolonged bed rest leads to bone atrophy that involves both organic and inorganic bone components. Increased urinary excretion of calcium and hydroxyproline as well as increased excretion of calcium in stool result in a decrease in total bone mass, especially from the weight-bearing bones. Osteoporosis due to immobilization is more marked in the subperiosteal region, in contrast to senile osteoporosis that develops from the marrow outward. In addition, disuse osteoporosis is most apparent in cancellous bone at the metaphysis and epiphysis, and later extends to the entire diaphysis. After 12 weeks of bed rest, bone density is reduced by 40–45%, and by 50% by the 30th week. Osteoporosis may lead to compression fractures of vertebral bodies and weight-bearing long bones with minor trauma, as well as predisposing the patient to hip fractures.

Metabolic Effects

Hypercalcemia

Marked hypercalcemia can occur several weeks after immobilization. This is most often seen in young adult males who were physically active prior to immobilization. It is associated with hypercalcemic metabolic alkalosis, and may lead to renal failure and ectopic calcification. It manifests clinically as headache, nausea, lethargy, constipation, and weakness. Renal function demonstrates a decrease in glomerular filtration, ability to concentrate urine, and increased excretion of phosphorous.

Cardiovascular System

Effects of immobility include increased sympathetic tone (adrenergic state), increased heart rate, decreased cardiac efficiency, postural hypotension, and phlebothrombosis.

Heart rate increases 1 beat per minute per 2 days of bed rest in healthy volunteers; blood volume decreases by 7% and maximum oxygen uptake (VO_2 max) decreases 27% after 20 days of bed rest. The combined effect of these factors is a reduction in cardiac efficiency and intolerance to upright posture, resulting in dizziness or faintness on attempting to stand. Difficulty in achieving upright posture interferes with functional activities.

Phlebothrombosis is a known risk. Lymphatic and venous stasis occurs in the lower limbs due to a lack of calf muscle pumping action as a result of inactivity. Other contributing factors usually associated with immobility include paralysis, postsurgical state, congestive heart failure, obesity, advanced age, and dehydration. All increase the risk of phlebothrombosis, and pulmonary embolus as a hypercoagulable state may result from these pathophysiological changes.

Respiratory System

Bed rest causes mechanical restrictive impairment as a result of decreased overall strength and a reduction of intercostal, diaphragmatic, and abdominal muscle excursion in supine breathing. The costovertebral and costochondral joints and the abdominal muscles may become fixed in an expiratory position, further reducing maximal inspiration, and resulting in a decrease in vital and functional respiratory capacities. This causes regional differences in ventilation/perfusion ratio, poorly ventilated as well as overly perfused areas, and arterio-venous shunts. If increased metabolic demand occurs, hypoxia results. Mucociliary function is also impaired; mucus secretions accumulate in the dependent respiratory bronchioli, leading to atelectasis and hypostatic pneumonia.

Digestive System

Anorexia and constipation are the result of decreased metabolic demand and endocrine changes, as well as decreased gastric and intestinal motility.

Skin

Skin atrophy results from inadequate nutrition. Pressure ulcers, a dreaded complication of immobility, are better prevented than treated. They occur over bony prominences such as the sacrum, ischium, trochanter, and heel. They result from prolonged pressure causing ischemic necrosis of soft tissue overlying the bony prominences. Edema, malnutrition, anemia, hypoalbuminemia, and paralysis are contributing factors.

■ Management of Complications

The best management of immobility is prevention. When this is not possible, the following management of potential complications is indicated.

Positioning of the patient in bed is extremely important. In the supine position, the trunk should align with the hips, knees, and ankles in a neutral position with the toes pointing towards the ceiling. The shoulders should be in 30 degrees of flexion and 45 degrees of abduction, the wrists in 20 to 30 degrees extension, and the hands in the functional position. This can easily be achieved with the use of pillows, trochanter rolls, or resting splints. Refer to Figure 10-1. A prone position or side-lying position may also be used. Position changes every 2 hours may be necessary in quadriplegic patients with insensate skin and in comatose patients. (Refer to Chapter 15, Pressure Ulcers.)

An appropriate bed has a 4-inch eggcrate mattress and footboard. Use knee- or thigh-high elastic stockings or elastic wraps in all bedridden patients. Consider use of external intermittent compression of the lower limbs. Low dosage heparin, 5000 to 8000 units subcutaneously every 8 to 12 hours, is indicated in patients at high risk for venous thrombosis. Adequate nutrition and proper hydration is essential. Prescribe a stool softener to prevent constipation.

Manage the bladder with an external catheter or intermittent catheterization, depending on the patient's needs. Give meticulous attention to skin care hygiene.

Physical therapy should begin at bedside and progress to the therapy department, emphasizing progressive mobilization. Passive and subsequently active assistive and active range of motion (PROM, AAROM, AROM) of all major joints is necessary, at least once daily.

Tilt-table conditioning should begin as soon as the pa-

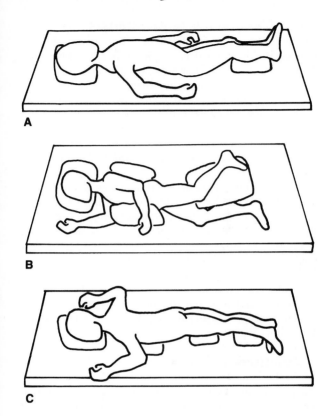

Figure 10-1. Appropriate Bed Positioning. (A) Supine: elevate the calves to remove pressure from the heels. (B) Side-lying: decrease trochanteric pressure by positioning the legs as shown. (C) Prone: provide pressure release for the iliac crests and knees by using the illustrated arrangement of pillows or foam. (From Donovan WH et al. Pressure ulcers. *In* DeLisa JA, *Rehabilitation Medicine,* 2nd ed., J.B. Lippincott, 1993, p. 726.)

tient is stable, beginning at a 30-degree tilt for 1 minute. Gradually increase the tilt 10 degrees every 3 to 5 days or earlier as tolerated, until the patient is able to tolerate a 70-degree tilt for 30 minutes. Then progress to standing, and finally, ambulation.

Osteoporosis can only be prevented by weight-bearing standing. Use a standing frame or tilt table with patients who are unable to stand unsupported. Begin a general endurance program, including strengthening and coordination exercises. Encourage functional activities if the patient is able to cooperate. Chest physical therapy with deep breathing exercises, incentive spirometer, assisted coughing, and/or chest percussion may be indicated, depending on the patient's needs. See Chapter 16, Pulmonary Rehabilitation. Teach independence in transfers and wheelchair propulsion to patients who are not ambulatory.

Make a referral to occupational therapy for activities of daily living (ADLs), application of splints, and upper limb care.

Avoid sensory deprivation; encourage the patient to interact with staff, other patients, and family members. Order recreational therapy for psychosocial integration, resocialization, and adjustment to independent functioning.

Carefully monitor the patient for signs and symptoms of hypercalcemia, pressure ulcers, urinary tract infection, or pneumonia, and treat the patient accordingly. Discuss all rehabilitative and medical treatment plans with the patient.

▮ Conclusion

The interventions that we as physiatrists use in the management of immobilized patients are numerous. However, all interventions are not necessary in all patients. In addition, other management may be indicated in specific patients. Interventions should be individualized; for example, in spastic patients, a more aggressive ROM exercise 3 to 4 times per day may be necessary, along with medical management of spasticity with medications, and/or nerve or motor point blocks. Consider using electrical stimulation and passive stretching to retard isolated muscle atrophy. Neuromuscular facilitation techniques may be helpful. Nurses or family members, after instructions, should be able to provide ROM for preventing contractures. Bed positioning changes may not be feasible in some patients; special beds may be necessary. See Chapter 15, Pressure Ulcers.

In some cases, bed rest is necessary for a short period of time, such as after acute myocardial infarction, cardiac dysrhythmia, or septic shock. Evaluate your patient from a rehabilitation standpoint, but obtain agreement from the referring physician prior to initiating an aggressive mobilization program. Problems related to immobility can, and should, be prevented.

Suggested Readings

Cardenas DD, Stolov WC, Hardy R. Muscle fibers numbers in immobilization atrophy. *Arch Phys Med Rehabil* 1977; 58:423–426.

Dietrick JE, Whedon GD, Shorr E. The effects of immobilization upon various metabolic and physiologic functions of normal man. *Am J Med* 1948;4:3–36.

Fournier A, Goldberg M, Green B, et al. A medical evaluation of the effects of computer-assisted muscle stimulation in paraplegic patients. *Orthopedics* 1989;7:1129–1139.

Haler EM, Bell KR. Contracture and other deleterious effects of immobility. *In* DeLisa JA, ed. *Rehabilitation Medicine: Principles and Practice.* Philadelphia: J.B. Lippincott, 1988, pp. 448–462.

Kottke FJ. The effects of limitation of activity upon the human body. *JAMA* 1966;196:117–122.

Muller EA. Influence of training and inactivity on muscle strength. *Arch Phys Med Rehabil* 1970;51:449–462.

Nicogossian AE: Overall physiologic response to space flight. *In* Nicogossian AE, ed. *Space Physiology and Medicine.* 2nd ed. London: Lea and Febiger, 1989, pp. 139–153.

Spencer WA, Vallbona C, Carter RE. Physiologic concepts of immobilization. *Arch Phys Med Rehabil* 1965;46:89–100.

Steinberg FU. The immobilized patient. *In Functional Pathology and Management.* New York: Plenum Publishing Co, 1980.

Tardin C, Tabary JC, et al. Adaptation of connective tissue length to immobilization in lengthened and shortened positions in cat soleus muscle. *J Physiology (Pare's)* 1982;78:214–220.

Vallbona C. Bodily responses to immobilization. *In* Kottke FJ, Stillwell GK, Lehmann JF, eds. *Krusen's Handbook of Physical Medicine and Rehabilitation.* 3rd ed. Philadelphia: W.B. Saunders, 1982.

Vallbona C. Immobilization syndrome. *In* Halstead LS, Grabois M, Howland CA, eds. *Medical Rehabilitation.* New York: Raven Press, 1985, p. 290.

Maureen R. Nelson

11

Neuromuscular Diseases

The neuromuscular diseases cover a wide spectrum of severity. The genetics of these various diagnoses are different, as is their outcome. The prototypical neuromuscular disease is Duchenne muscular dystrophy (DMD), one of the group of rapidly progressive neuromuscular diseases on which much of neuromuscular disease research has been based. See Chapter 13, Pediatric Rehabilitation, for a review of DMD. Other neuromuscular diseases include other dystrophies, lower motor neuron diseases, multiple sclerosis, diseases affecting the neuromuscular junction, polyneuropathies (see Chapter 14, Peripheral Neuropathy and Plexus Injury), inflammatory myopathies, metabolic diseases and Guillain-Barré syndrome. See Table 11-1 for specific diseases in these categories.

Neuromuscular diseases have in common the symptom of weakness. However, they differ in the muscle groups involved, as well as in the onset and pattern of weakness.

▓ Lower Motor Neuron Diseases

Motor neuron diseases include amyotrophic lateral sclerosis (ALS), spinal muscular atrophy (SMA), and polio. SMA is divided into acute infantile spinal muscular atrophy (SMA Type I, Werdnig-Hoffman disease); chronic childhood spinal

Susan J. Garrison (Ed.): *Handbook of Physical Medicine and Rehabilitation Basics.* First Edition. Copyright © 1995 J. B. Lippincott Company

Table 11-1. Examples of Neuromuscular Diseases

Lower motor neuron diseases
Amyotrophic lateral sclerosis (ALS)

Spinal muscular atrophy (SMA)

 Acute infantile SMA, SMA Type I—Werdnig-Hoffmann
 disease
 Chronic childhood SMA Type II
 Late onset juvenile SMA Type III—Kugelberg-Welander
 disease

Post-polio syndrome (PPS)

Multiple sclerosis

Myopathies

Dystrophies
Becker muscular dystrophy (BMD)

Duchenne muscular dystrophy (DMD)

Fascioscapulohumeral (FSH)

Limb girdle

Myotonic muscle dystrophy (MMD)

Toxic
Alcohol
 acute
 chronic

Vincristine

Endocrine
Hyperthyroid

Hypothyroid

Exogenous corticosteroids

Inflammatory
Polymyositis

Dermatomyositis

(*continued*)

Table 11-2. (*Continued*)

Metabolic diseases
Periodic paralysis

Glycogen storage diseases

Neuromuscular junction diseases
Myasthenia gravis (MG)

Eaton-Lambert syndrome (ELS)

Guillain-Barré syndrome (GBS)

muscular atrophy (SMA Type II); and late-onset juvenile spinal muscular atrophy (SMA Type III, Kugelberg-Welander disease). Each is described in detail, as follows.

Amyotrophic Lateral Sclerosis (ALS)

Definition

ALS is an adult onset, asymmetrical, painless weakness with muscular atrophy, hyperreflexia, and relentless progression. The median age of onset is approximately 66 years. ALS patients demonstrate symptoms that are associated with degeneration of motor nerve cells throughout the body. Lower motor neuron signs include wasting and weakness of muscles that lose their innervation; upper motor neuron signs include spasticity and hyper-reflexia. Symptoms of ALS include patchy, often distal weakness; bulbar symptoms, including dysarthria and dysphagia, the presenting complaint in approximately one third of patients; leg cramps; and muscle fasciculations. A paucity of fasciculations suggests slow progression of disease, but more fasciculations do not mean more severe disease. Fasciculations are believed to indicate anterior horn cell degeneration; however, they are not uncommon in healthy persons in whom they are not associated with weakness or atrophy. Pseudobulbar palsy is seen, particularly in patients with bulbar symptoms, along with involvement of

higher levels of the brain stem or cerebral cortex. As the
disease progresses, it spreads to most muscles within months,
causing weakness and atrophy. Speech and swallowing problems follow bulbar weakness; extraocular movements usually
remain intact. Cranial nerves X, XI, and XII are most frequently involved, with cranial nerves V and VII somewhat
less frequently. Bowel, bladder, and sexual functions are usually preserved, as is sensation.

Epidemiology

The incidence of ALS is 1 to 2 per 100,000 with a prevalence
of 2 to 7 per 100,000. It affects whites more than blacks; the
male to female ratio is 1.8 to 1. Approximately 5% to 10% of
patients with ALS have a positive family history. Those with
a positive family history generally have an earlier age of
onset, and there is an equal male to female ratio in this
group.

Risks/Etiology

The etiology and risk factors of ALS are unknown.

Pathology

In ALS, there is a degeneration of large motor neurons, and
changes are found in the axons of anterior horn cells as well as
the anterior horn cells themselves.

Evaluation

A careful history and physical exam is vital. Signs and symptoms of both upper motor neuron and lower motor neuron
dysfunction are indicative of ALS. Mild elevations or normal
levels of cerebral spinal fluid (CSF) protein are found on lab
exam. Creatine kinase (CK) levels are normal or within two

to three times the normal range. Electromyographic (EMG) studies can be performed to help with this diagnosis and serial EMGs may be of benefit. Studies of affected muscles reveal positive sharp waves and fibrillations (some small), as well as fasciculations. Clinical severity correlates with the distribution and magnitude of fibrillations. Motor unit potentials show increased amplitude, duration and polyphasicity. Muscles that show electrical abnormality with no clinical involvement of the limb, particularly in multiple spinal segments, help confirm the diagnosis. Muscles which may be of particular assistance in diagnosing ALS are those in the tongue, cranial nerve innervated muscles, and the sternocleidomastoid. Sensory nerve conduction studies are usually normal. Motor nerve conduction studies are normal early with a mild slowing later in the disease. Repetitive stimulation studies may show decremental responses, more often in atrophic muscles. This is believed to be a negative prognostic factor, possibly indicating rapid motor neuron loss. Single fiber EMG (SFEMG) may demonstrate increased fiber density in affected muscle, with abnormally increased jitter and blocking, and may show abnormalities prior to the standard EMG exam. Abnormal EMG findings in at least three limbs involving different nerves and roots should be present for a diagnosis; however, no findings are pathognomonic. Serial EMG and nerve conduction studies (NCVs), along with the course of the disease, help in confirming the diagnosis and following disease progression.

Treatment

Various medications are used in the treatment of ALS; however, they are currently unproved and unsuccessful. Education is an important aspect of treatment, including discussion of unfounded fears such as loss of mentation, and providing medical information so that the patient and family can make plans for disease progression. Intervention such as gastrostomy and assisted ventilation should be discussed as early as possible. Assistive devices should be used as needed. Oxygen at night may be of assistance early. Respiratory depressants should be avoided, including alcohol. Additionally, these patients should be immunized against pneumococcal and influenza infections. Range of motion (ROM) exercises should be taught to the patient and family and used daily to prevent contractures.

Complications

The loss of motor function as well as inability to talk and swallow is part of the progression of ALS. There are problems with frozen shoulder and loss of ROM in other joints.

Prognosis, Outcome, and Follow-Up

Approximately 50% of patients with ALS are alive 3 years after diagnosis, 20% after 5 years, and an occasional patient will live 20 years after diagnosis. Death generally results from respiratory failure. Patients are usually mobile, using wheelchairs approximately 1 to 1½ years after diagnosis, and later bedridden. The subsequent disease course is loss of ability to move, talk, swallow and then respiratory failure.

Spinal Muscle Atrophy (SMA)

Definition

SMA Type I, known as Werding-Hoffman disease, is a degenerative disease of the anterior horn cells and the motor nuclei of some of the cranial nerves. The clinical onset is generally by age 3 to 6 months, with approximately one third of cases apparent early in life through decreased fetal movements and sometimes arthrogryposis at birth. The classic description is that of an alert child with active facial expressions, frog leg position, thin chest, and paradoxical thorax movement with breathing. Often they have feeding difficulties, as well as a poor cry, due to their weakness. Approximately 50% of these children demonstrate tongue fasciculations. They are unable to lift their heads or sit up. Weakness is most severe proximally. Reflexes are absent or very decreased. Sensation is normal.

SMA Type II has a more insidious onset, beginning from approximately age 3 to 15 months. This is often first noticed when an infant fails to reach motor milestones, such as the ability to roll over, a skill attained in approximately one third of these babies. A loss of milestones can also indicate this disease. Very few of these children are able to maintain sitting or standing positions for any length of time. Weakness in the legs is generally more severe than in the arms. The children are usually able to chew and swallow, and respiratory muscles are spared. Hand tremors are often present. Reflexes are decreased or absent.

SMA Type III, termed Kugelberg-Welander disease, generally has an onset at approximately 5 to 15 years of age and follows a slowly progressive course. Generally, hip weakness is noticed first and then a waddling gait, progressing to difficulty with stairs, to using a Gowers' maneuver for rising from the floor, and weakness of the shoulders. Additionally, increased lordosis and eversion of feet appear. Coarse tremor of trunk and arms may be present, and less commonly, bulbar findings. Approximately 20% of these patients demonstrate pseudohypertrophic calves, but it is unusual to see toe-walking or early contractures of the gastrocnemius. Most of these patients walk for 10 to 30 years after onset of the disease, but generally use a wheelchair by age 30 years. Fasciculations may be noted in about half of these patients at some stage of the disease, especially in the shoulder and hip region. Muscle atrophy is common, as well as decreased reflexes. Kyphoscoliosis and contractures are often present in later stages of the disease.

Epidemiology

SMA Type I has an incidence of 1 in 15,000 to 25,000 live births. Approximately 30% of all cases of spinal muscular atrophy are of the Type I variety. This disease is usually inherited as an autosomal recessive. It is believed that SMA Type II is probably part of a spectrum between Werdnig-Hoffman disease and Kugelberg-Welander disease; most of the cases are believed to be autosomal recessive. SMA Type III is occasionally autosomal dominant.

Risks/Etiology

The etiology of SMA is unknown.

Pathology

Histological studies of SMA Type I show marked abnormalities of the large anterior horn cells in the spinal cord, along with a reduced number of these cells. Degeneration of large thalamic neurons as well as large bundles of glial tissue extended into spinal nerve roots have been noted. Muscle biopsy demonstrates atrophic fibers, both Type I and Type II fibers, mostly round, as well as hypertrophic fibers. The intermediate form of SMA shows changes of denervation, as does SMA Type III. SMA Type III often shows some fiber type grouping and an increase in Type II fibers, which may sometimes be present in SMA Type II.

Evaluation

The history focuses on the time frame and progression of the disease, in order to distinguish between the types described above. The exam in SMA should include particular attention to facial expression, cognitive status, sensory evaluation, reflexes, and strength. Laboratory studies should include CK and aldolase levels, which are normal or slightly increased in SMA Type I. CK levels are normal or elevated up to 5 times normal, increasing as the disease advances, in SMA Type II. In SMA Type III, CK in about half of the patients is from 2 to 10 times normal, also increasing with the progression of the disease. Neurodiagnostic studies reveal the underlying degeneration of anterior horn cells with denervation of muscle fibers in all SMA types. Reinnervation by collateral sprouting appears in SMA Type III more than in Type II. Electrodiagnosis reveals reduced number of motor unit potentials of increased duration and amplitude. These may, however, decrease in amplitude as the disease progresses and motor units degenerate. Fibrillations and fasciculations are believed to be caused by motor neuron irritability and are more frequently seen in SMA Type III than in Types I or II. On nerve conduction study, sensory evaluations are normal. Motor nerve conduction studies reveal slightly slowed or normal values. In SMA Type I, there have been reports of spontaneous, regularly discharging potentials in relaxed muscles at 5 to 15 per second which persist even in sleep. There is also decreased recruitment, or absence of, motor units in the weakest muscles.

Treatment

There is no cure for SMA. Therefore, treatment is directed toward maximizing function at each level of progression and minimizing complications, including assisting in allowing normal cognitive and social development for the children and the family unit. In growing children, emphasize ROM exercises, particularly to prevent kyphoscoliosis and flexion contractures. Braces and surgery are more frequently used in SMA Type II and Type III.

Complications

Respiratory problems are frequent in SMA. Arthrogryposis may be present in SMA Type I; problems with skeletal deformities are common with disease progression in the other types of SMA.

Prognosis/Follow-Up/Outcome

Patients with SMA Type I generally die prior to age 2, but occasionally survive to the age of 3 years. Respiratory failure is the usual cause of death. Patients with SMA Type II have a variable course, at times demonstrating static weakness, and at other times experiencing alternating periods of weakness and stability of symptoms. Patients with SMA Type III may walk for 10 to 30 years after the onset of disease, but most use wheelchairs by the age of 20 to 30. These patients may survive to adulthood and generally die of respiratory failure.

Post-Polio Syndrome

Definition

Post-polio syndrome (PPS) is a collection of signs and symptoms appearing decades after acute onset of polio and after decades of stable function. PPS includes the three major complaints of new pain, weakness, and fatigue. The term progressive post-poliomyelitis muscular atrophy (PPMA) is used to describe new onset weakness and atrophy. PPMA includes new muscular atrophy, pain, weakness, fasciculation, respiratory and bulbar symptoms, and sleep difficulties. Muscles that were originally weakened by polio, as well as those subclinically affected, are commonly involved. Progression is slow, with a reported decrease in strength of approximately 1% to 2% per year.

Epidemiology

There are approximately 250,000 polio survivors in the United States today. Predictions are that 25% of these people will have symptoms of PPS beginning approximately 30 to 40 years after the original onset of polio, with a mean latency of 36 years.

Risk Factors

Major factors associated with the development of PPS appear to correlate with the severity of the original disease. Polio patients who originally required ventilatory assistance and those who experienced involvement of all four extremities are more likely to develop PPS. Patients who were over 10 years of age at onset are also at risk.

Pathology

PPMA is now thought to be secondary to the degeneration and atrophy of neuromuscular connections, nerve cell, and muscle fibers. This can appear in muscles that were already weakened as well as in those affected subclinically in which weakness was not previously noted. Research suggests that motor units enlarged by reinnervation in recovery from polio may experience disintegration with aging. The degeneration of the very large motor unit resulting from such reinnervation has a much greater functional impact than the degeneration of a normal-sized motor unit. The decline in the number of anterior horn cells, a normal part of the aging process, could also be more functionally apparent in a person with borderline muscle capacity.

Assessment

Obtain a complete history emphasizing the severity of the original disease, need for ventilatory support, and age at onset. Focus on current respiratory symptoms. Evaluate complaints of new pain, weakness, nocturnal shortness of breath, and day-time sleepiness. Perform a careful assessment of the amount of functional impairment and discomfort as a result of pain. Obtain baseline spirometry measures in all patients; carefully follow those with a history of respiratory involvement. Scoliosis, as well as respiratory muscle weakness, can have adverse affects on respiratory status. Blood gas analysis during sleep can be used to screen for respiratory dysfunction.

Evaluate the patient's orthotic devices. An inappropriate or unused orthosis may contribute to pain and decreased function. Evaluate muscular strength as objectively as possible. Fatigue is more difficult to evaluate objectively, but should be tested as much as possible. Evaluate performance of all daily functions, including housework and transportation. Document psychosocial status, because extreme functional changes occurring after decades of physical stability can create stress. Dysphagia, reported in approximately 20% of post-polio patients, can also be a significant stressor. Ask specific questions about difficulty with swallowing. Evaluation may include a modified barium swallow.

Laboratory evaluation is generally unremarkable. CK levels in some patients have been elevated approximately 4 times normal; however, this seems prevalent in patients who over-exert themselves physically. It is therefore not a diagnostic measure, but can be one method of following compliance in a rehabilitation program. Muscle biopsy cannot distinguish between patients with stable polio and those with new weakness. SFEMG studies reveal unstable neuromuscular connections with increased jitter and blocking.

Treatment

Treatment must be individualized for PPS patients. Limb pain secondary to chronic overuse, degenerative arthritis, or muscular strain may be relieved by use of nonsteroidal anti-inflammatory drugs (NSAIDs), limited rest, or bracing. Reduction of abnormal stress on joints as well as weight reduction are also factors in pain management.

For weakness, it appears that a short-term, resistive exercise program may improve function in many muscle groups, and thereby increase the general level of activity. Research continues to evaluate exact parameters for exercise; therefore, if a short program, for example 6 weeks, is to be performed, it should be with careful monitoring. Endurance training programs have also been undertaken in experimental groups with polio with beneficial results. They have demonstrated subjective decrease in fatigue, although it has been noted that a few patients do display muscle overwork changes. Therefore, close monitoring is essential. Modify gait patterns using gait training to obtain the most efficient bio-mechanically appropriate motion. This may include use of appropriate orthotic devices, such as ankle foot orthoses (AFOs), as well as assistive devices. Patients who did not use orthoses or gait assistive devices earlier in the course of the disease may benefit from their use over time. Be aware of the increased risk of carpal tunnel syndrome (CTS) with the use of assistive devices. If CTS is diagnosed, treat with NSAIDs and night-time splinting.

Treatment of respiratory difficulties must be a major focus. Monitor vital capacity regularly. With increasing scoliosis and decreasing respiratory muscle function, respiratory assist frequently is necessary. Consider and discuss assisted ventilation early with such patients. Use intermittent positive pressure via nasal or oral interface for assisted night-time breathing support; intermittent abdominal pressure ventilation can be performed during the day. (See Chapter 16, Pulmonary Rehabilitation.) Some patients require late tracheostomies for ventilatory assistance. Careful and close evaluation when using oxygen therapy is imperative, due to the risk of increased carbon dioxide retention, hypersom-nalence, and possible respiratory arrest.

Patient education is necessary; PPS patients should learn to modify activities to simplify work and minimize energy consumption. Encourage the use of assistive devices and environmental adaptation. Ongoing general medical care is vital. Suggest patient support groups and family counseling as indicated.

Complications

Joint pains may be secondary to increased weakness, muscle imbalance, and chronic biomechanical stress. Nerve compression syndromes, with symptoms of pain and paraesthesias, may result from repetitive stress or change in position.

Muscle pain can be related to overwork or muscle substitution. Increased weakness with over-exercise can be a complication of strengthening or endurance programs. Pulmonary complications have been described previously.

Prognosis, Outcome, and Follow-Up

PPS is usually a slowly progressive disease; weakness increases approximately 1% to 2% per year. Therefore, follow-up is usually every 2 years, but more frequently if needed. The PPS patient should be seen immediately if any new respiratory problems arise. When respiratory compromise is identified, monitoring is indicated at least every year. If the patient requires ventilatory assistance, monitor every 3 months. Prognosis depends on each patient's general health, as well as individual symptoms.

Multiple Sclerosis

Definition

Multiple sclerosis (MS) is a neuromuscular disease affecting mostly young adults. MS is characterized by symptoms that wax and wane. For a diagnosis of MS, there must be at least two areas of the central nervous system (CNS) demonstrating abnormalities separated by time and physical location. Common initial symptoms are paresthesias, visual loss, and gait disturbance. Additionally, diplopia, vertigo, fatigue, hemiparesis, and dysarthria can be initial symptoms. See Table 11-2 for categorization of the four general types of MS by course.

Anatomy

MS is primarily a disorder of myelin, although serum factors may be involved. The myelin of the brain and spinal cord is predominately affected, although peripheral nerves may show

Table 11-2. The Four General Types of Multiple Sclerosis*

Type of Course	Characteristics	Approximate Frequency
Benign	Mild or completely remitting attacks with long symptom-free periods	20%
Relapsing/ remitting	Periodic acute onset of symptoms followed by partial or complete recovery, with plateaus of stable impairment	25%
Relapsing/ progressive	Exacerbations with modest recovery and significant residual impairment; there is a slow "stepwise" deterioration of function	40%
Chronic/ progressive	continuous functional deterioration over months or years with risk for life-threatening complications	15%

*Reprinted with permission by the National Multiple Sclerosis Society. For more information, call 1-800-FIGHT MS.

minimal changes. The neurological functions that are impaired depend on the location of the myelin abnormality in the CNS.

Epidemiology

MS is a common neurological disease in the temperate climate above the 40th north parallel. This includes persons from the north who move south after the age of 14 years.

There is a prevalence of approximately 1 in 1,000 in some northern areas of the United States. MS is 2 to 4 times more common in the northern half of the United States than in the south. MS affects approximately 250,000 persons in the United States. Age of onset is generally between 20 and 40 years. The ratio of females to males is 2 to 1. The mortality rate, however, is slightly higher in males. The risk increases when immediate family members are affected. Risk for an identical twin of a patient with MS having the disease is 20%; non-identical twins have a risk of 15%. There is some histocompatibility linked antigen (HLA) association. It is believed that susceptibility to MS is inherited, but that environmental factors also play a role. One theory is that MS is caused by a virally induced immunoregulatory problem involving an improper immune response against the myelin in the CNS.

Pathology/Physiology

Initially there is swelling of the myelin; subsequently, the myelin sheath is destroyed and replaced by a sclerotic plaque.

Assessment

Diagnosis of MS is made over time. A new diagnosis must include two affected CNS areas that are separated in time and location, without other neurological explanation for the symptoms. Because the myelin damage occurs in various areas of the CNS, diverse symptoms may be present. These include paraesthesias, visual changes, gait disturbance, diplopia, vertigo, fatigue, hemiparesis, dysarthria, spasticity, incoordination, bowel or bladder problems, tremor, mental disturbances, pain, dizziness, convulsions, and dysphagia.

Laboratory work-up includes CSF studies of oligoclonal bands and myelin basic protein. Myelography or magnetic resonance imaging (MRI) can be performed to rule out spinal cord tumors or other lesions. Additionally, computerized tomography (CT) or MRI can evaluate for any type of changes in the brain itself. Evoked potentials are also commonly performed to look for new, distinct, previously unidentified lesions. The visual evoked response is the most sensitive for changes in MS patients, followed by somatosensory evoked potentials. Brain stem auditory evoked potentials best document an individual lesion in a patient with minimal symptoms.

Complications

At different times during the course of the disease, most MS patients will experience varying degrees of weakness. This can involve any part of the body, but most prominently the legs. Spasticity is often associated with weakness and may interfere with walking or other daily activities. Spasticity, however, may be useful in the patient who has severe weakness as it substitutes for muscular strength. Movement disorders include lack of coordination as well as ataxia, dystonia, and tremors. Fatigue is a common symptom, particularly apparent after the patient uses an extremity excessively or exercises. Prolonged exercise or work may cause more generalized weakness or incoordination of the body.

Urinary symptoms may be present at some point in the course of the disease. Proper urological work-up followed by appropriate treatment is vital. Due to the variable course of this disease, frequent re-evaluations and urodynamic studies as needed are appropriate, along with conservative treatment. Bowel problems, particularly constipation, are common; however, fecal incontinence may occur in patients with decreased sensation in the rectal vault.

Visual problems, including optic neuritis, are present in many patients. This may be the presenting symptom, ranging from a blind spot to nearly total blindness, sometimes associated with pain. Optic neuritis is associated with a relatively good prognosis when it is the only symptom at onset. Most cases of optic neuritis, however, do not lead to MS. Diplopia can also be seen as symptom of brainstem demyelination.

Sensory symptoms such as dysaesthesias, tingling, and numbness are frequent. Sensory symptoms also suggest a better prognosis if they are present at the onset of MS.

Dysarthria is commonly noted, secondary to involvement of the muscles used in speech. Due to the same difficulty, dysphagia may also be a problem.

Treatment

Treatment of MS depends on the various symptoms and individual disease course. Baseline and follow-up functional assessments are very helpful. In general, patients with stable neurological status do well with home exercise programs and regular physician follow-ups. Group exercise programs are also beneficial. During periods of relapse in exacerbating-remitting MS, treatment is aimed at restoring the previous baseline functional level. Specific treatment continues until the previous baseline or until 2 to 3 weeks of stable, though lesser function is achieved.

Carefully follow psychological and social issues. Anxiety about the patient's medical status is common, due to the presenting symptoms and uncertainty surrounding the diagnosis of MS. Counseling is often beneficial for the patient and family. Depression, usually a reactive type, is common. Euphoria and emotional lability may occur in the later stages. Denial is also common.

The rehabilitative treatment plan varies with the degree of disease progression and specific symptoms. Ambulation is often a problem. Canes, walkers, and AFOs may be helpful. As the disease progresses, a wheelchair or electric cart may be required for mobility. If weakness becomes extreme, stretching and range of motion exercises may be necessary to prevent contractures. Strengthening exercises must be very carefully performed because overexertion can lead to a functional decline. Treat spasticity with exercises to increase ROM. Oral medications for spasticity include dantrolene (Dantrium), diazepam (Valium), and baclofen (Lioresal). The medications all have side effects that must be monitored. (Refer to Chapter 17, Spinal Cord Injury.) Motor point injections also decrease spasticity locally. Treatment of spasticity may unmask weakness, so that overall the patient's functional status may actually decrease. For incoordination and tremor, use of weights on the limbs or walker, or wrist may be helpful. A wheelchair may also be useful for safety and mobility. Medications used to improve coordination include isoniazid (INH), propranolol (Inderal), and clonazepam (Klonopin). Discontinue the medication if there is no improvement after a 4 to 6 week trial.

Fatigue can be a severe problem; rest is the treatment of choice. Many patients adjust their work and activity schedule so they have a mid-day rest to enable them to increase their activity level. For patients with diplopia, the usual treatment is eye patching. Patients with sensory abnormalities, including pain, are often treated with a trial of carbamazepine (Tegretol). When using this, monitor blood count for possible bone marrow suppression. Avoid the use of narcotics for pain or other sensory abnormalities. Treat urinary problems as indicated by urodynamic studies. Intermittent catheterization or oxbutynin (Ditropan) is commonly used. Constipation is generally treated by a high-fiber diet, increased fluids and a bowel program. Speech therapy is indicated for dysarthria and dysphagia. (See Chapter 17, Spinal Cord Injury.)

In MS many symptoms' exacerbation or onset is thought to be secondary to physical and emotional stress. Therefore, attempt to minimize stress via counseling or decreasing lifestyle pressures. Psychological problems and depression are often treated by counseling. At times, tricyclic antidepressants are used and are particularly helpful when associated with insomnia or, at times, with pseudobulbar palsy. Also, in some patients hot environmental or body temperatures worsen symptoms. Short courses of steroids and adrenocorticotrophic hormone (ACTH) are sometimes used in an attempt to reduce the severity and duration of an exacerbation. These have not been proved to affect the long-term outcome of the disease.

Complications

Dramatic, acute complications may occur with elevation in
environmental and body temperature. Advise patients to
avoid hot showers and baths. Overexertion can lead to excessive fatigue, resulting in a decrease of overall functional status; therefore overexertion should also be avoided.

Prognosis, Outcome, and Follow-Up

Patients with benign-type MS usually have few functional
problems. Patients with exacerbating-remitting type lose
function during the exacerbations; they experience a variable
return to their previous level of function during remissions.
Patients with the progressive form of MS generally deteriorate more rapidly, and quickly become more disabled than
other patients. However, the remitting-exacerbating type
may change to the progressive form. Generally, a more severe
prognosis is found in patients whose MS begins over age 35,
who have slow onset of disease, have more initial symptoms,
have presented with motor symptoms, and are unable to
ambulate. In such patients, follow-up should be every 6 to 12
months due to the possibility of a change in the clinical
picture.

▨ Myopathies

Definition

Myopathies are a group of primary muscle diseases whose
common, principal symptom is weakness, usually proximal.
This is manifested by difficulty in climbing stairs, rising
from a chair, or using the arms to work over the head. The
primary groups of myopathies include the muscular dystrophies, toxic, endocrine, inflammatory, and metabolic myopathies. Each group will be described.

Muscular Dystrophies

The muscular dystrophies can be further divided into specific diseases including DMD (Chapter 13, Pediatric Rehabilitation), Becker muscular dystrophy (BMD), fascioscapulohumeral (FSH) dystrophy, limb girdle dystrophy (LGD), and myotonic muscular dystrophy (MMD).

Anatomy/Epidemiology

BMD displays anatomical findings of proximal weakness, toe walking, and pseudohypertrophy of the calves. The incidence is approximately 1 in 50,000 male births. FSH dystrophy manifests itself by weakness primarily in the face, shoulder girdle, and the anterior portion of the legs. The incidence is approximately 3 to 10 per million people. LGD is manifested by shoulder and hip weakness. MMD is characterized by more distal than proximal weakness, which is generally symmetrical. The face may also be involved, including the temporalis and masseter muscles, making the face appear hollow. Cardiac muscle is also affected; cardiac conduction disturbances are found in over $\frac{1}{2}$ of these patients. The prevalence of MMD is 3 to 5 per 100,000 population.

Risks/Etiology

BMD is an X-linked recessive disorder at the Xp21 locus. FSH is inherited by autosomal dominance with complete penetration but variable expressivity, so that there are both mild and severe cases possible in the same family. If this disease begins in infancy, a more severe case ensues, but most cases actually begin in the mid-teens and have a slow progressive course. LGD may have a variety of etiologies but is usually transmitted as an autosomal recessive trait. MMD is autosomal dominantly inherited, with a defective chromosome 19.

Pathology

BMD shows an abnormal quality and quantity of the muscle protein dystrophin; however, BMD demonstrates less severe abnormalities in both the quality and quantity of dystrophin than does DMD.

Assessment

Increased CK levels and pseudohypertrophy of the calves appear in BMD. The onset is generally in the second decade and disease progression is slow. BMD is evaluated by distribution of weakness, age at onset, and progression. Mental retardation, contractures, and EKG abnormalities are less common than in DMD. The EMG is myopathic, but complex repetitive discharges may be seen as well. Biopsy may show inflammatory changes and abnormal dystrophies.

FSH generally first appears in the early teen years with facial weakness and weak hips and shoulders. There is atrophy of neck and facial muscles, resulting in "smooth face," and shoulder weakness, frequently sparing the deltoid. Patients may be unable to drink with straws or do pushups. The forearms are generally stronger than the proximal muscles of the upper limbs, but wrist extensors may be weak. Hip weakness may lead to a compensatory lordosis. Additionally, weakness of the tibialis anterior and peroneal muscles may be present. CK levels are normal, as is early EMG; myopathic changes occur later. Progression is gradual, with some periods of more rapid decline in strength.

LGD generally occurs at 20 years of age, with weakness at the hips noticed first and shoulder weakness soon thereafter. Neck flexor and extensor weakness may also occur. Biceps weakness and atrophy are present. CK and lactic dehydrogenase are elevated up to ten times the normal level. EMG may show small, polyphasic motor units and complex repetitive discharges. Muscle biopsy reveals varied fiber size, increased internal nuclei, fiber splitting, and "moth-eaten" whorled fibers.

In MMD, an insidious onset generally occurs in early adulthood. The patient's voice becomes more nasal in quality.

Myotonia, muscle contraction with characteristic slow relaxation, also presents, and may be noted in voluntary muscle movement or with percussion of muscle. Myotonia becomes less pronounced with more severe atrophy and with repetition, and generally worsens in cold. Dysarthria and swallowing problems may be present over the disease course. Cardiac evaluations must also be performed in MMD because cardiac conduction disturbances are found in over $\frac{1}{2}$ of patients. Pulmonary hypoventilation may be present; care must be taken in the use of general anesthesia. Endocrine abnormalities may be present, including testicular atrophy. Cataracts are found in approximately 90% of patients. Mild mental retardation and denial of symptoms may both also be present. EMG is distinctive for the myotonic or dive-bomber type discharges that sound like a motorcycle revving its engine. This is very distinctive and easily distinguished with waxing and waning of motor unit amplitude and frequency. Muscle biopsy may show internal nuclei and atrophy of Type I fibers. In patients with childhood-onset disease, education is a part of the functional evaluation. Psychosocial and leisure activities also are areas of emphasis and possible assistive intervention.

Treatment

There is no cure for the muscular dystrophy group of diseases. However, there can be rehabilitative intervention to minimize the complications and the secondary impact of the disease.

BMD is treated with ROM, exercise, and assistive devices as needed. BMD generally requires much less intervention than DMD. FSH is treated similarly. Occasionally surgical intervention to fix the scapula to the chest wall is required, so that the FSH patient may raise his/her arm above the horizontal.

Management of MMD occasionally includes pharmaceutical treatment for the myotonia if it becomes problematic. If the patient has a cardiac conduction disturbance, certain medications for treatment of myotonia, such as quinine and procainamide hydrochloride (Procan), which prolong the PR interval, should not be used. Phenytoin (Dilantin) and carbamazepine (Tegretol) may be used to treat myotonia. The cardiac conduction disturbances are sometimes treated with insertion of a pacemaker. Use cardiac drugs with caution since propranolol (Inderal) exacerbates myotonia. Treatment is available for cataracts. Respiratory therapy may be indicated, particularly as disease advances. Care must be taken with anesthesia. Orthotics such as AFOs or wrist hand orthoses (WHOs) may be beneficial for distal weakness.

Prognosis/Outcome

With BMD, there is a favorable prognosis and a slow progression of disease, with most patients ambulating into their teens and surviving into middle age. FSH shows a normal life span and prolonged ambulation. In LGD, weakness frequently progresses so that ambulation is minimal or absent after a period of 20 years of disease progression. Death from cardiopulmonary complications may occur. MMD progresses slowly, particularly with later onset. There can be cardiac failure and sudden death secondary to the cardiac conduction disturbances, however. Cardiorespiratory failure may occur about age 50.

Follow-Up

When the cardiac conduction disturbance is present, follow-up should be frequent. The more slowly progressive diseases such as BMD and FSH can be less frequently, though still regularly, followed.

Toxic Myopathy

Anatomy/Epidemiology

Toxic myopathies include those caused by alcohol, diuretics, and vincristine as well as other medications. Alcohol is the most common cause of toxic myopathy. It can present in two ways—acute or chronic. The acute form generally follows a binge of drinking alcohol and the chronic form slowly progresses over years.

Risks/Etiology

The risks with the toxic myopathies depend on exposure to the toxins.

Assessment

Acute alcohol toxic myopathy is usually revealed by muscle pain, swelling and weakness, usually involving thigh musculature. Chronic alcohol toxic myopathy is exhibited by progressive proximal weakness.

Functional Evaluation

Functional evaluation for each of these groups of patients is approximately the same, although it varies with the degree of muscle weakness, severity, and age of the patient. Evaluate mobility; it may worsen over time from independent ambulation to unsteady gait, to use of assistive devices, and finally to a wheelchair. Evaluate transfers in wheelchair users and those who have poor balance. Upper limb function, such as lifting items above the head, is pertinent for evaluation, as is swallowing ability. Bathing, toileting, and dressing are specifically evaluated in each of these patients as well.

Treatment

Toxic myopathies are treated by removing the toxin when possible.

Prognosis/Outcome

Toxic myopathies are reversible with removal of the toxin as noted above, although there may be residual weakness.

Follow-Up

Toxic myopathies are noted to be generally reversible with the removal of the toxin. Of these, however, chronic alcohol myopathy, with its proximal weakness, often requires monitoring for some time.

Endocrine Myopathy

Anatomy/Epidemiology

Endocrine myopathies include those secondary to hypothyroidism, hyperthyroidism, and corticosteroids. Myopathy due to hyperthyroidism is generally a very minor and often overlooked proximal weakness that may include some atrophy. The quadriceps and shoulder musculature are classically involved and there is commonly extraocular muscle abnormality. Myopathy due to hypothyroidism may be manifested by stiffness, cramps, and hypertrophy of the muscle, in addition to myoedema. Corticosteroid endocrine myopathy may result from either endogenous or exogenous sources.

Risks/Etiology

Endocrine myopathies include corticosteroid myopathy, most commonly seen in the exogenous form after use of high-dose, long-term corticosteroids. These patients generally show recovery after decreasing or discontinuing the medication.

Assessment

In patients with hyperthyroid myopathy, the quadriceps and shoulder muscles may show weakness and atrophy. Additionally, there may be exophthalmic ophthalmoplegia which is associated with extraocular muscle abnormality, specifically tethering of the muscles. In hypothyroid myopathy, there may be a change in muscle contractility manifested by a slow relaxation phase. In more severe cases, there may be stiffness, cramps, hypertrophy, and myoedema of the muscles. Knowledge of thyroid profiles and medications used are vital in the evaluation of both of these cases.

Treatment

Endocrine myopathies are improved by treating the underlying endocrine disease. With removal of the use of exogenous corticosteroids, improvements have been shown.

Prognosis/Outcome

Since endocrine myopathies are treated by managing the primary disease, improvement occurs as the primary disease resolves.

Follow-Up

Endocrine myopathies require a short-term follow-up, with requisite physical exam and thyroid lab studies.

Inflammatory Myopathy

Anatomy/Epidemiology

Inflammatory myopathies are classically represented by polymyositis and dermatomyositis. Neck and proximal lower limb muscles are the most affected. Incidence is approximately 5 to 10 per million per year.

Risks/Etiology

Polymyositis and dermatomyositis are acquired acute or sub-acute inflammatory muscle diseases which are most common in children or in the 40 to 50 year age group. They frequently follow a systemic disease.

Assessment

In patients with polymyositis, approximately $\frac{1}{2}$ will complain of pain. The patients who do so describe a deep aching in the muscle with a type of soreness that improves with rest. There may be swelling in the muscles, particularly in the proximal lower extremities, which may also be tender to palpation. The course may progress over days to weeks, showing first proximal limb and anterior neck weakness and then spreading distally. Neck muscular weakness is often quite prominent. Dysphagia may be present.

In dermatomyositis, the muscle symptoms are generally the same. There may also be systemic symptoms including fever, malaise and GI discomfort. Dermatomyositis is known for a rash on the skin which may be present before, after, or during the muscular problem. Purple, sometimes swollen eyelids and puffiness around the eyes are often seen. There can be an erythematous rash of the chest and neck and the thickened skin over the elbows and knees. Hands often reveal the rash. Improvement in response to steroids may be diagnostic, particularly in polymyositis. There may be association of dermatomyositis in adults with neoplasms, especially carcinomas, and in children there may be an association with vasculitis. Both of these may be associated with connective tissue disorders.

Lab studies demonstrate increased CK and myoglobin levels during the acute event. The EMG classically shows a triad of positive sharp waves and fibrillations, polyphasic potentials, and complex repetitive discharges. Biopsy shows inflammation in about 70%, with "ghost fibers" sometimes present and perifascicular atrophy in dermatomyositis.

Treatment

In polymyositis and dermatomyositis, there may be a therapeutic response to steroids or to immunosuppression. Preserving passive ROM is vital during the acute stage. Gradually increase activity to promote strength and endurance.

Prognosis/Outcome

Inflammatory myopathies generally show improvement over time, though this varies.

Follow-Up

Inflammatory myopathies require follow-up through the period of active involvement and recovery. Thereafter, the need is less frequent.

Metabolic Myopathy

Anatomy/Epidemiology

Metabolic myopathies include periodic paralysis and glycogen storage diseases. There are ten well-described glycogen storage diseases, with four of these demonstrating significant muscular involvement, including Types II, III, V, and VII. Periodic paralysis is characterized by episodic periods of weakness that vary in severity and frequency, sparing extraocular and respiratory muscles. It may be due to hyperkalemia or hypokalemia.

Risk/Etiology

Glycogen storage diseases produce myopathies because of the patient's inability to utilize muscle glycogen. Many metabolic myopathies are secondary to genetic disorders.

Assessment

In patients with periodic paralysis, a family history is very important, along with a history of episodic weakness sparing extraocular muscles and respiratory muscles, with recovery between episodes. Glycogen storage disease muscle problems present in one of two ways. One manner, with progressive muscle weakness, is shown in acid maltase deficiency (Type II) and debranching enzyme deficiency (Type III). The other mode of presentation is with exertional cramps and myalgias. This occurs in McArdle's disease (phosphorylase deficiency, Type V) and phosphofructokinase deficiency (Type VII). The ischemic forearm exercise test is used to show the muscle's ability to utilize glycogen in ischemic conditions.

Functional Evaluation

See Toxic Myopathy, page 221.

Treatment

The metabolic myopathies are treated by managing the underlying metabolic disease.

Prognosis/Outcome

Progress of the metabolic myopathies depends on the underlying disease and varies.

Follow-Up

Metabolic myopathy should be followed by the primary caregiver for treatment of the metabolic disease. Exercise must be carefully monitored.

■ Neuromuscular Junction Diseases

Myasthenia Gravis

Definition

Myasthenia gravis (MG) is an autoimmune disorder characterized by a reduced number of functional acetylcholine (ACh) receptors post-synaptically, with antibodies blocking nerve transmission. There is a fluctuating weakness which improves with rest. Eye and facial muscles are frequently involved.

Anatomy

The reactive post-synaptic area is decreased in size with fewer folds and clefts. Some areas have IgG or complement bound instead of ACh. The pre-synaptic area, including the size and number of synaptic vesicles, is normal.

Epidemiology

MG has an incidence of 1 in 20,000 and is most common in females in their twenties and males in their forties and fifties. Female to male ratio is 3 to 2; about 5% of cases are familial. MG is considered an autoimmune disease, with a close relationship to thymic hyperplasia (70%), as well as other immune disorders.

Etiology

MG is presumed to be among the group of immune diseases. Many patients have positive antinuclear antibody (ANA) or other immune disorders along with histocompatability-linked antigen (HLA) pattern commonalities.

Pathology

Post-synaptic simplification, along with a decrease in functional receptors due to antigen antibodies, reduce the patient's ability to generate action potentials with prolonged effort. This results in increased weakness with increased work.

Evaluation

Laboratory testing includes serum acetylcholine receptor antibody levels, elevated in 80%. Administration of intravenous edrophonium (Tensilon) shows repair of weakness, uniformly beginning in 1 minute and lasting about 5 minutes. This is specifically used more for facial than limb weakness. A control injection is also done. Electrodiagnostic testing typically shows a normal or slightly decreased motor amplitude in nerve conduction studies (NCS). The remarkable finding in about 75% of patients is a decremental response in affected muscles to repetitive stimulation at low rates of 2 to 3 Hz. A decrement of at least 10% from the first to the fifth response in two or more muscles is considered significant. The area must be immobilized to minimize movement artifact. Proximal muscles give a higher yield of positive findings. Brief, voluntary exercise for 30 seconds should show repair of the response, then post-tetanic exhaustion 2 to 4 minutes later will show increased decrement. EMG shows a variability in the amplitude and duration of motor units, and fibrillations may be noted. Single fiber EMG (SFEMG) is more sensitive than EMG or repetitive stimulation. SFEMG will show increased jitter, as well as blocking in later stages, even in clinically normal muscles. Evaluate for thymoma.

Functional Evaluation

Physical difficulties include ptosis and diplopia that fluctuate. Chewing, swallowing, and speaking may also be impaired. All symptoms worsen with fatigue and improve with rest. Weakness of the neck flexors is common, while proximal limb muscles are less often involved. Lifting the head off a pillow and reaching above the head may thus be difficult.

Treatment

Medications traditionally used are anticholinesterases, generally pyridostigmine or neostigmine bromide. Dosage is titrated to minimize side effects. Steroids are used for symptomatic control, and anticholinesterase medications may often be decreased as Prednisone is increased. Azathioprine and plasmapheresis are also used at times for severe exacerbations. Thymectomy is often performed, as remission is more likely in patients who have had this procedure. Recommendations are also made to avoid excessive heat, alcohol, some medications (particularly antibiotics ending in "mycin"), and emotional stress, as these have exacerbated the condition. Resting at regular intervals and avoiding excessive physical stress are advised.

Complications

Exacerbations of the disease can be devastating. Myasthenic crisis may cause the patient to require urgent care, including respiratory assistance. This may be incited by illness or a need for anticholinesterase adjustment. Cholinergic side effects of the anticholinesterase medications may be a problem, and weakness may be a side effect.

Follow-Up

Following the status of the thymus, the general medical condition, and an awareness of the connection with other immune diseases are important. The physical state will vary over time and this will determine care plans.

Eaton-Lambert Syndrome/Myasthenic Syndrome

Definition

Eaton-Lambert syndrome (ELS)/Myasthenic syndrome is a disease presenting variable weakness, often associated with a malignancy.

Anatomy

There is severe weakness of proximal muscles, especially of the lower limbs, which improves after exercise and spares the facial, neck, and extraocular muscles.

Epidemiology/Etiology

ELS is associated with a malignancy in 75% of men and 25% of women affected. Either the ELS or the cancer may be noted first. The classic connection is with small cell bronchogenic carcinoma. The male to female ratio is 2–5:1 and most of those affected are over 40 years old.

Pathology

There is an increased complexity of the post-synaptic membrane, with release of a decreased number of ACh quanta with nerve depolarization. There is a decreased readily available store of quanta, and also a decreased number of active zones on the post-synaptic membrane.

Evaluation

Nerve conduction studies (NCS) demonstrate a very small motor amplitude response to nerve stimulation with normal sensory studies. Low rate (2–3 Hz) repetitive stimulation shows a decrement or no change. High rate (20–50 Hz) stimulation shows dramatic motor amplitude incremental response, as does brief voluntary exercise, with amplitude increased by 50% to 200%. This will decrease in 20 seconds and be below baseline in 2 to 4 minutes. SFEMG shows increased jitter and blocking which worsens with rest and improves with exercise.

Function

Patients with ELS show most weakness on waking, with improvement throughout the day until fatigue sets in. Hip weakness is generally first noted, with difficulty rising from a chair or climbing stairs. Proximal arm muscle weakness may lead to difficulty with overhead activities. Facial muscles are generally spared.

Treatment

Treatment for ELS usually begins with the malignancy; when it is found and treated, the symptoms may improve. The possibility of malignancy, if none is found, should be evaluated approximately every 6 months due to the high association. Medications include corticosteroids and immunosuppressives.

Outcome/Follow-Up

This is primarily determined by the malignancy associated with ELS.

Guillain-Barré Syndrome

Definition

Guillain-Barré Syndrome (GBS) is an acute, inflammatory, demyelinating polyneuritis affecting any level of the peripheral nervous system. It progresses rapidly from the lower limbs, often worse proximally, to the upper limbs and often, the face. Respiratory muscle involvement is present in about 25%.

Anatomy

Weakness of the lower limbs, then upper limbs and face is noted. Decreased or absent reflexes are noted. There may be loss of sensation in distal aspects of the limbs, often involving proprioception, vibration, or pain. Autonomic abnormalities may be present.

Epidemiology

GBS follows a viral illness, most commonly a respiratory infection ($\frac{1}{2}$ to $\frac{2}{3}$ of patients). It may also follow surgery, immunization, or other illness.

Etiology

There is an inflammatory attack on the myelin, with axonal damage often present as well. Pathologic studies may reveal edema of the nerves or roots.

Evaluation

CSF usually shows elevation of protein levels with normal cells. Reflexes are decreased or absent. Proximal muscle strength decreases, the legs before the arms, and the face may be weak. NCS show decreased conduction velocity of about 35%, though this may be normal for the first several weeks. Prolonged or absent H-reflex or F-waves may be noted early due to proximal nerve involvement. Amplitudes may be decreased in NCS and EMG. Sensory studies may be abnormal, except the sural nerve is often spared. EMG may show fibrillations and positive sharp waves about 3 weeks after onset.

Function

Respiratory function is the most serious potential problem; ongoing monitoring of respiratory status is vital. Weakness can range from mild lower limb weakness to quadriplegia and bilateral facial palsy.

Treatment

GBS treatment is primarily supportive. Any respiratory loss is compensated for, depending on its severity. Ventilator-dependent status is not unusual during the most severe phase of the disease. No treatment is specific and curative. Plasmapheresis is commonly used, as are steroids. Physical therapy is important, with ROM exercises in severely affected patients, progressing to gentle strengthening as improvement occurs.

Complications

The most serious complication in GBS is respiratory insufficiency, treated with mechanical ventilation. Deep venous thrombosis (DVT) and pulmonary embolism (PE) are risks due to immobility, as are pressure ulcers. Refer to Chapter 10, Immobility, and Chapter 15, Pressure Ulcers.

Prognosis

Prognosis in GBS varies with the severity of disease. Most patients have a self-limited course with maximal physical deficit at 2 to 4 weeks. After a variable plateau period, improvement occurs. In patients who require ventilatory assistance and have all four limbs involved, recovery is longer and may be incomplete.

■ Suggested Readings

Brooke MH, ed. A Clinician's View of Neuromuscular Diseases. Baltimore: Williams & Wilkins, 1986.

Cogrove JL, Alexander MA, Kitts EL, et al. Late effects of poliomyelitis. *Arch Phys Med Rehabil* 1987;68:4–7.

Currie DM, Nelson MR, Buck B. Electrodiagnostic evaluation and follow-up of children with Guillain-Barré Syndrome. *Arch Phys Med Rehabil* 1990;71:244–247.

Daube JR. EMG in Motor Neuron Disease: Monograph 18. *AAEM,* 1982.

Einarsson G. Muscle conditioning in late poliomyelitis. *Arch Phys Med Rehabil* 1991;72:11–14.

Einarsson G, Grimby G. Disability and handicap in late poliomyelitis. *Scand J Rehabil Med* 1990;22:113–121.

Fowler WM, Jr., Johnson ER, Yang CCS. Management of medical complications in neuromuscular diseases. *In:* Fowler WM, Jr., ed. *Physical Medicine and Rehabilitation State of the Art Reviews.* Philadelphia: Hanley and Betts, Inc., 1988; 2:4:597–616.

Greenspun B, Stineman M, Agri R. Multiple sclerosis and rehabilitation outcome. *Arch Phys Med Rehabil* 1987;68:434–437.

Johnson E., ed. *Practical Electromyography.* 2nd ed. Baltimore: Williams & Wilkins, 1988.

Kimura J, ed. *Electrodiagnosis in Diseases of Nerve and Muscle: Principles and Practice.* Philadelphia: F.A. Davis, 1983.

Lord J, Behrman B, Varzos N, et al. Scoliosis associated with Duchenne muscular dystrophy. *Arch Phys Med Rehabil* 1990;71:13–17.

Molnar GE, ed. *Pediatric Rehabilitation.* 2nd ed. Baltimore: Williams & Wilkins, 1992.

Rudick RA, Schiffer RB, Schwartz KM, et al. Multiple sclerosis: the problem of incorrect diagnosis. *Arch Neurol* 1986;43:578–583.

Schneitzer L. Rehabilitation of patients with multiple sclerosis. *Arch Phys Med Rehabil* 1978;59:430–437.

12

Susan J. Garrison

Osteoporosis

■ Definition

Osteoporosis is loss of skeletal bone which may result from a variety of factors.

Any person who is immobilized over a prolonged period will experience some degree of osteoporosis. Refer to Chapter 10, Immobilization. Advanced age is a factor in osteoporosis. Remarks here will mainly address postmenopausal osteoporosis, but overall concepts may be applied to most situations.

■ Anatomy

Trabecular bone is more affected than cortical bone. Spinal vertebrae are usually affected first. Typically, these are the lower thoracic and upper lumbar (T6-L1). If lesions are higher than this, neoplasm must be considered. Thoracic vertebrae sustain wedge-shaped fractures, while crush fractures are common in lumbar vertebrae. See Figure 12-1.

Thoracic wedge fractures create the typical "dowager's hump" of kyphoscoliosis. The arms and legs lose their normal proportion to the axial skeleton and appear to be longer. Loss of height due to vertebral collapse may be as much as 5 to 8

Susan J. Garrison (Ed.): *Handbook of Physical Medicine and Rehabilitation Basics.* First Edition. Copyright © 1995 J. B. Lippincott Company

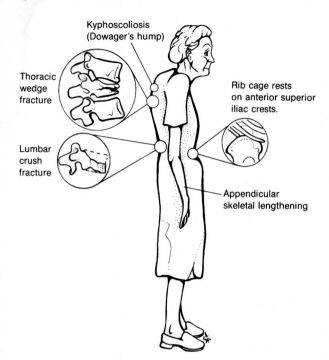

Figure 12-1.   Skeletal changes of postmenopausal osteoporosis.

inches. This phenomenon may progress until the lower rib cage rests upon the anterior iliac crests. Again, see Figure 12-1.

■ Epidemiology

In the U.S., osteoporosis affects one in four women over age 60, and virtually all white women by the age of 90. At that age, a white woman has at least a 30% chance per year of hip fracture. Estimated costs are 4 to 10 billion dollars per year for patients with symptomatic fractures. In many instances, death results from complications related to hip fracture; the

Table 12-1. Risk Factors for Osteoporosis

> Fair-skinned, white female
>
> Positive family history
>
> Thin, small-framed
>
> Surgical removal of ovaries/early menopause
>
> Over age 35
>
> Smoking
>
> Alcohol ingestion
>
> High-protein diet
>
> Sedentary lifestyle

mortality rate of those affected in the first year post fracture are 12% to 20% higher than for matched populations without fracture.

Some of the risk factors for postmenopausal osteoporosis are listed in Table 12-1. Premenopausal peak bone mass may be related more directly to premenopausal estrogen exposure and genetic predisposition than to environmental factors.

▪ Etiology/Pathophysiology

Normally, 10 to 30% of the skeleton is remodeled yearly by the process of bone mineralization. See Table 12-2.

Reduced bone mineralization is ubiquitous with age. Un-

Table 12-2. Bone Mineralization Process

1. Osteoclasts absorb bone

2. Osteoblasts produce collagen matrix

3. Calcium and phosphorus crystals laid down in matrix

til early adulthood, more bone is built than absorbed. By the fourth decade, both males and females experience a gradual loss of bone. However, after menopause, females are 6 times more affected than males. Women lose 0.5% to 1% of their peak bone mass yearly for approximately 20 years after menopause. The rate of bone loss slows after the age of 65 years.

Estrogen protects against bone loss by reducing plasma calcium, thereby stimulating parathyroid hormone (PTH). This increases the formation of 1,25 dihydroxycholecalciferol through the kidneys, and thus increases the tubular reabsorption of calcium and intestinal calcium. In this way calcium is maintained in plasma.

An inadequate dietary intake of calcium may contribute to osteoporosis. Premenopausal calcium needs are considered to be 800 to 1000 mg/day, while postmenopausal needs are 1200 to 1500 mg/day. Secondary hyperparathyroidism may result from reduced absorption or increased excretion of calcium. Vitamin D deficiency also is a factor.

Parathyroid hormone (PTH) levels increase when dietary calcium is deficient, calcium absorption is defective, or estrogen is absent. PTH maintains constant calcium plasma levels by depleting skeletal stores.

■ Assessment

Routine radiographic evaluation is not helpful in the detection of osteoporosis, because bone loss must exceed 30% before it becomes apparent. Bone mass measurement may be accomplished through the use of photon absorptiometry, which measures low energy gamma rays of radionuclide through bone. Single photon absorptiometry is used to evaluate the wrist or heel (cortical bone). Dual photon absorptiometry (DPA) is used for spinal vertebrae assessment. Ultrasound of the patella has been shown to measure a property of bone fragility that is distinct from bone mass; it is less expensive than DPA but is not widely utilized. CT scanning using a phantom device for comparison is more appropriate, but has drawbacks of expense, radiation exposure, and availability. There is as yet no standard for bone mass measurement, and little to be gained by obtaining routine lateral X-rays of the thoracic and lumbar spine.

Diagnosis is usually made on symptoms of gradual or sudden onset backache and/or change in bodily habitus. It may take up to 4 weeks for an acute compression fracture to become apparent on routine X-ray. It is important that a timely diagnosis be made, so that bone trauma and resultant pain can be minimized, family members at risk can be followed, and other causes of bone loss such as osteomalacia can be eliminated. See Table 12-3.

▦ Evaluation

On physical examination, note general bodily habitus, kyphoscoliosis and any other scoliosis. Usually there will not be tenderness directly over the vertebral spinous process. Cervical or lumbosacral paravertebral muscles may be in chronic spasm. Observe gait for shuffling or poor balance. A patient who has sustained a recent vertebral fracture may be unable to sit or stand for a prolonged period because of pain. This pain may be radicular in a thoracic pattern related to the level of the fractured vertebrae.

Table 12-3. Other Causes of Bone Loss

Osteomalacia
Hyperparathyroidism
Hyperthyroidism
Immobilization
Multiple myeloma
Metastatic carcinoma
Chronic anemia

Treatment

Treatment encompasses two aspects: medications for those known to be at risk, and rehabilitative management of the patient who has general back pain or who has experienced an acute spinal vertebral fracture.

Drug Therapy

The two main objectives are to decrease the rate of bone loss and increase the rate of new bone formation.

Estrogen replacement, given as cyclic therapy (0.635 mg of conjugated estrogens for 21 days, followed by 7 days of progestin) is recommended in the perimenopausal period. However, the protective effect may last only 2 to 3 years. There is little evidence that it is helpful in osteoporotic women over age 65. The risk of endometrial cancer must be considered; however, progestins may have a protective effect against breast cancer.

Calcitonin reduces bone turnover by inhibiting osteo-clasts. Salmon calcitonin, given as 50 to 100 units intra-muscularly daily, or human calcitonin, 0.5 mg intra-muscularly every other day, is commonly used. An intranasal calcitonin spray may soon be available in the United States. Calcitonin is used for therapy of diagnosed osteoporosis; its use in prevention is under investigation.

Use of supplemental calcium is controversial. Typical di-ets do not provide the 1500 mg/day postmenopausal require-ment. Caution must be used in patients who are known to form kidney stones. There may be poor intestinal absorption of sufficiently provided dietary calcium in the aged patient.

Vitamin D should be supplemented only if the patient is deficient. Do not use combination calcium/Vitamin D tab-lets; the ratio may lead to Vitamin D toxicity. Avoid more than 5000 units vitamin D per day. Some sources advocate 5 to 10 minutes of sunshine 3 times per week, rather than supplementation. Use of calcitrol, the biologically active Vitamin D metabolite, is controversial, and requires further research.

Fluoride therapy is used to stimulate new bone formation and inhibit resorption. Given as sodium fluoride, 40 to 100 mg/day, the larger doses result in fragile bone formation, more likely to fracture. Side effects include GI disturbances, inflamed joints, recurrent vomiting, and anemia. Do not use this as a routine treatment.

Etidronate (Didronel) administered orally on an intermittent, cyclic basis has been shown in some studies to increase bone mineral content and decrease the rate of new vertebral fractures. Coherence therapy, known as ADFR (activate, depress, free, repeat) involves use of oral phosphate as an activator of bone remodeling, followed by etidronate, and finally a drug-free period of several weeks. The cycle is then repeated. This method is still undergoing study.

In hypertensive females at risk, another consideration is the use of thiazide diuretics that lead to tubular reabsorption of calcium. Adequate studies have not yet established the role of these medications.

Use of anabolic steroids for osteoporosis requires further study and should be avoided, due to androgenic effects as well as problems associated with liver function and plasma lipoproteins.

Rehabilitative Treatment

Chronic back pain may result from compression fractures or kyphotic/scoliotic changes. Posture can be addressed by several means. A Posture Training Support (PTS) by CAMP may be used to improve posture in an effort to prevent or lessen osteoporotic skeletal problems. See Figure 12-2. For more involved cases, a back support device can be used, such as a semi-rigid dorsolumbar support with shoulder straps, or a custom-made jacket. Proper back exercises emphasize extension and omit flexion maneuvers. See Figures 12-3 and 12-4. Chronic pain management techniques may be helpful. See Chapter 8, Chronic Pain.

Acute back pain secondary to osteoporotic vertebral frac-

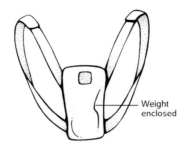

Posture Training Support

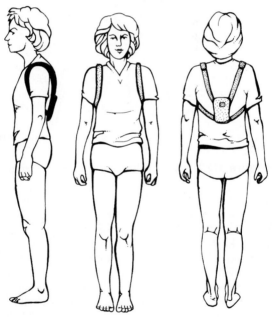

Figure 12-2. Posture Training Support, by CAMP.

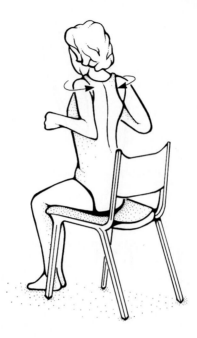

Figure 12-3.   Seated position: back extension exercise.

ture follows a typical course, shown in Table 12-4. General preventive measures are shown in Table 12-5.

Severe kyphotic posture causes fatigue easily due to ligamentous stretch and reduced vital capacity. A back support device should be worn. Stooping should be discouraged. Chest expansion may be improved by deep breathing exercises, pectoral stretching, and thoracic spine extension.

■ Outcomes

The typical postmenopausal osteoporotic female is at great risk for fracture-related complications. However, these can be minimized with patient education and appropriate drug therapy where indicated. Women at risk should be followed

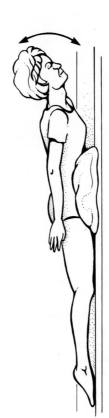

Figure 12-4. Prone position: back extension exercise.

Table 12-4. Acute Back Pain

Bed rest (position of comfort) 7–14 days

Hospitalization not usually required

Analgesics, including oral narcotics for severe, or nonsteroidal anti-inflammatory drugs for mild to moderate pain

Modalities: heat, massage, TENS

Back support

Cane in opposite hand if pain unilateral

perimenopausally to assess the need for estrogen replacement. Encourage young women to routinely perform weight-bearing exercises and obtain sufficient daily amounts of dietary calcium.

Follow-Up

The patient with postmenopausal osteoporosis requires intermittent follow-up for management of sporadic acute injuries, prescription of therapies, and instruction in appropriate exercises. Routine plain radiographs are not indicated. Ongoing patient education and psychological support is necessary.

Table 12-5. Osteoporosis: General Preventive Measures

Avoid heavy lifting and bending

Proper shoes: rubber heels or cushion soles; avoid high heels

Use cane for stability

Weight-bearing exercise throughout life (walking, bicycling)

Appropriate drug therapy

Proper nutrition

■ Suggested Readings

Ambrus JL, Hoffman M, Ambrus CM, et al. Prevention and treatment of osteoporosis. One of the most frequent disorders in American women: a review. *J Med.* 1992;23:369–388.

Armamento-Villareal R, Villareal DT, Avioli LV, Civitelli R. Estrogen status and heredity are major determinants of premenopausal bone mass. *J Clin Invest.* 1992;90:2464–2471.

Avioli LV. Osteoporosis syndromes: patient selection for calcitonin therapy. *Geriatrics.* 1992;47:58–67.

Avioli LV. Significance of osteoporosis: a growing international health care problem. *Calcif Tissue Int* 1991;49:S5–7.

Brixen K, Nielsen HK, Charles P, Mosekilde L. Effects of a short course of oral phosphate treatment on serum parathyroid hormone (1–84) and biochemical markers of bone turnover: a dose-response study. *Calcif Tissue Int* 1992;51:276–281.

Felson DT, Sloutskis D, Anderson JJ, et al. Thiazide diuretics and the risk of hip fracture. *JAMA* 1991;265:370–373.

Heaney RP, Avioli LV, Chesnut CH, et al. Osteoporotic bone fragility. *JAMA* 1989;261:2986–2990.

Melton LJ, Chrischilles EA, Cooper C, et al. Perspective: how many women have osteoporosis? *J Bone Miner Res* 1992;7:1005–1010.

National Institutes of Health Consensus Development Panel: Osteoporosis. *JAMA.* 1984;262:799–802.

Pacifici R, McMurtry C, Vered I, et al. Coherence therapy does not prevent axial bone loss in osteoporotic women: a preliminary comparative study. *J Clin Endocrinol Metab* 1988;66:747–753.

Simmons JW, Norwood SM. Calcitonin and osteoporosis new mechanisms of pathophysiology. *Orthop Rev* 1987;16:718–725.

Sinaki M. Osteoporosis. *In* DeLisa JA, Gans BM, eds. *Principles and Practice of Rehabilitation Medicine,* 2nd ed. Philadelphia: J.B. Lippincott, 1993.

Sinaki M, Nicholas JJ. Metabolic bone diseases and aging. *In* Felsenthal G, Garrison SJ, Steinberg FU, eds. *Rehabilitation of the Aging and Elderly Patient.* Baltimore: Williams & Wilkins, 1994, pp. 107–122.

Sinaki M, Wahner HW, Offord KP, Hodgson SF. Efficacy of nonloading exercises in prevention of vertebral bone loss in postmenopausal women: a controlled trial. *Mayo Clin Proc* 1989;64:762–769.

Storm T, Thamsborg G, Steiniche T, et al. Effect of intermittent cyclical etidronate therapy on bone mass and fracture rate in women with postmenopausal osteoporosis. *N Engl J Med* 1990;322:1265–1271.

Barry L. Bowser
Itzel S. Solis

13

Pediatric Rehabilitation

▌ Introduction

Some of the more frequently encountered disabling conditions of childhood are cerebral palsy, muscular dystrophy, spina bifida, developmental delays, and hypotonia.

Keep in mind the following aspects of rehabilitation that are unique to treating children:

- Do not treat children as though they are little adults; it is the job of parents and society to help children, including those with handicaps, grow into mature adults capable of independent living. This responsibility should be shared by the health professionals concerned with their care.
- Because children are largely products of their environment, educate parents about what would constitute a therapeutic environment for their children.
- Rehabilitation of children, in contrast to that of adults, often does not mean relearning lost skills, but rather, learning appropriate motor and social skills for their age or developmental level under adverse conditions.
- Knowledge of normal motor learning, growth, and development is essential for therapeutic intervention in the growing child. Understanding the emotional needs of the child at various ages is equally important.

Susan J. Garrison (Ed.): *Handbook of Physical Medicine and Rehabilitation Basics*. First Edition. Copyright © 1995 J. B. Lippincott Company

   Treatment must take into consideration decelerated bone growth in weakened extremities, compared to the strong stimulus for bone growth in extremities with normal muscle activity. Asymmetrical muscle involvement may produce significant leg and arm length discrepancies. The child's bone age can be monitored by radiographic studies. Carefully timed surgical procedures can lengthen shortened extremities or slow the growth rate of normal extremities.

Cerebral Palsy

Definition

Cerebral palsy is paralysis resulting from nonprogressive brain damage that occurs any time before the brain has reached maturation, from conception to age 5 or 6 years. It has an incidence of approximately 5.5 per 1000 live births and is distributed equally between the sexes, among the races, and across national boundaries.

   To be classified as cerebral palsy, the brain damage must result in loss or impairment of control over voluntary muscles. The symptoms of cerebral palsy vary greatly, ranging from extremely mild and barely detectable to almost total lack of voluntary motor functions and profound retardation. Therefore, specification of the type and distribution of motor disturbance, the degree of involvement (mild, moderate, or severe), and the etiology, if known, is important before planning rehabilitation management. Table 13-1 describes the motor disturbances most commonly associated with cerebral palsy.

Etiology

The etiologies of cerebral palsy encompass all the causes of brain damage in the fetus, newborn, and young child. They can be divided into congenital (prenatal and perinatal factors) and acquired (postnatal factors) as in Table 13-2.

text continues on page 253

Table 13-1. Motor Disturbances Associated with Cerebral Palsy

Disturbance	Lesion Site	Characteristics*
Spasticity	Motor cortex, area VI, pyramidal system	Increased muscle tone, hyperactive reflexes, easily elicited stretch reflexes, increased resistance to full range of motion of joints
Athetosis	Basal ganglia, extrapyramidal system	Slow, involuntary, continuous writhing movements of the extremities, trunk, face
Ataxia	Cerebellum or cerebellar tracts	Wide-based, unsteady gait; dysmetria; intention tremor in upper extremities; truncal titubation
Tremor	Basal ganglia	Often hereditary; fine tremulousness of musculature similar to that of parkinsonism; not seriously disabling
Rigidity	Diffuse; basal ganglia, cortex	Muscles contract slowly and stiffly; increased resistance to passive movement of muscle throughout range of motion; slow, laborious voluntary movements
Hypotonia	Motor cortex, area IV	Markedly decreased muscle tone, hyperelasticity of joints; hyperactive deep-tendon reflexes despite diminished muscle tone (if central in origin)

*With the exception of concurrent spasticity and hypotonia, mixtures of any of these motor manifestations are possible.
From Bowser BL, Solis IS. Pediatric rehabilitation. *In* Halstead LS, Grabois M, Howland CA, eds. *Medical Rehabilitation.* New York: Raven Press, 1985, p. 266.

Table 13-2. Etiology of Cerebral Palsy*

Congenital		Acquired
Prenatal	Perinatal	Postnatal
Anoxia	Anoxia	Trauma
Maternal anemia shock	Respiratory obstruction	Skull fracture
Placental disturbances	Atelectasis	Brain contusion
Rh incompatibility	Placenta previa	Infections
	Premature separation of placenta	Meningitis
Maternal infection	Over-sedation	Encephalitis
Rubella	Breech delivery	Cerebrovascular
Toxoplasmosis		accident
Cytomegalovirus	Trauma	
Herpesvirus	Cephalopelvic disproportion	Anoxia
Syphilis		Shock
	Cesarean section	Poisoning
Trauma		Near drowning
	Prematurity	
Metabolic factors		Brain tumor
Brain malformation		

* In many cases, more than one etiological factor is present.

text continued from page 250

Diagnosis/Assessment

Diagnosing cerebral palsy may be extremely difficult in early infancy. Spasticity may not manifest until 6 to 9 months of age; athetoid movements may not occur until the second year of life. Comprehensive evaluation of the cerebral palsy patient is multidisciplinary. It requires an assessment of physical growth, developmental level of the child, and motor and neurological skills; a psychological evaluation for intellectual level or potential; and speech, visual, and hearing evaluations. In addition, the older child should receive language and learning assessments.

Taking a careful history of pregnancy, labor, delivery, and the immediate neonatal period, and repeating developmental assessments of the infant are essential for arriving at a diagnosis of cortical damage. In general, a diagnosis of cerebral palsy is suggested by failure to accomplish motor milestones at the expected time, persistence of primitive reflexes beyond the time at which they are expected to disappear, paucity of movement in affected extremities, and inappropriate muscle tone in affected extremities.

Viral antibody titers from the mother and infant for toxoplasmosis, syphilis, rubella, cytomegalovirus, and herpesvirus may identify prenatal infections as a possible cause. A CT scan of the brain may show cortical abnormalities or areas of damage.

Medical Management

Anticonvulsant medication may be necessary if the child has an associated seizure disorder. Spasticity may be reduced by carefully titrated doses of diazepam (Valium), baclofen (Lioresal), or dantrolene sodium (Dantrium). Although these drugs do not abolish spasticity, they may reduce it to the point where increased voluntary control of spastic muscles is possible.

Rehabilitation Management

Birth to Three Years of Age:

For the normal child, this is the age period when intense motor learning and basic language development occur. Accordingly, this is the time that intervention by physical therapy, occupational therapy, and/or speech therapy can be most beneficial in promoting the development of normal motor patterns (gross, fine, and oral), and perhaps inhibiting abnormal patterns. With a good program of early intervention, surgery is rarely necessary in this age group.

Therapists must teach the parent or caretaker specific play activities so that the child's daily environment encourages independence. In addition, exercise programs are necessary to stretch tight muscles and prevent deformity (Figure 13-1). Special positioning may be needed to support weak muscles and prevent deformity from the unopposed force of gravity. Special feeding techniques enable the child to learn to chew and develop better control of the oral musculature so that speech will be possible at a later age.

Three to Seven Years of Age:

Bracing rarely is required before 3 years of age, unless the child is standing or ambulating with severe leg, ankle, or foot deformity. Bracing is used to augment weak muscles and oppose strong muscles, thus preventing deforming forces on the bones and joints.

Minimal bracing is indicated; an ankle foot orthosis (AFO) will stabilize the ankle and prevent extreme plantar flexion of the foot. In some cases, the foot and ankle cannot be properly braced until the Achilles tendon is lengthened. For severe adductor spasticity causing scissoring during ambulation, long leg braces (knee ankle orthoses or KAOs) with a pelvic band may be necessary to control the lower extremities of children when surgery is contraindicated or otherwise not desired.

If functional ambulation without or with minimal brac-

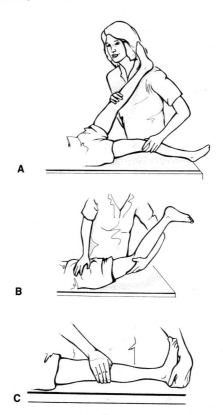

Figure 13-1. Passive stretching of the lower limb. (A) hamstrings (stabilize opposite limb) (B) iliotibial band (stabilize pelvis) (C) heel cord (keep knee extended). (Adapted from Vignos PJ. Rehabilitation in progressive muscular dystrophy. *In* Licht S, ed. *Rehabilitation and Medicine.* New Haven, CT: Elizabeth Licht, 1958.)

ing has not been achieved by 5 to 7 years of age, refer the child to orthopedics for surgical release or lengthening of spastic muscles. This may reduce the amount of bracing and promote more efficient patterns of ambulation. An appropriate surgical candidate has the balance, voluntary motor control, and motivation to walk. Dislocation or subluxation of the hip is a frequent problem associated with adductor and flexor spasticity. The mean age of occurrence of dislocation in the spastic child is 7 years. When this occurs, reduction of the dislocation can be maintained only if it is accompanied by surgical release of the spastic muscles. Complete dislocation can be monitored by periodic hip X-rays starting at two years of age so that surgical management can be minimized (only soft tissue releases).

The occupational therapist is concerned with improving fine motor control and independence in feeding, dressing, grooming, and toileting, as well as preventing deformities and enhancing function of the upper extremities and trunk balance. A wrist hand orthosis (WHO) may be used at night to maintain muscle length of the wrist flexors and small muscles of the hand. Functional WHOs may be used during the day to improve position of the hand and facilitate fine motor function of the fingers, such as writing and eating.

Speech therapy should continue during this period to stimulate language development and overcome articulation problems.

Eight Years of Age to Adulthood:

Periodic monitoring of children or adults with cerebral palsy is necessary to prevent or correct deformity before permanent damage or pain results. If functional ambulation has not been achieved by 8 years of age, despite adequate therapeutic intervention, it is probably not a realistic goal.

Physical therapy should be limited to a maintenance program for preventing contractures and deformity and promoting independence at the wheelchair level. This will allow the child to direct energies toward academic and social learning in order to acquire the intellectual and social skills needed for competition in the adult world. Occupational therapy may still be necessary to enable the child to reach an optimal level of independence in activities of daily living (ADLs) in accordance with abilities and limitations.

If speech has not developed by age 8, further speech therapy is probably not indicated. Alternate forms of communication should be developed. In early to mid teens, assessment and counseling will be necessary to help the patient set realistic goals for employment and financial independence, if possible.

Selective Posterior Rhizotomy:

This is a surgical procedure that reduces excessive muscle tone in spastic cerebral palsy. The L1-S2 posterior roots are divided into rootlets which are electrically stimulated. If the stimulation results in a sustained muscle contraction or spread to muscles innervated by another segmental level, the rootlet is sectioned.

This procedure reduces tone to normal or to hypotonia in the lower extremities, without persistent sensory impairment. Ideal candidates are 3 to 14 years of age with normal intelligence and some form of ambulation. Athetosis is a contraindication for the procedure.

Complications

In addition to the obvious motor dysfunction, approximately 50% of all children with cerebral palsy exhibit mental retardation. Seizures are present in approximately 40%, speech and language problems in 80%, visual problems in 40%, and diminished hearing in 20%. Almost 100% have significant dental problems, and a significant number may have leg length discrepancies. All of these aspects must be considered and intervention made at appropriate times.

Muscular Dystrophy

The term muscular dystrophy applies to a group of relentlessly progressive diseases of voluntary muscle, characterized by increasing weakness and eventual loss of voluntary

Table 13-3. Classification of Muscular Dystrophies

Diagnosis	Percentage	Genetic Transmission	Age at Onset
Duchenne	30%	Sex-linked recessive	3 to 5 years
Fascioscapular-humeral	10%	Autosomal dominant	Second or third decade
Limb-girdle	±5%	Mixed; most are autosomal recessive	First to third decade
Myotonic	50%	Autosomal dominant	Second to third decade

From Bowser BL, Solis IS. Pediatric rehabilitation. *In* Halstead LS, Grabois M, Howland CA, eds. *Medical Rehabilitation.* New York: Raven Press, 1985, p. 270.

motor power in the muscles affected. While all muscular dystrophies are genetically transmitted, they differ primarily in their mode of inheritance, age at onset of clinical symptoms, rate of progression, and muscles first affected, as indicated in Table 13-3.

Incidence and Mode of Inheritance

Duchenne muscular dystrophy (DMD) is the most common of the muscular dystrophies seen in childhood, and the most rapidly progressive. Comments on diagnosis and management will be directed mainly at this type of muscular dystrophy. Although the other dystrophies progress at a much slower rate, the principles of management are the same as for DMD.

DMD usually affects only male children because of its X-linked recessive mode of inheritance. The mother is an asymptomatic carrier of the recessive gene. Each of her male offspring has a 50% chance of receiving the affected gene and thus manifesting the disease; each of her female offspring has a 50% chance of receiving the affected gene and being an asymptomatic carrier of the disease. DMD may occur in females with Turner's syndrome or with a translocation at the Xp21 site of the X chromosome.

Diagnosis/Assessment

History

An affected boy is usually normal at birth and reaches his motor milestones at the appropriate times. It is not until between the ages of 2 and 4 years that, compared to his siblings or peers, the child seems to fall more often and have more difficulty negotiating stairs and curbs, and rising from the floor unassisted. A family history of affected males on the mother's side is extremely helpful, but not necessarily present, in diagnosing DMD.

Physical Examination

The first signs and symptoms of DMD involve increased fatigue and weakness of the hip girdle muscles. However, a routine physical examination is unlikely to reveal such manifestations early in the disease. Deep tendon reflexes are still normal early in the disease and are maintained until extreme muscle weakness occurs. Increased lumbar lordosis and hypertrophy of the calves may make the child look stronger than he actually is. Other subtle signs include flatfootedness and a slightly waddling gait that is accentuated by having the child walk fast. These children also rise on their toes when they walk, which becomes more pronounced as the disease progresses. Signs of muscular dystrophy are best revealed by watching the child in motion, walking, rising from the floor, or stepping up on a low stool or chair.

Laboratory Examinations

In DMD, there is marked elevation of the creatinine phosphokinase (CPK) level in the blood, usually 30 to 60 times normal, and a slightly elevated CPK level in other forms of dystrophy. The electromyogram (EMG) can help differentiate weakness caused by primary muscle disease from weakness resulting from anterior horn cell disease. Muscle biopsy with histochemical staining also is helpful in differentiating the dystrophies from neuromuscular atrophy and congenital infections, and from metabolic myopathies. See Chapter 11, Neuromuscular Diseases. Abnormal or absent muscle protein dystrophin is evident on biopsy.

Management

There is currently no treatment that will cure or arrest the disease. The basic philosophy of management is to maintain ambulation as long as possible, maintain maximum muscle strength by encouraging the family to allow the child to do as much as he can for himself, avoid immobilization and prolonged bed rest, and delay joint contractures and respiratory impairment by appropriate therapeutic interventions.

Surgical Intervention

Percutaneous tenotomies at hips, knees, and ankles on carefully selected patients may significantly prolong ambulation.
These procedures must be followed by ambulation on the day
after surgery using lightweight casts. To continue ambulating after the casts are removed, the patients are placed
in lightweight, plastic long leg braces. After surgery, these
patients are only able to walk with their knees locked in
KAOs.

Genetic Counseling

All families of patients with muscular dystrophy should have
genetic counselling as soon as the diagnosis is made. Since
the mode of inheritance differs considerably among the various dystrophies, it is important that an accurate diagnosis be
made. Search for carriers throughout the family, and inform
family members of the risk factors and options available to
them. Genetic counseling is available free of charge through
clinics sponsored by the Muscular Dystrophy Association
(MDA). The gene for this disease is located on the short arm
of the X chromosome. It is known to produce a protein called
dystrophin. This protein is markedly decreased in patients
with DMD.

Rehabilitation Management

Management of the patient during the ambulatory phase of
the disease is directed at maintaining functional ambulation
and muscle strength for as long as possible. Parents are instructed in range of motion (ROM) exercises for the lower
extremities, with gentle muscle stretching to delay joint contractures (see Figure 13-1, p. 255). The child is encouraged
to sleep on his abdomen to prevent hip flexion contractures.
In addition, before ankle dorsiflexion becomes limited, the
child may be placed in night splints with maximum dor-

siflexion at the ankles to help delay ankle contractures. Use of long leg night splints that incorporate the knees is more appropriate, but seldom tolerated. Specific exercise programs are unnecessary in ambulatory patients because their daily activity level is usually adequate to maintain muscle strength at an optimal level for their disease state. When ambulation becomes too slow and laborious to be functional, or the patient suffers frequent falls or fractures, consider surgical treatment or use of a wheelchair.

Management of the patient confined to a wheelchair is directed primarily at maintaining spinal alignment and maximum respiratory function. Lower limb contractures develop quickly; to delay them, encourage the child to spend some time out of the wheelchair, on his abdomen on the floor at home crawling around as long as he can. Early in the period of wheelchair confinement, some children may delay the development of flexion contractures of the hips and knees by remaining upright in a standing table for several hours a day in school and at home.

Watch the spine closely for signs of scoliosis. Fitting the child with a thoracolumbar corset with metal stays helps maintain good posture in the wheelchair. Even while the child is in the corset, however, evidence of scoliosis may appear and progress. Only surgical stabilization can halt progression of scoliosis. It must be carefully timed so that vital capacity is sufficient when surgery is performed in order to preven pulmonary compromise.

Vital capacity must be monitored carefully. Breathing exercises, as well as postural drainage and assisted cough should be taught to the child and family in order to manage respiratory secretions. Intermittent positive pressure breathing (IPPB) is used to maintain compliance of the thorax and lungs. Respiratory infections must be treated promptly and adequately. As the disease progresses, patients may exhibit evidence of CO_2 retention, manifested by morning headache and lethargy. Many patients need assistive respiratory devices when sleeping. Adequate respiratory treatment is critical; the cause of death in children with DMD is usually respiratory infection and failure.

Psychosocial Adjustment

A high rate of emotional disturbance and some intellectual impairment, particularly verbal, is associated with DMD. Intellectual impairment, affecting from 8% to 30% of these patients, is nonprogressive. Passivity related to confinement to a wheelchair may produce self-image problems and agitated, aggressive, almost paranoid behavior. The latter is most common in patients who survive after age 20 and feel they are living on borrowed time, yet not fit vocationally for continued life. Typical personality traits of DMD patients include superficial brightness, hysteria, and apathy. Minor dementia and other organic changes may result from pulmonary insufficiency associated with respiratory muscle weakness and scoliosis, with anoxic cerebral changes secondary to hypercapnia and infection. Typically, the I.Q. of the patient with DMD hovers at about 85+.

Parental distress is most marked on diagnosis because usually the child had appeared normal during infancy, only to begin deteriorating suddenly from 2 to 6 years of age. The parents are then faced not only with the physical handicaps of their disabled child, but also with the need to acquire educational assistance, keep up with numerous medical appointments, become familiar with frequently changing assistive devices and appliances, and understand the language of the various medical disciplines involved in order to supervise the child's home treatment. As a result, families often become so overwhelmed that they fail to prepare the child to cope with not only the ordinary events of childhood, such as school, but also the knowledge of probable premature death. Inadvertently, parents may interfere with the child's development of autonomy and associated persistence of effort, initiation of activity, and motivation to participate in interpersonal relationships. Lack of practice in applying steady effort and diligence toward completing a task often causes disabled children to perceive that they have less control over their environment than they actually have. Thus, they may avoid trying to perform some independent functions they could eventually master with effort.

■ Spina Bifida

Definition

Spina bifida is defined as the separation of the vertebral elements in the midline. The three major classifications, occulta, manifesta, and aperta, are described in Table 13-4. Associated congenital anomalies are listed in Table 13-5.

There is a polygenically inherited predisposition to this malformation. It is probably caused by environmental factors, which may or may not be specific, acting on a genetically susceptible embryo around the 28th day of gestation.

The incidence of this disease in the United States and England is 1:1000 when there are no other family members affected; 5.5:100 after one affected child; 13:100 after two affected children; and 20.6:100 after three affected children.

Table 13-4. Classification of Spina Bifida

Type	Description	Manifestations
Occulta	Epithelialized skin covers hidden lesion	Hair tuft or skin dimple
Manifesta	Skin is incompletely epithelialized	Cystica: vertebral elements covered by poorly epithelialized membrane
		Meningocele: cystic lesion of meninges only, with or without dysplasia of neural contents
		Meningomyelocele: meninges around malformed neural tube
Aperta	No cover of neural tissue	Myeloschisis: neural tube is completely open

From Bowser BL, Solis IS. Pediatric rehabilitation. *In* Halstead LS, Grabois M, Howland CA, eds. *Medical Rehabilitation.* New York: Raven Press, 1985, p. 272.

Table 13-5. Associated Congenital Anomalies in Spina Bifida

Micropolygyria

Abnormalities of the aqueduct

Arnold Chiari malformation

Vertebral wedges (anteroposterior and lateral)

Myelovertebral disproportion

Large fontanelles

Shallow posterior fossa

Large foramen magnum

Prenatal Diagnosis

Prenatal diagnosis is possible by measuring serum alpha-fetoproteins from the pregnant woman. If elevated, measurements are then obtained from fetal amniotic fluid by amniocentesis. Fetal ultrasound can also be used in making the diagnosis.

Management

The patient with spina bifida must often consult many different specialists in order to receive adequate treatment. It is not unusual for such patients to require the services of a neurosurgeon, pediatrician, orthopedist, urologist, ophthalmologist, and physiatrist. These patients may also require physical therapy and occupational therapy. Ideally, they should be treated in a multidisciplinary clinic where all of these services are provided. Such clinics allow specialists to share information and coordinate treatment.

Table 13-6. Complications of Spina Bifida

Hydrocephalus
Paralysis
Hip dislocations
Knee flexion contractures
Foot and ankle deformities
Sensory loss
Spinal deformities
Neurogenic bladder
Neurogenic bowel

Complications

There are numerous complications associated with spina bifida. Refer to Table 13-6.

Hydrocephalus

Hydrocephalus develops toward the end of intrauterine life. It is present in the first days or weeks of life in 90% of children affected with spina bifida, even though the fronto-occipital circumference is normal. There is some incidence of spontaneous arrest of the hydrocephalus.

A shunting procedure (ventriculoperitoneal or ventriculoatrial) is necessary in the management of progressive hydrocephalus. Complications of shunting may include obstruction and ventriculitis, which are associated with a drop in I.Q. Intelligence is below average in children with spina bifida without hydrocephalus, slightly lower in those with arrested hydrocephalus, and significantly lower in those with spina bifida severe enough to require a ventricular peritoneal shunt.

Paralysis

There may be no motor weakness associated with lesions affecting the sacral segments, or motor weakness may be considerable, as in the case of higher lesions in the thoracic and thoracolumbar segments. Paralysis may be either complete or incomplete. The deformities most often associated with paralysis and/or weakness are hip dislocation, knee contractures, and foot deformities. Back anomalies such as kyphosis and scoliosis are common. The management of weakness or paralysis includes the prevention of complications and bracing to improve function and enable ambulation. Figure 13-2 compares the motor development of the normal child and the child with spina bifida, indicating recommended assistive devices at each age level.

Hip Dislocations

Hip findings in spina bifida include decreased abduction, shortening of one leg, asymmetry of gluteal folds, and Ortolani click (felt when femoral head slides over acetabular rim). Hip dislocations can be present with lesions at any level, but are more common when there is hip flexor function but no hip extensor function. Unilateral dislocation should be treated; however, there is much discussion as to whether bilateral dislocations should be treated. This is a decision that must be reached on an individual basis. The treatment can be conservative, using traction and casting, or surgical.

Knee Flexion Contractures

Knee flexion contractures may occur due to spasticity of the hamstrings in the case of weak or absent quadriceps function. They also affect children who are flaccid across the knee and do not receive daily PROM exercise. In mild cases, stretching

text continues on page 270

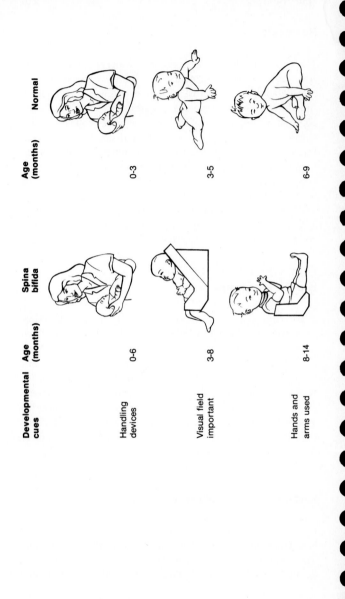

Developmental cues	Age (months)	Spina bifida		Age (months)	Normal
Handling devices	0-6			0-3	
Visual field important	3-8			3-5	
Hands and arms used	8-14			6-9	

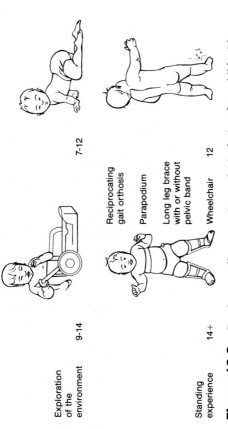

Exploration
of the
environment   9-14   7-12

Reciprocating
gait orthosis

Parapodium

Long leg brace
with or without
pelvic band

Standing
experience   14+   Wheelchair   12

Figure 13-2. Developmentally appropriate orthotic devices for a child with moderate spina bifida, compared to a normal child. (Adapted from Motloch W. Orthotic philosophies of treatment. *Clin Prosthet Orthot* 1984;8:10.)

text continued from page 267

of the hamstrings (see Figure 13-1) provides sufficient treatment. In more severe cases, surgical procedures for lengthening or dividing the hamstrings are indicated. Knee hyperextension (genu recurvatum) can then be a problem in patients with poor quadriceps function.

Foot and Ankle Deformities

Those associated with spina bifida include equinovarus, calcaneovalgus, vertical talus, and pes cavus foot deformities, as well as valgus deformity of the ankle (Figure 13-3). Mild conditions can be treated with conservative methods such as casting; however, most cases require surgical correction.

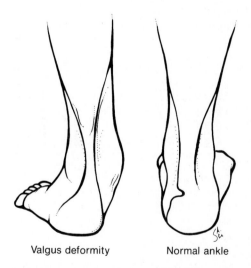

Valgus deformity   Normal ankle

Figure 13-3. Valgus deformity of the ankle in a child with spina bifida. (Adapted from Schafer MS, Dias LS. *Myelomeningocele: Orthopaedic Treatment.* Baltimore: Williams & Wilkins, 1983.)

Sensory Loss

Sensory impairment in spina bifida depends on the level of involvement. The patient and family must be aware of the area of decreased or absent sensation in order to avoid complications such as burns and pressure ulcers.

Spinal Deformities

About 5% to 20% of children with myelomeningocele are born with some degree of kyphosis. This is due to abnormalities of the vertebral bodies and weakness of dorsal muscles. Surgical removal of atypical vertebral bodies may be necessary in the neonatal period to allow closure of the skin defect. In milder cases, surgery may be delayed. Scoliosis may be congenital and, in the case of spina bifida, associated with hemivertebra. Conservative management using a Milwaukee brace may be adequate for correction of smaller curves if there is sufficient skin coverage to tolerate the brace. Correction of large curves requires surgical intervention.

Neurogenic Bladder

Neurogenic bladder is present in more than 90% of patients with spina bifida aperta. The neurogenic bladder may be either upper motor neuron or lower motor neuron type. The type of bladder may change as the child grows. If saddle anesthesia is present, there will be some disturbance of the child's bladder. The physical examination should include observation of the pattern of unaided micturition. Investigations during the neonatal period should include urine cultures and excretion pyelography.

Treat urinary tract infections promptly while avoiding overdistention. Some useful techniques for managing neurogenic bladder in children include early intermittent catheterization, often the ongoing treatment of choice; vesicotomy; or Crede's maneuver, a technique of emptying a flaccid bladder by exerting pressure over the lower abdomen (to be avoided in children with vesiculouretheral reflux).

Neurogenic Bowel

There is a high incidence of neurogenic bowel in patients with spina bifida aperta. Common problems include constipation, overdistention, incontinence, and rectal prolapse. As in neurogenic bladder, neurogenic bowel may be either upper or lower motor neuron type.

Management includes the following:

- Obtain stool history and diary.
- Avoid overdistension.
- Individualize each child's program.
- Individualize stool consistency.
- Modify the diet by increasing fluids or adding bulk.
- Use stool softeners.
- Sit child on toilet at a certain time every day and have him or her strain.
- Use digital stimulation, suppositories, or enemas if and when necessary.

Upper Extremity Involvement

There may be upper motor neuron involvement of the upper extremities due to hydeocephalus. This often ignored complication may be significant. Typical manifestations include difficulties with fine motor coordination, muscle weakness, spasticity, and increased reflexes. Management includes strengthening exercises and activities to improve coordination.

▉ Developmental Delay

Even a single disability may produce problems in different areas of the child's development; the effects of multiple disabilities on development are exponential rather than additive. A child born prematurely should not be considered developmentally delayed if development is normal for gestational age. Possible causes of developmental delay include the following:

- Mental retardation.
- Lack of stimulation, occurring sometimes in institutions or some homes.
- Chronic illness, such as congenital heart disease.
- Early neuromuscular disease, or peripheral nerve injuries such as brachial plexus injuries, resulting in weakness (paresis).
- Disease associated with alteration of muscle tone and abnormal movements, such as cerebral palsy.
- Hearing deficits.
- Visual deficits.

Occasionally, a specific cause for developmental delay cannot be determined.

Diagnosis

The diagnosis of delayed development requires a complete examination on more than one occasion, since normal development occurs over time. Screening tests are of great value. There are several that offer different degrees of reliability. It is better to select screening tests that occasionally mislabel some uninvolved children as delayed than tests that fail to identify some delayed children. Preferred tests also divide rather than combine different areas of behavior. One of the more reliable tests is the Developmental Screening Inventory, which is standardized to 18 months of age. Unfortunately, there are presently no well-standardized tests that screen children beyond this age, although some are being devised.

The areas of behavior that should be measured are as follows:

- Personal-social: the response of the child to cultural habitat.

- Adaptive: the child's use of resources in problem solving.
- Speech: forms of communication, not exclusively language.
- Gross motor: head control, trunk control, standing balance, and ambulation.
- Fine motor: the child's use of a hand to manipulate objects.

The child may be referred to a developmental clinic, a pediatric neurologist, or physiatrist for follow-up.

Rehabilitation Management

In planning treatment, remember that tests of early development have poor correlation with future cognitive function; the child who performs poorly on these tests during infancy will not necessarily remain behind peers in school. Nevertheless, parents will need support as well as information regarding the implications and prognoses of their child's condition after the diagnosis is made.

Most communities offer numerous programs for stimulating infants (less than 1 to 3 years) and young children (3 to 5 years). These programs provide the following kinds of help:

- Support for parents and children.
- Experiences appropriate to the child's maturity level.
- Ways for parents to structure the child's activities.
- Techniques for handling destructive behavior.
- Reviews of parenting techniques.

However, such developmental programs have two main disadvantages. Overenthusiastic personnel may imply to parents that the programs are failure-proof, and that if the child does not "catch up" with his or her peers, it is because the parents have not worked hard enough. This burdens parents who already may feel guilty about their child's problem. Second, the techniques used in developmental programs may not alter the ultimate performance of the child. There is evidence, however, that institutionalized children decline in their intellectual functioning or do not progress as well as comparable children from supportive homes. Ultimately, learning can be compared to a pyramid; the top of the pyramid, or the child's total knowledge capacity, is determined by the width of the bottom of the pyramid, or the breadth of the child's early experience.

Hypotonia

Hypotonia refers to decreased resistance to passive movement, sometimes including unusual postures and excessive joint mobility. It is often difficult to evaluate. The etiology of this condition is varied, as shown in Table 13-7.

Only those children who improve and who exhibit normal enzyme studies, EMG findings, and muscle biopsy results should be diagnosed as having benign congenital hypotonia.

Table 13-7. Causes of Hypotonia

Central nervous system disorder
    Perinatal brain insult
    Metabolic disorders
    Chromosomal abnormalities (e.g. Down's syndrome)

Peripheral nervous system
    Werdnig-Hoffman disease
    Myasthenia gravis
        Neonatal
        Transient

Congenital myopathies

Glycogen storage disease

Connective tissue disorders
    Ehler-Dahnlos syndrome
    Marfan's syndrome

Congenital spinal cord injury

Rehabilitation Management

In general, hypotonia may be managed in the following ways:

* Genetic counseling when the diagnosis has been established.
* PROM exercises to prevent contractures, especially when the hypotonia is associated with weakness.
* Bracing, when indicated, to improve function or to prevent deformity.
* Instructing the caretaker in techniques of handling, including developmental stimulation programs (see Developmental Delay).

In cases of hypotonia resulting from congenital spinal cord injury, management will be complicated by neurogenic bladder and bowel, decreased or absent sensation, respiratory difficulties (even in the presence of normal phrenic nerves), and poor body temperature regulation.

■ Suggested Readings

Brooke MH, ed. *A Clinician's View of Neuromuscular Disease.* Baltimore: Williams & Wilkins, 1986.

Brooke MH, Carroll JE, Ringell SP. Congenital hypotonia revisited. *Muscle Nerve* 1979;2:84–100.

Downey JA, Low NL. *The Child with Disabling Illness.* 2nd ed. New York: Raven Press, 1982.

Keele DK. *The Developmentally Disabled Child: A Manual for Primary Physicians.* Oradell, NJ: Medical Economics Books, 1983.

Levine MS. Cerebral palsy diagnosis in children over age 1 year: standard criteria. *Arch Phys Med Rehabil* 1980;61:385–389.

Levitt S. *Treatment of Cerebral Palsy and Motor Delay.* Boston: Blackwell Scientific, 1982.

Menelaus MB. *The Orthopedic Management of Spina Bifida Cystica.* 2nd ed. New York: Churchill Livingstone, 1980.

Molnar GE, ed. *Pediatric Rehabilitation.* 2nd ed. Baltimore: Williams & Wilkins, 1992.

Motloch W. Spina bifida: orthotic philosophies of treatment. *Clin Prosthet Orthot* 1984;8:9–11.

Rutten M. The long-term effects of early experience. *Dev Med Child Neurol* 1980;22:800–815.

Schafer MF, Dias LS. *Myelomeninogocele: Orthopaedic Treatment.* Baltimore: Williams & Wilkins, 1983.

Scherzer AL, Tacharnuter I. *Early Diagnosis and Therapy in Cerebral Palsy: A Primer on Infant Developmental Problems.* New York: M. Dekker, 1982.

Thompson GH, Rubin IL, Bilenker RM, eds. *Comprehensive Management of Cerebral Palsy.* New York: Grune and Stratton, 1983.

14
Katie Irani
Michael J. Vennix
Anjali Jain

Peripheral Neuropathy and Plexus Injury

▪ Peripheral Neuropathy

Definition

The terms peripheral neuropathy, polyneuropathy, or polyneuritis refer to an illness marked by disordered function of
peripheral nerves.

Etiology and Pathophysiology

Peripheral nerves consist of a bundle of axons; the large and
medium-sized axons are usually covered with a layer of myelin and the small diameter fibers are often unmyelinated.
Most peripheral nerves are mixed nerves carrying both incoming sensory information (afferent fibers), and outgoing
motor and autonomic impulses (efferent fibers). Large-
diameter afferent fibers convey vibration and position sense;
large-diameter efferent fibers innervate the muscles. Pain and
temperature sensation and autonomic information is carried
by small-diameter unmyelinated fibers.

Peripheral neuropathies result from diseases which affect
either the axons, their myelin sheaths, or both. Axonal neuropathies are the result of processes that primarily affect the

Susan J. Garrison (Ed.): *Handbook of Physical Medicine and Rehabilitation
Basics.* First Edition. Copyright © 1995 J. B. Lippincott Company

cell body or the axon; demyelinating neuropathies result from involvement of the myelin sheath. Regardless of the initial pathological process, secondary changes are produced because of the interdependence between myelin and axon. Mixed pathological changes with evidence of both demyelination and axonal degeneration are seen on biopsy.

The clinical presentation distinguishes the three major types of peripheral nerve diseases: mononeuropathy, mononeuropathy multiplex, and polyneuropathy. Mononeuropathy is a lesion of an individual nerve root or peripheral nerve, usually due to local causes such as trauma, entrapment, or compression. Multifocal neuropathy or mononeuritis multiplex refers to involvement of two or more discrete nerves which are usually affected sequentially in different limbs. This is commonly the result of multifocal nerve infarctions due to occlusion of the vasa nervorum, and is seen in systemic diseases causing vasculitis, such as periarteritis nodosa and diabetes.

Peripheral neuropathy (polyneuropathy) occurs in diseases which affect the peripheral nerves symmetrically, usually distally. The longer and larger axons are affected earlier and more severely than the shorter ones. In the demyelinating type, this occurs because the longer axons have more potential sites for demyelination; in the axonal type, the longer, larger axons do not have adequate nutritional support. Therefore, the symptoms tend to appear in the feet before the hands. Many polyneuropathies affect both the sensory and motor fibers indiscriminately. However, at times either the sensory or motor fibers are primarily affected, either clinically or pathologically.

Pathophysiologically, there are three types of nerve lesions:

- Neuropraxia: Both axon and myelin sheath are intact with minimal changes seen in paranodal region. There is physiological loss of function.
- Axonotmesis: There is degeneration of the axon with Schwann's sheath intact.
- Neurotmesis: Complete severance of the nerve.

Assessment/Evaluation

Patients with polyneuropathy often present with complaints of paresthesias, a pins and needles sensation, in the feet. Other symptoms are loss of sensation, sometimes accompanied by pain; weakness; muscle cramps; coldness; heaviness; and symptoms of autonomic dysfunction such as impotence, urinary retention or overflow incontinence, diarrhea or constipation, and orthostatic hypotension.

The major signs of peripheral neuropathy are loss of sensation, weakness, muscle atrophy, and loss of tendon reflexes. The most common sensory modalities affected are vibration and pain in a glove and stocking distribution. If position sense or proprioception is markedly affected, the patient may manifest unsteadiness or ataxia. Often the weakness is noted distally, affecting the small intrinsic muscles of the feet. The patient has difficulty spreading the toes and walking on uneven surfaces. With long-standing peripheral neuropathies, imbalance of muscles results in claw toes and high, arched feet. Eventually there is atrophy of the tibialis anterior muscle with prominent tibia. The hands show atrophy of the intrinsics and develop clawing. Tenderness of the soles and palms is typical in neuropathies such as nutritional, alcoholic, arsenic, and porphyric neuropathies, in which pain is a major feature.

There are many etiologies of peripheral neuropathies. During the patient's examination, recognizing distinctive features may suggest a particular diagnosis. When taking the history, include questions regarding alcohol intake, nutritional status, symptoms of diabetes and collagen vascular disease, exposure to toxic substances, and current medications. Try to determine possible patterns of repeated trauma in vulnerable areas. Refer to Table 14-1.

The chronology of presenting symptoms is an important consideration. Mononeuropathies are often acute in onset and sometimes have obvious causes, such as trauma. The most common acute polyneuropathy is Guillain-Barré syndrome. Some other acute polyneuropathies are caused by infections such as diphtheria, toxins, or metabolic processes. Most toxic and metabolic neuropathies develop somewhat slowly, within

Table 14-1. Activities and Resulting Nerve Trauma

Activity	Nerve Injury
Scrubbing, vacuuming, typing, sewing, or knitting	Carpal tunnel syndrome
Repetitively resting elbows on hard surfaces, or prolonged positioning with elbows flexed and pronated	Ulnar palsy
Crossing legs while seated or prolonged squatting	Peroneal palsy
Carrying heavy loads on shoulder	Suprascapular palsy

weeks. Chronic neuropathies are associated with diabetes mellitus and alcoholism, and are also found in hereditary disorders such as Charcot-Marie Tooth disease.

Cranial nerve involvement is common in acute idiopathic polyneuropathy, in neuropathies associated with porphyria, diabetes, sarcoidosis, and periarteritis nodosa. It is unusual to find cranial nerve abnormalities in alcoholic, arsenic, and other toxic neuropathies.

On physical examination, note the pattern of involvement. In mononeuropathy, motor and sensory involvement in the distribution of a single root or peripheral nerve is usually found. Most polyneuropathies produce both motor and sensory involvement. Predominantly motor involvement suggests Guillain-Barré syndrome, recurrent inflammatory polyneuropathy, porphyritic, lead, diphtheritic, or a hereditary neuropathy. Predominantly sensory involvement is commonly found in diabetic, alcohol, cancer, and nutrition-related neuropathies. Occasionally dissociated sensory losses are seen. The patient has diminished pain and temperature sensation with preservation of other modalities; this is typical in small fiber neuropathies. When pain is preserved but position sense is lost, consider vitamin B_{12} deficiency or the rare Friedreich's ataxia. These neuropathies affect the posterior columns, leading to the involvement of fibers conveying joint position. Predominant autonomic involvement is found in diabetes, amyloidosis, dysproteinemia, and dysautonomia.

Laboratory Investigations

Many common causes of peripheral neuropathy such as diabetes, hypertension, and alcoholism can be evaluated by routine lab tests including complete blood count (CBC), erythrocyte sedimentation rate (ESR), serum glucose, blood urea nitrogen (BUN), and thyroid function tests. There are innumerable rare conditions associated with polyneuropathy; an extensive screening process is unnecessary and expensive. History and physical examination can point to an appropriate test, such as that for lead, or a particular toxin, for example, suspected in occupational exposure.

Electrophysiologic Studies

Nerve conduction studies are very helpful in establishing the involvement of peripheral nerves as the site of pathology. Such testing can distinguish a peripheral neuropathy from myopathy or anterior horn cell disease. It can also document predominantly motor or sensory involvement, and distinguishes between primary axonal or demyelinating processes. The site of involvement in cases of entrapment or compression neuropathies can be revealed in many cases, such as ulnar neuropathy at the elbow or common peroneal neuropathy at the fibular head.

Electromyography (EMG) is useful in detecting or confirming evidence of denervation in distal muscles that can be seen in axonal peripheral neuropathies. Abnormalities on needle examination can also indicate the course of the peripheral neuropathy in the acute period following injury. Amplitude of abnormal spontaneous activity is large and decreases as the process becomes chronic. The configuration of the motor unit also can reflect chronic changes in reinnervation.

Nerve Biopsy

Avoid obtaining a nerve biopsy on a routine basis. It should be done only in cases for which a histological diagnosis is a possibility, such as vasculitis or amyloidosis.

Treatment

In general, the treatment of neuropathies aims to maintain range of motion (ROM) of the joints, prevent contractures, reeducate the patient in skilled activities, and maximize residual function.

Treatment of mononeuropathies depends upon the focal deficit noted. If there is a complete lesion of the nerve, employ techniques to substitute for the loss of musculature. Use orthotic devices to prevent contractures, support weak muscles, or substitute for paralyzed muscles. Educate the patient to prevent complications from the lack of sensation.

Contractures. Peripheral neuropathies cause paralysis of muscles with decrease in, or loss of, muscle tone; therefore, contractures are easily prevented if range of motion exercises are performed routinely. Educate the patient in appropriate ROM exercises. If contractures are present, use heat followed by stretching. Try prolonged stretching over 20 minutes. Adequate stretching to increase the range of motion means that the joint is taken past the point of pain.

Weakness. Exercising weak muscles with significant denervation must be done in moderation. Experimental evidence suggests that long duration, low-intensity activity, meaning high-repetition, low-weight, does not damage the muscle. Discourage patients who have significant partial denervation from engaging in moderate to severe intensity, prolonged exercises.

Teach patients with acute polyneuropathy such as Guillain-Barré syndrome to limit their activities in the early recovery period to prevent the possibility of an exacerbation. When recovery has progressed to fair to good muscle strength, patients may resume full activities.

In cases of chronic neuropathy, use maximum isometric or progressive resistive exercises to increase muscle strength.

Orthoses. Orthoses may be used to support an unstable joint, to prevent overstretching of a muscle in an elongated position, or to substitute for the function of paralyzed muscles. Wrist hand orthoses (WHOs) are used commonly for short periods of time in the upper limbs which do not significantly improve; WHOs actually may interfere with hand function. They may be used indefinitely for the lower limbs, such as an ankle foot orthosis (AFO).

Temperature. Cold may cause temporary weakness, a heavy feeling, and decreased strength in patients with peripheral neuropathies. Advise patients to wear warm clothes and avoid exposure to cold. Assure them that the weakness is a temporary response to cold.

Electrical Stimulation. Electrical stimulation has not been shown to enhance reinnervation in a denervated muscle. However, electrical stimulation does retard atrophy. It can be used to maintain the contractility and bulk of the muscle, but is not a very practical treatment, as it must be performed intensively for a prolonged period of time.

Functional Retraining. Teach compensating mechanisms in order to maximize function. Avoid abnormal habit patterns. Teach substitutions when primary movers are paralyzed, such as using the finger extensors to extend the wrist. Teach the patient to contract isolated muscles to strengthen and prevent disuse atrophy.

Sensory Reeducation. Order sensory reeducation for nerve injuries involving the hand. Initiate therapy when vibratory sensation returns.

Pain. Pain may be present in the distribution of the nerve with mononeuropathy, or in a more diffuse manner distally in the hands and feet. The pain is usually a burning type, and the area may be hyperesthetic or dysesthetic. Try tricyclic antidepressants in small doses, such as amitriptyline (Elavil) 50 to 75 mg orally at bedtime, or antiseizure medications such as carbazepine (Tegretol) and phenytoin sodium (Dilantin). Maintain good nutritional status, including vitamin supplementation, especially Vitamin B. Use a trial of transcutaneous electric stimulation (TENS) over the proximal location of the offending nerve(s) or over the painful area. Cover the painful area with a light elastic garment or an adhesive plastic such as Op-Site, Tegeaderm, or Second Skin. Advise the patient to avoid exposure to cold.

Surgery.   Surgical treatment includes nerve suturing following nerve injury; decompression and/or transposition in nerve entrapment; and tendon transfers, if there are muscles of sufficient strength to be utilized for transfer.

Postoperatively, immobilize the part for 4 to 6 weeks; avoid any tension on the repaired site. Then initiate a gradual stretching and mobilization program. At times, tendon transfers are performed acutely after a complete nerve injury. Usually, however, they are done when the patient's functional recovery has significantly slowed. Preoperatively, strengthen the muscles to be transferred. A transferred muscle looses its strength by one grade. Postoperatively, train the patient to perform the new activity of the transferred muscle. Biofeedback may be useful in retraining. Later, use strengthening exercises.

Complications

Complications are usually due to lack of sensation. Commonly, ulceration of the feet occurs, along with secondary infection. Hand ulcers are rare, but burns occur. Prevent these problems through patient education. Encourage meticulous foot care and use of appropriate shoes. If an ulcer has already formed, prevent further trauma by avoiding weight-bearing on the affected foot. A total contact cast may be used until the ulcer heals.

With severe sensory loss, Charcot's joint, a severe form of osteoarthritis with pronounced disruption and disorganization of the midtarsal and tarsometatarsal joints, may develop. This can be associated with loss of pain sensation, proprioception, or a combination of both.

Outcome/Follow-Up

Patients with acute peripheral neuropathy such as Guillain-Barré syndrome usually experience complete recovery in 12 to 18 months.

Chronic neuropathies, for example, diabetic neuropathy, may require periodic evaluation for any deterioration in function and for necessary rehabilitation intervention.

▎ Brachial Plexus Injury

Brachial plexus injury often presents major problems in diagnosis and management. It commonly occurs with trauma to multiple systems, such as from motorcycle accidents, so that concern for preservation of life or limb obscures its presence.

Anatomy

The brachial plexus is usually formed by the union of anterior rami of the last four cervical nerve roots and the first thoracic root. Refer to Figure 14-1. Often there is contribution from the C4 to C5 root (termed prefixed), or rarely, from the T2 to T1 root (postfixed). Proceeding distally, the plexus consists of trunks, divisions, cords, and finally, peripheral nerves. The five segmental roots form three trunks, upper (C5–C6), middle (C7), and lower (C8–T1). Each trunk separates into anterior and posterior divisions. The anterior divisions of the upper and middle trunks unite to form lateral cord; the anterior division of the lower trunk forms the medial cord, and the posterior divisions of all three trunks form the posterior cord. Most of the peripheral nerves originating in the plexus derive from the three cords. Exceptions are the long thoracic and dorsal scapular nerves that arise directly from the spinal roots and innervate muscles around the scapula. The only significant nerve that originates from the trunk is the suprascapular nerve (C5–C6).

Etiology

There are many possible causes of brachial plexus injury. Direct trauma is the most common; others are local compression, tumor, idiopathic, radiation, postoperative, and birth injury.

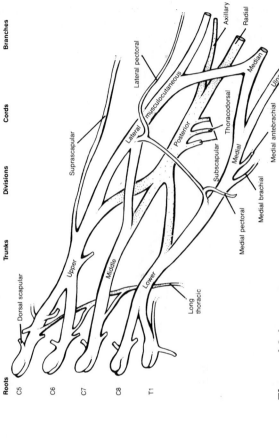

Figure 14-1. The brachial plexus.

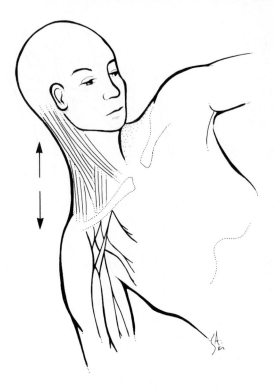

Figure 14-2. Forces producing injury to the upper portion of the brachial plexus.

Direct trauma accounts for more than half of brachial plexus injuries and is usually due to vehicular accidents. The most common mechanism of damage is traction injury. The most frequently seen traction injury is normally produced by a forceful distraction of the head from the shoulder, resulting in Erb's paralysis, as shown in Figure 14-2. In this injury, C5, C6, and occasionally C7 nerve roots are injured, leaving a nonfunctional shoulder, with good distal muscular function of the affected limb. Less commonly, a pull on an abducted arm results in Dejerine-Klumpke's paralysis, in which C8, T1, and occasionally C7 roots are damaged, with subsequent

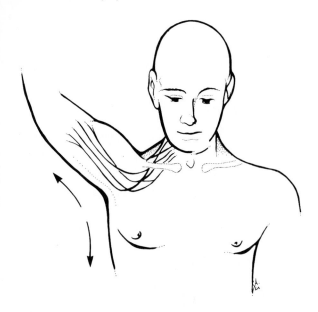

Figure 14-3.   Forces producing injury to the lower portion of the brachial plexus.

loss of hand and forearm function. Refer to Figure 14-3. Clinical experience shows that multiple level injuries are common; segmental classification is frequently impossible.

Evaluate the patient systematically in order to make an accurate diagnosis and prognosis for both neurologic and functional recovery.

An accurate history and physical examination is imperative. Record a detailed manual muscle test and sensory examination at the initial evaluation; update it during each subsequent visit.

Review radiographic examinations such as X-rays of the cervical spine and shoulders, myelogram, CT scan, and MRI to appreciate the extent of the lesion.

Use electromyography (EMG) to demonstrate objectively the extent of pathology. Serial studies provide a more accu-

Table 14-2. Interpretation of Electromyography (EMG)

- **Normal muscle**
  At rest: electrical silence

  Minimal effort: biphasic and triphasic motor unit potentials

  Maximal effort: complete recruitment pattern

- **Denervated muscle**
  At rest: spontaneous potentials, i.e. fibrillations and positive sharp waves

  Minimal effort: fast firing motor unit if present

  Maximal effort: incomplete or absent recruitment pattern

- **Signs of reinnervation**
  At rest: decreasing number of fibrillations and positive sharp waves

  Minimal effort: nascent small polyphasic potentials, increasing number of motor unit potentials

  Maximal effort: increasing recruitment pattern; polyphasic potentials

- **Signs of neuropraxia 14–21 days after injury**
  At rest: no spontaneous potentials

  Minimal effort: absent or occasional motor unit potentials

  Maximal effort: absent recruitment

rate method of prognosis than does a single study. See Table 14-2.

Sensory nerve action potential (SNAP) is helpful in distinguishing preganglionic (root avulsion) lesions from postganglionic lesions. Refer to Figure 14-4. SNAP shows a normal response if the lesion is preganglionic, meaning that the sensory ganglion is intact. A positive SNAP in an area of anaesthesia or with a negative sensory evoked potential (SEP) is an almost definite indication of a nerve root avulsion. Distinguish between pre- and postganglionic lesions, because prognosis and management are different. Refer to Table 14-3.

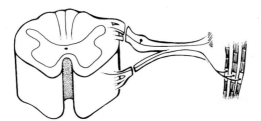

Preganglionic injury

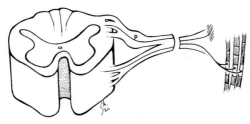

Postganglionic injury

Figure 14-4. Preganglionic and postganglionic injuries.

Evaluate associated injuries; most patients sustain multi-system trauma, particularly if injured in vehicular accidents.

Recognize social and psychological problems. Sudden loss of all or part of a limb is psychologically and economically catastrophic.

Table 14-3. Signs and Symptoms of Cervical Root Avulsion

Burning pain

Horner's sign

Loss of serratus, rhomboids, and pectorals

Fracture of transverse process

Positive myelogram

Negative SEPs with positive SNAP

Address vocational aspects. The largest single group of patients are motorcyclists, who tend to be manual laborers. The alteration in their potential for making a living or simply performing daily activities is dramatic.

Management

From a rehabilitation standpoint, patients with brachial plexus injuries are best managed by a multidisciplinary approach. Physicians, physical and occupational therapists, psychologists, social workers, and vocational counselors all have patient care responsibilities.

Major deficits resulting from brachial plexus injuries include motor paralysis, causing loss of function and secondary deformities such as joint stiffness, muscle contractures, and edema; sensory loss; and pain.

Initiate conservative treatment as soon as possible after injury. Instruct the patient to wear a sling to lessen shoulder subluxation and to decrease the possibility of further traction injury to the neurovascular bundle.

Begin physical therapy early for passive range of motion (PROM) to joints of the affected limb, in order to prevent contractures. Also, teach a self-ranging exercise program and active exercises of those muscles that are capable of voluntary movement.

Prevent edema, which can increase stiffness and contractures, by use of PROM and elevation. Consider elastic support of various types, such as Jobst garments and Isotoner gloves, but avoid a tourniquet effect. Electrical stimulation of paralyzed muscle remains controversial; no objective studies have demonstrated that it is effective.

When reinnervation occurs, strengthen the muscles using a full program of resistive exercises.

The occupational therapist trains patients in one-handed activities as well as in use of orthoses. Prevent secondary complications such as injuries or burns that may result in soft tissue infection or osteomyelitis by teaching the patient to protect the anaesthetized limb and fingers.

Management of pain in brachial plexus injury patients is

difficult. Use a trial of TENS, properly applied, early in treatment. Medication management includes use of phenytoin (Dilantin), carbamazepine (Tegretol), amitriptyline (Elavil), and nonsteroidal anti-inflammatory medications. (Refer to Chapter 2, Acute Pain). Neurosurgical intervention, such as brachial plexus exploration and lysis, is usually not helpful for pain reduction, although nerve blocks may be used in specific cases.

Surgical Management

While it is generally accepted that neural reconstructive surgery is indicated for brachial plexus injuries, there is controversy about appropriate candidates, timing of surgery, and specific levels of intervention. Commonly used procedures are neurolysis, excision and grafting, and neurotization.

Peripheral reconstructive surgery, such as Steindler flexor plasty, restoration of elbow flexion with pectoral and other muscle transfers, has been used to enhance function. Occasionally, a shoulder fusion with amputation is done in a flail limb and a prosthesis is used.

Following all reconstructive surgeries, intensive rehabilitation for many weeks is necessary to reeducate the muscle.

Lumbosacral Plexus Injury

Anatomy

The lumbosacral plexus originates from all of the nerve roots inferior to and including the T12 nerve root. Refer to Figure 14-5. The lumbar plexus is formed by the L1–L4 nerve roots with a small communication from the twelfth thoracic nerve root. The L1 root, having received this branch from T12, divides into iliohypogastric and ilioinguinal nerves which travel down the inferior portion of the abdominal wall. Small branches from the L2–L4 nerves merge to form the obturator nerve. Remaining branches exit the ventral rami of the L2–

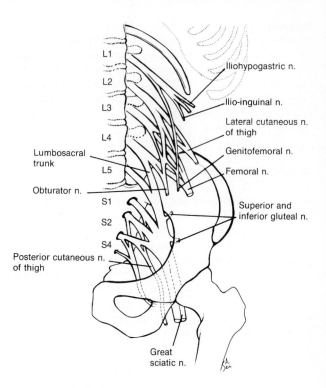

Figure 14-5. The lumbosacral plexus.

L4 nerves and combine to form the largest peripheral nerve originating from the lumbar portion of the plexus, the femoral nerve. The L4 root usually divides into two parts, one contributing to the obturator and femoral nerves of the lumbar plexus, and other contributing to the sacral portion of the plexus. In the sacral plexus anterior branches from the L4–S3 roots join to form the tibial nerve, while posterior branches from the L4–S2 roots form the peroneal nerve. These two nerves travel together down the thigh within a connective tissue sheath as the sciatic nerve. Other posterior branches from the sacral plexus combine to form the superior and inferior gluteal nerves.

Etiology

As a group, lumbosacral plexus injuries occur much less commonly than injuries to the brachial plexus. As with the brachial plexus, there are many causes for injury to the lumbosacral plexus. Although the term lumbosacral plexus is used here, simultaneous injury is less common than involvement of the lumbar plexus or the sacral plexus. Carcinomas of the rectum, prostate, or cervix can, by direct extension, invade the lumbosacral plexus. Metastatic and lymphomatous infiltrates of the plexus can produce a painful paralysis which develops over a long period of time. Less commonly a hematoma within the psoas muscle can cause a compression plexopathy.

Diagnosis

Electrodiagnostic studies as well as imaging studies and radiographic evaluations are important in differentiating a lumbosacral plexopathy from a radiculopathy, a lesion of the cauda equina, or proximal mononeuropathy.

Treatment

Similar principles of muscle strengthening and pain control are utilized for lumbosacral plexus injuries as for those already discussed in this chapter in the section on brachial plexus injury.

▣ Suggested Readings

Brown WF, ed. *The Physiological and Technological Basis of Electromyography.* Boston: Butterworth, 1984.

Brown WF, Bolton CF, eds. *Clinical Electromyography.* Boston: Butterworth, 1993.

Chaudry V, Glass JD, Griffin JW. Wallerian degeneration in peripheral nerve disease. *Neurol Clin* 1992;19(3):613–26.

Donofrio PD, Albers JW. Polyneuropathy: classification by nerve conduction studies and electromyography. AAEM Minimonograph #34. *Muscle Nerve* 1990;13:889–903.

Dyck PJ, Thomas PK, eds. *Peripheral Neuropathy,* 2nd ed. Philadelphia: W.B. Saunders, 1993.

Herbison GJ, Jaweed MM, Ditunno JF. Exercise therapies in peripheral neuropathies. *Arch Phys Med Rehab* 1983;64:201–205.

Josifek IF, Bleecker ML. Chapter 84. *In* Dyck PJ, Thomas PK, eds. *Peripheral Neuropathy*, 2nd ed. Philadelphia: W.B. Saunders, 1993.

Parry GJ. Mononeuropathy multiplex. *Muscle and Nerve* 1985;8:493–498.

Kimura J. Diseases of the root and plexus. *In* Kimura J. *Electrodiagnosis in Diseases of Nerve and Muscle: Principles and Practice,* 2nd ed. Philadelphia: F.A. Davis, 1989.

Sabin TD. Classification of peripheral neuropathy: the long and the short of it. *Muscle and Nerve.* 1986;9:711–719.

Sibley W. Polyneuritis-Symposium in Clinical Neurology in Medical Clinics of North America. Vol 56, No. 6, Nov. 72.

T'sairis P. Differential diagnosis of peripheral neuropathies. *In* Dyck et al. *Peripheral Neuropathy,* 2nd ed. Philadelphia: W.B. Saunders, 1993.

15

Susan L. Garber
Susan L. Blair
Thomas Krouskop

Pressure Ulcers

Definition

Pressure ulcers are localized areas of cellular necrosis. In general, they are characterized by an open wound in which tissue necrosis has occurred in response to externally applied pressure. Although the terms pressure ulcer, decubitus ulcer, pressure sore, and bedsore are used interchangeably, "pressure ulcer" is the term currently accepted by the U.S. Department of Health and Human Services, Public Health Service, Agency for Health Care Policy and Research, and the National Pressure Ulcer Advisory Panel.

Anatomy

Pressure ulcers usually occur over bony prominences (Figure 15-1). They are classified by stages according to the degree or extent of tissue damage (Figure 15-2).

Stage I. nonblanchable erythema of intact skin, the heralding lesion of skin ulceration. Do not confuse with reactive hyperemia.

Stage II. partial thickness skin loss involving epidermis and/or dermis.

Stage III. full thickness skin loss involving damage or ne-

Susan J. Garrison (Ed.): *Handbook of Physical Medicine and Rehabilitation Basics.* First Edition. Copyright © 1995 J. B. Lippincott Company

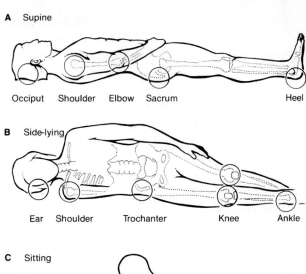

A Supine

Occiput   Shoulder   Elbow   Sacrum   Heel

B Side-lying

Ear   Shoulder   Trochanter   Knee   Ankle

C Sitting

Scapula

Sacrum
Ischium

Heel   Ball
        of foot

Figure 15-1. Typical locations of pressure ulcers.

crosis of subcutaneous tissue that may extend down to, but not through underlying fascia.

Stage IV. full thickness skin loss with extensive destruction, tissue necrosis, or damage to muscle, bone, or supporting structures.

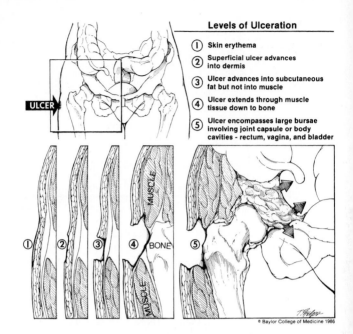

Figure 15-2. Pressure ulcer grade according to depth of tissue involvement. (From Donovan WH, Pressure ulcers. *In* DeLisa JA, *Rehabilitation Medicine: Principles and Practice,* 2nd ed. Philadelphia: J.B. Lippincott, 1993, p. 722.)

Identification of Stage I pressure ulcers may be difficult in persons with darkly pigmented skin. Furthermore, when eschar is present, accurate staging of the pressure ulcer is not possible until the eschar has sloughed or the wound has been debrided.

Epidemiology

It is difficult to determine accurately the incidence and prevalence of pressure ulcers, due to variations in data-gathering from acute care hospitals, rehabilitation centers, long-term

Table 15-1. Risk Factors for the Development of Pressure Ulcers

Immobility and altered activity

Incontinence

Nutritional deficiencies

Altered level of consciousness

Altered mental status

Altered or absent sensation

Psychological stress and depression

facilities, and home care settings. It has been estimated, however, that the incidence of pressure ulcers in hospitals ranges from 3% to 29%; in chronic or long term care facilities, the incidence could be as high as 45%.

Risk factors for the development of pressure ulcers are in Table 15-1.

Individuals at risk include those with spinal cord injury, the elderly disabled, bed- or chair-bound persons in nursing homes or at home, and persons hospitalized following a stroke, hip fracture, or surgery.

■ Etiology/Pathology

The normal structure of skin and physiological processes involved in maintaining healthy tissue are fairly well understood. However, the exact causes and mechanisms of soft tissue breakdown resulting in pressure ulcers are not as clear.

Three major factors contribute to the formation of pressure ulcers: biomechanical, biochemical, and medical factors.

Biomechanical Factors

These include pressure, shear, friction, moisture, and temperature. Normal activities such as sitting, lying, and leaning against another surface, cause small volumes of flesh to be compressed between the internal bony skeleton and an external surface. This results in extremely high tissue stresses. Classically, pressure ulcers are assumed to be caused by pressure-induced vascular ischemia as a result of tissues being deprived of oxygen and nutrients as the nonrigid walls of blood and lymph vessels collapse under pressures that are higher than those of the fluids inside. Also, mechanical deformation of flesh due to high levels of sustained load, or more moderate and repetitive forces, produce tissue damage. Shear forces play a significant part in the occlusion of blood vessels, but large compressive forces must also be applied for suitable shear conditions to develop.

Incontinence and excessive perspiration contribute to skin breakdown. Moist skin is susceptible to maceration through direct trauma or exposure to pressure. Wet skin may adhere to clothing and bed linen, causing shearing. Fecal incontinence causes chemical irritation of the epidermis, which can result in infection.

Biochemical Factors

Associated factors include fat distribution, circulation, collagen metabolism, heterotopic ossification, and anemia (with low serum iron and low serum iron binding).

Poor nutrition results in weight loss and reduced padding over bony prominences. Normal tissue integrity is dependent on correct nitrogen balance and vitamin intake. Hypoproteinemia leading to edema causes the skin to become less elastic and more susceptible to inflammation.

Slight changes in skin temperature, particularly an elevation with resulting perspiration, can increase metabolic demands of cells in a local region. This is also a potential factor in skin breakdown.

Medical Factors

A large number of diagnostic-specific medical and clinical factors are associated with pressure ulcers. Potential risk factors for an individual with spinal cord injury include level and completeness (motor and sensory) of injury, spasticity, ethnicity, employment, level of education, and socioeconomic factors. Anyone who is immobile as a result of trauma, illness, or disease is at high risk, especially if there is associated malnutrition, anemia, infection, spasticity, contractures, edema, and/or psychological problems such as depression. The skin of the elderly loses its elasticity, may become more dry, and is more fragile.

▧ Assessment/Evaluation

Risk Assessment

1. Use a validated risk assessment tool (such as the Braden Scale or the Norton Scale) to identify factors predisposing a person to the development of pressure ulcers. Use of these tools ensures systematic evaluation of individual risk factors, primarily mobility and activity levels.
2. Assess skin at admission to the hospital, nursing home, rehabilitation facility, or at home, and at regular intervals.
3. Document all risk assessments.

Skin Inspection:

1. Inspect skin at least once a day. Pay particular attention to tissue over bony prominences.
2. Document the results of skin inspection.
3. Note potential signs of tissue breakdown. (Table 15-2)

Skin Care

1. Cleanse at time of soiling and at routine intervals.
2. Minimize friction and forces applied to the skin.
3. Individualize the frequency of routine skin cleansing.
4. Use care in positioning, turning, and transferring patients.
5. Avoid massage over bony prominences.

Table 15-2. Potential Signs of Tissue Breakdown

Color variation

Blisters

Rashes

Swelling

Temperature variation

Pimples and ingrown hairs

Bruises

Surface breaks

Dry, flaky skin

Treatment

Prevention

Prevention is the most cost-efficient approach to pressure ulcer management. Essential elements of an effective prevention program include an integrated team management approach emphasizing good medical and nursing care, proper training and education of patients, family, and caregivers, encouragement of patient compliance, and the proper prescription of support surfaces.

Skin Inspection

Skin inspection is the basis of prevention. A rigid schedule must become part of the patient's daily routine. Examine the skin regularly each morning and evening and each time the patient is turned or receives a specific treatment. Any sign of redness, skin discoloration, irritation, or abrasion is an indication of impending ulcer formation. Remove all pressure from the area immediately. Teach the patient and family the importance of these skin checks and reinforce these behaviors.

Skin Maintenance

Keep the skin clean and dry at all times. Wash areas where perspiration or body fluids collect several times daily with mild soap, rinse with warm water, and pat dry. Apply a lotion or cream after washing. Massage it well into the skin. Avoid leaving any moist areas that may result in irritation and maceration.

Traditionally, prevention and management of pressure ulcers focused on frequent patient repositioning to relieve pressure and maintain capillary blood flow. Currently, the management of pressure ulcers is divided into three steps: reduction of pressure, treatment of any predisposing factors, and care of the wound.

Pressure Reduction: Turning, Transfers and Positioning

Turn high-risk patients every 2 hours around the clock: 2 hours on the side, 2 hours on the back, and 2 hours on the other side regardless of the type of support surface. Use care in transferring patients. DO NOT drag the patient across the bed. Use a draw sheet under the patient and have two people lift the patient for transfers. Use therapeutic mattress surfaces to minimize pressure on vulnerable areas of the body; use pillows to support extremities so that pressure is reduced where knees and ankles may oppose each other. Teach a patient in a wheelchair to shift his weight or elevate himself for approximately 15 seconds out of every 30 minutes. This pressure relief allows the person to continue sitting for several hours at a time without the risk of developing a pressure ulcer.

Pressure Reduction: Support Surfaces

There are more than 140 different support surface products on the market today. Some are recommended for comfort only; some assist with the task of turning patients or eliminate the need for it; some are technologically sophisticated and are intended to reduce significantly the pressure between the body and the support surface. In choosing a support surface for a patient, either for wheelchair or bed, consider the following characteristics:

* Minimizes pressure under bony prominences
* Controls pressure gradient in tissue
* Provides stability
* Does not interfere with weight shifts
* Does not interfere with transfers
* Controls the temperature at the tissue interface
* Controls moisture at the skin surface
* Lightweight
* Low cost
* Durable

Obviously, no one product fulfills all of these requirements all of the time. Support surfaces are rapidly outdated as a result of technological advances. Examples provided only represent a category, which is not limited to those brands specifically mentioned. Choose the appropriate product to meet individual patient needs, recognizing the advantages, disadvantages, and limitations of the different surfaces. Use the most sophisticated technology for the most difficult cases, such as multiple ulcers, severe contractures, and inability to tolerate the prone position.

BEDS AND MATTRESSES

Pressure relief devices for beds are categorized as therapeutic mattress surfaces, mattress overlays, or pressure relief beds. (See Tables 15-3 and 15-4.)

Therapeutic Mattress Surface or Overlay. The overlay is placed directly on top of regular mattress; its design and material determine effectiveness in relieving pressure.

Replacement Mattress. The replacement mattress has an overlay incorporated into it, which must be evaluated over time for effectiveness in relieving pressure. Check the warranty on materials and workmanship.

Air Flotation Bed. The air flotation bed is used in severe or high-risk cases, when contractures preclude appropriate

Table 15-3. Support Surfaces: Mattresses and Beds

Mattress	Mattress Overlay	Air Flotation Bed
"Replacement"	Convoluted foam	Air-fluidized
Gel and foam	Solid foam	Low-air-loss
Water beds	Alternating air	
Foam	Static air	

Table 15-4. Air Flotation Beds

Air-fluidized Bed	Low-air-loss Bed
Description	
A support system in which a high volume of air is forced through a fine granular material so that the material behaves like a liquid with a high density	A support system composed of air-filled pillows that leak air slowly, and a pump that is used to keep the pillows filled to the desired firmness
Advantages	
Ease of operation	Comfortable
Fail-safe	Control of skin maceration
Control of skin maceration	Can change from lying to sitting or semi-Fowler's position without foam components
Disadvantages	
Requires foam for positioning in sitting or semi-Fowler's position	Requires skilled setup
	Not fail-safe
Heavy	

From Donovan WH, Dinh TA, Garber S, et al. Pressure ulcers. *In* DeLisa JA, ed. Rehabilitation Medicine: Principles and Practice, 2nd ed. Philadelphia: J.B. Lippincott, 1993, p. 728.

positioning, and when there is limited access to skilled nursing care. It can be used at home, but only after consultation with a physician, therapist, or nurse.

Wheelchair Seating: Pressure-Relief and Positioning

Wheelchair cushions reduce the risk of pressure ulcers in persons with physical disabilities. Cushions function to:

*   relieve pressure in vulnerable anatomical areas by providing an additional protective layer between the seating surface and the body;
*   distribute the body's weight away from bony prominences; and
*   stabilize the body for balance and functional positioning.

Wheelchair seating is classified by function: postural control or pressure relief. Positioning and postural alignment are important considerations during wheelchair sitting. Special back cushions and total seating systems are available to enable a person in a wheelchair to maintain the most functional position while reducing the risk of pressure ulcers.

Seating surfaces for pressure relief are categorized as either dynamic or static devices. Dynamic wheelchair cushions are designed to produce alternating high and low pressures at any point on the sitting surfaces of the body. Dynamic cushions depend on an external power source, such as battery or wall socket, which may limit mobility and interfere with functional independence. In static wheelchair cushions, pressure reduction is determined by the material and/or design of the cushion. There are three major categories of static wheelchair cushions: air-filled, flotation, or foam. Each category has distinct advantages and disadvantages, as described in Table 15-5.

■ Treating Predisposing Factors

Patients with pressure ulcers often have problems with wound healing due to inadequate nutrition. Evaluate and treat nutritional deficiencies so that underlying tissues re-
text continues on p. 310

Table 15-5. Characteristics of Static Wheelchair Cushions

Category	Definition	Advances	Disadvantages
Air-filled	An inflatable membrane filled with air	Lightweight	Subject to puncture; not easily repaired.
		Easy to clean	Requires monitoring of air pressure
		Can be customized: multiple heights	May cause balance or transfer problems
		Can be compartmentalized: multiple valves	
Flotation-filled	Chemically treated water or other liquid within plastic or rubber membrane	Adjusts to body movement	Heavy
		Easy to clean	May leak of punctured
			Difficult to transfer
Flotation-gel	Plastic-like material that simulates body fat tissue	Adjusts to body movement	Same as flotation-filled
	Ideally, compression of one area of flotation cushion allows liquid or gel to flow into noncompressed areas	Acts as a shock absorber	

Table 15-5. (*Continued*)

Category	Definition	Advances	Disadvantages
Polyurethane foam	Solid blocks or layers of foam	Readily available	Wears out quickly (average, 6 months)
	Compression of one area has little effect on other areas.	Lightweight	Cannot be washed or cleaned
		Can be cut into any size, shape, or thickness	Subject to changes in temperature
	Pressure distribution depends on design and firmness	Easy to transfer	Should not be exposed to direct sunlight
		Provides stability and good balance	

From Donovan WH, Dinh TA, Garber S, et al. Pressure ulcers. *In:* DeLisa JA, ed. Rehabilitation medicine: Principles and Practice, 2nd ed. Philadelphia: J.B. Lippincott, 1993, p. 729.

ceive an adequate supply of amino acids, calories, and other nutrients.

Protein

Protein must be available for wound granulation to occur. Begin aggressive protein feeding if the patient's serum albumin drops below 3.1 g/dl, and total lymphocyte count (TLC) falls below 1200 mm.

Ideally, protein is given by mouth in the form of complete food, but oral supplements or even tube feedings may be utilized. If pressure ulcers are present, the individual's protein requirements may rise to between 1.2 and 2.0 g/kg of ideal body weight to maintain positive nitrogen balance and promote protein synthesis for healing. Fever, infection, and wound drainage all increase protein demands. Protein must be available for wound granulation to occur.

Deficiencies Causing Anemia

Presence of anemia also influences prevention and healing of pressure ulcers. Although not always related to diet, anemia can be caused by various nutritional deficiencies as shown in Table 15-6.

Patients with pressure ulcers often have hemoglobin levels of 10g/100ml or lower because of decreased appetite, loss of serum and electrolytes from the ulcer, infection, and generalized debilitation. Low hemoglobin levels cause a lower blood oxygen content and therefore a decrease in oxygen

Table 15-6. Nutritional Deficiencies Relating to Anemia

Iron

Folic acid

Vitamin B_{12}

Vitamin B_6

Some trace minerals, such as copper

delivered to the tissues. Deficiencies of various nutrients cause malformed red blood cells, which further aggravate the problem.

Other Nutritional Deficiencies

Vitamin C and zinc also have an essential role in wound healing. Vitamin C promotes intracellular "cement," supporting collagen in capillaries and various connective tissues. Stress conditions and wound healing cause increased loss of body stores of vitamin C. Zinc is recognized as the primary mineral directly involved in wound healing. Twenty percent of the body's zinc is stored in the skin.

▨ Wound Care

Cleaning

Preparation of the wound is the first stage of wound care. A dressing cannot be applied without first cleaning the wound and removing necrotic tissue; otherwise ineffective and even harmful results, such as infection, can occur. Many cleansing agents are available, as described in Table 15-7.

Necrotic Tissue Removal

Necrotic tissue can be removed from a pressure ulcer surgically, mechanically, or chemically. Usually a combination of methods is used.

Surgical Debridement

Surgical debridement is mandatory if the ulcer is covered by a hard black eschar, which can shield the wound from any other type of treatment.

Table 15-7. Wound Cleansing Agents

Cleansing Agent	Possible Detrimental Effects
Normal saline 0.9%	
Savlodil (chlorhexidine gluconate 0.015%, centrimide 0.15%)	Toxic to fibroblasts, key cells responsible for laying down the collagen-based scar in soft tissue repair
Eusol (chlorinated lime 1.2%, boric acid 1.25% in water)	Debriding action is not specific to necrotic tissue; can lead to increased urea and acute oliguric renal failure
Hydrogen peroxide	May be caustic to the surrounding skin

Mechanical Debridement

Mechanical debridement consists of packing the ulcer with saline-soaked gauze which is allowed to dry for 6 to 8 hours and is then removed. Necrotic tissue will adhere to the gauze and be extracted with it. Whirlpool is a useful modality for mechanical debridement. Necrotic tissue is softened, agitated loose, and washed from the area.

Chemical Debridement

Chemical debridement (topical medications) has value in limited circumstances. If properly used, it can remove the superficial layers of an ulceration. However, its ability to penetrate an eschar or to remove devitalized tissue is not proved. Enzymatic agents used for debridement of pressure ulcers include collagenase, papain, urea, chlorophyllin, and sutilains.

Mixtures that are effective in dissolving fibrin and liquefying pus but have no effect on the dissolution of necrotic tissue include streptokinase, fibrinolysin, and deoxyribonuclease.

None of these chemical agents will remove large amounts of devitalized collagenous tissue, penetrate thick eschar, affect a well-established bursa or sinus tract, or penetrate a deep wound. Some may actually impair drainage.

Wound Dressing

For most cases, use an occlusive dressing of the clean wound as the primary dressing. These dressings provide an optimal wound environment, and protection from outside contamination. The moist environment they create allows epithelial cells to migrate. Occlusive dressings are gas permeable, providing healing tissue an adequate oxygen supply. Many synthetic occlusive dressings are available and can be divided into four groupings, each with its advantages and disadvantages (see Table 15-8).

Table 15-8. Synthetic Occlusive Dressings

Dressing	Advantages	Disadvantages
Hydrocolloid (e.g. Duoderm)	Easy to apply; good retention of moderate exudate; water-impermeable; self-adhesive	Leakage and displacement with high exudate wounds
Polyurethane (e.g. Tegaderm®)	Good on superficial wounds	May be difficult to apply; poor adherence; minimal absorption
Biodressings (e.g. Spenco Second Skin®)	May be used on friable tissues	Suitable for superficial lesions only; difficult to maintain over wound
Gels	Same as biodressings	Same as biodressings

Avoid use of an occlusive dressing if:

* The pressure ulcer shows clinical signs of infection
* A culture yields greater than 10^5 organisms per gram of tissue
* There are exposed tendons or bones
* There are draining sinus tracts

Topical Antibiotics

There are no conclusive data on the superiority of topical antibiotics over wet-to-dry saline dressings. Topical antibiotics do not penetrate the depths of wounds or affect bacterial growth in granulation tissue. They may cause localized tissue sensitivity and may also have a detrimental effect on healing.

Surgical Management

Physiatric expertise should be combined with the plastic surgeon's skills for optimal pressure ulcer management. The patient with a pressure ulcer often has complex medical problems, and requires physiatric input from a functional standpoint throughout the entire course of hospitalization and treatment.

Spasms

Spasms are short, sudden, involuntary and uncontrollable muscle contractions that often occur in patients with spinal cord or head injuries. Because the spastic movements may rub the body against bedsheets, clothing, bedrails, or adaptive equipment, patients with spasms have a tendency to develop pressure ulcers. The most effective medications for control of spasticity are sodium dantrolene (Dantrium) and baclofen (Lioresal). Prior to surgery, make every effort to reduce or eliminate spasms; otherwise, surgery will inevitably be unsuccessful.

Surgical Closure

Grade III and IV ulcers heal faster and generate less scar tissue when treated surgically. Surgery for pressure ulcers includes excision of the ulcer, scar tissue, and usually the bony prominence, followed by closure of the defect through one of the procedures discussed below.

The primary procedures are standard, safe, time-tested techniques, used the first time a pressure ulcer develops and while there is still adequate skin, subcutaneous tissue, and muscle in the adjacent area. They include primary closure, skin grafts, skin flaps, and skin flaps plus muscle interposition.

PRIMARY CLOSURE

Primary closure consists of excision of the ulcer margin and conversion of the wound into an ellipse. The wound is then closed in layers to obliterate the dead space. The skin margins are opposed and sutured. Occasionally, a drain is required. Primary closure can usually be completed as an outpatient procedure in a day surgery unit. Keep pressure off the area for 2 weeks following the closure; begin sitting after the second week, depending upon the case. Remove sutures in the third week. With this form of treatment, the patient loses a minimum of time and can remain reasonably active.

SKIN GRAFT

A skin graft is a segment of dermis and epidermis that is completely separated from its blood supply at the donor site and transferred to the surface of a wound. There are two kinds of skin grafts: full-thickness skin grafts (FTSG) containing the epidermis and all of the dermis, and partial-thickness or split-thickness skin grafts (STSG), which consist of the epidermis and only a portion of the underlying dermis. The STSG is the more likely of the two to survive on the recipient site because it accepts a longer phase of plasmatic absorption, and therefore can survive longer before vascularization occurs. STSGs do not contain dermal appendages (sweat glands and hair follicles), and therefore need continuous lubrication.

SKIN FLAP

Skin flaps, the mainstay of pressure ulcer surgery, are used when wounds are too extensive for primary closure and loss of tissue mass precludes grafting. A skin flap is a "tongue" of tissue detached from surrounding tissue except for a pedicle or base, through which blood supply is maintained. It consists of full thickness of skin and underlying subcutaneous tissue, and can be elevated and moved to another area of the body within the limits of its vascular pedicle. If a defect requires a flap, the patient must be prepared for a major operative procedure and anticipate 4 to 6 weeks of hospitalization. Usually, only ischial, trochanteric, or sacral ulcers necessitate flaps. The musculocutaneous flap is the most commonly used. A composite of skin, subcutaneous tissue, and underlying muscle, its blood supply derives from the major vascular leash (artery and veins), which enters the proximal undersurface of the muscle and is elevated along with the muscle. In order to mobilize the flap, the fascia and subcutaneous tissue are sutured together to avoid disrupting the perforating vessels in the loose, gosamerlike, areolar tissue at the interface of these two layers. Transfer of a musculocutaneous flap leaves a deep donor site which must be covered by a skin graft in most cases. Occasionally, it can be closed primarily.

OTHER PROCEDURES

Secondary procedures are used after multiple breakdowns have occurred. Adequate tissue is not then available immediately adjacent to the new pressure ulcer, either because of scarring from previous ulcers or surgical procedures, or because the surrounding subcutaneous tissue has atrophied and decreased in volume.

Tertiary procedures are reserved until both primary and secondary procedures have been attempted. The most common tertiary method is unilateral or bilateral amputation and fillet (removal of bone) of the lower extremity.

■ Complications

There are different types of medical complications that can result from the development of pressure ulcers as well as subsequent treatment.

Use of an air-fluidized bed can cause multiple problems, which can usually be avoided. Severe dehydration occurs in 3% to 4% of patients because of increased insensible fluid loss caused by the continuous flow of warm, dry air through the filter sheet. Extra fluid intake is necessary. Dry scaly skin may develop, especially in the elderly. The low relative humidity of the bed environment causes drying of the nasal mucosa, potentially resulting in epistaxis. Hypernatremia may occur, as well as hypophosphatemia and hypocalcemia with chronic use, due to prolonged periods in a weightless environment. The sensation of floating can lead to confusion and disorientation. New pressure ulcers may develop, especially at the heels. Turn the patient and perform frequent skin checks. The patient's cough mechanism may be rendered ineffective because of the lack of a firm back support; therefore, pulmonary hygiene is an essential measure in patients with restricted mobility. Leakage of particles may cause eye injury to the patient and caregivers. Inspect the filter sheet frequently for tears; replace as necessary.

Osteomyelitis

There is a 10% incidence of osteomyelitis related to pressure ulcers. Additionally, sepsis secondary to pressure ulcers can be a serious and sometimes fatal complication. There may be difficulty differentiating osteomyelitis underlying the pressure ulcer from soft-tissue infection. Surgical debridement of the ulcer combined with broad-spectrum antibiotics is needed in soft-tissue infection. The presence of osteomyelitis will indicate the extent of ostectomy and can modify the length of antibiotic treatment.

Radionuclide bone scanning has been proposed as a sensitive diagnostic tool for osteomyelitis. However, a significant problem with false-positive results has been recognized. Needle biopsy of the underlying bone is the most accurate method for diagnosis of osteomyelitis. However, if any test is positive, recent studies have advocated use of a plain X-ray, white cell count ($\geq 15,000/mm^3$), and erythrocyte sedimentation rate (≥ 120) as the most sensitive, specific, and cost-effective workup for osteomyelitis.

Amputation

Amputation and the fillet procedure are reserved for those
patients who have extensive ulceration, with or without underlying osteomyelitis, and cannot be treated successfully
with any of the primary or secondary procedures previously
described. The procedure can consist of an above-knee amputation, fillet (removal of the femur) and use of the entire
thigh for flap coverage. A more extensive and formidable
technical procedure comprises amputation at the level of the
ankle and fillet of the entire leg. This provides the largest
possible amount of muscle and subcutaneous tissue to cover
the defects. This technique must be classified as a tertiary
procedure and only performed when all other procedures have
proved unsuccessful.

The psychological aspects of amputation surgery yield
several major problem areas. Life for the amputee has been
disrupted in a profound manner. The psychological consequences of having an obvious disability may also be significant.

▨ Summary

There is no ideal method for managing and preventing pressure ulcers. However, by considering advantages and disadvantages of the many techniques available, decisions can be
made about the most effective and economical support surfaces and methods of treatment to meet the unique needs of
each patient.

▨ Suggested Readings

Agris J, Spira M: Pressure ulcers: prevention and treatment.
Clin Symp 1979;31(5):2–32.

Allman RM, Walker JM, Hart MK, et al.: Air-fluidized beds
or conventional therapy for pressure sores: a randomized trial.
Ann Intern Med 1987;107:641–8.

Alpert SH: The psychological aspects of amputation surgery. *Orth and Prosth* 1982;36(4):50–56.

American Academy of PM&R Handbook. Chicago: American Academy of PM&R, 1989: Appendix 7–10.

Bergstrom N, Braden BJ, Laguzza A, Holman V: The Braden Scale for predicting pressure sore risk. *Nursing Research* 1987;36(4):205–210.

Constantian MB: *Pressure Ulcers: Principles and Techniques of Management.* Boston: Little, Brown and Company, 1980, p. 146.

Donovan WH, Dinh TA, Garber SL, et al.: Pressure ulcers. *In* DeLisa JA, ed. *Rehabilitation Medicine* 2nd ed. Philadelphia: J.B. Lippincott, 1993, pp. 716–732.

Kosiak M: Etiology of decubitus ulcers. *Archives of Physical Medicine and Rehabilitation* 1961;42:19–28.

Krasner D: *Chronic Wound Care: A Clinical Source Book for Health Care Professionals.* King of Prussia, PA: Health Management Publications, 1990, pp. 74–77, 152–56.

Krouskop TA: Selecting a support surface. *CAET Journal* 1990;9:5–10.

Krouskop TA, Noble PC, Garber SL, Spencer WA: The effectiveness of preventive management in reducing the occurrence of pressure sores. *Journal of Rehabilitation R&D* 1983; 20(1):74–83.

Lewis VL, Baily MH, Pulawski G, et al.: The diagnosis of osteomyelitis in patients with pressure sores. *Plast and Reconst Surg* 1988;81(2):229–32.

Nimit K: Guidelines for home air-fluidized bed therapy. *Health Technology Assessment Reports* 1989;5:1–11.

Pressure Ulcers in Adults: Prediction and Prevention. Clinical Practice Guideline Number 3. Rockville, MD: US Dept of Health and Human Services, publication AHCPR 92–0047.

Seiler WO, Stahelin HB: Recent findings on decubitus ulcer pathology: implications for care. *Geriatrics* 1986;41:47–57.

Webster JG: *Prevention of Pressure Sores: Engineering and Clinical Aspects.* Bristol, Philadelphia, and New York: Adam Hilger, 1991, pp. 208–212.

Woolsey RM, McGarry JD: The cause, prevention, and treatment of pressure sores. *Neuro Clin* 1991;9:797–808.

S. Ann Holmes

16

Pulmonary Rehabilitation

Definition

According to the American College of Chest Physicians, pulmonary rehabilitation is "the art of medical practice wherein an individually tailored, multi-disciplinary program is formulated which, through accurate diagnosis, therapy, emotional support, and education, stabilizes or reverses both the physical and psychopathological aspects of pulmonary diseases." Although a comprehensive rehabilitation program may have little effect on the rate of progress of the underlying disease, a number of beneficial effects have been documented, including reduction in the average number of hospitalization days per year and subjective improvement in symptoms and quality of life. The primary goal is to return the patient to the highest possible functional capacity despite the pulmonary disease.

Epidemiology

Chronic respiratory diseases are a leading cause of major limitation in activity, loss of work days, and premature retirement due to disability. Chronic obstructive pulmonary disease (COPD) is the fifth leading cause of death in the United States, and its incidence has doubled since 1970. Cigarette

Susan J. Garrison (Ed.): *Handbook of Physical Medicine and Rehabilitation Basics.* First Edition. Copyright © 1995 J. B. Lippincott Company

smoking is the major risk factor in the development and clinical course of COPD. Studies indicate that physician-delivered smoking intervention can be effective, and that smoking cessation results in lowering the excessive rates of lung functional loss associated with smoking. Therefore, tell your patients not to smoke.

Pulmonary disease is the most common cause of early death in traumatic quadriplegia and neuromuscular disorders.

▦ Anatomy and Physiology

There are four groups of muscles of respiration. The diaphragm, which is innervated by the phrenic nerve (C3, C4, and C5), is the principal muscle of respiration. The chest wall muscles include the internal and external intercostals, the scalenes, and the accessory muscles of respiration (sternocleidomastoid, trapezius, and pectoralis major). The abdominal muscles enhance the mechanical advantage of the diaphragm during inspiration and are the primary expiratory muscles. The muscles of the upper airway are important for keeping the upper airway open; they include the muscles of the mouth, tongue, uvula, palate, and larynx.

During quiet breathing, diaphragmatic contraction forces the abdominal contents away from the thorax and elevates the ribs in a bucket-handle fashion resulting in inspiration. Subsequently, the elastic recoil of the thorax produces expiration, a passive process in normal quiet breathing. With increased ventilatory demand the chest wall, abdominal, and accessory muscles actively contribute to the respiratory effort. Expiratory muscles participate in the mobilization of secretions during coughing and sneezing. Chest wall structure and compliance as well as airway resistance are important determinants of respiratory function.

▦ Control of Respiration

The respiratory center in the medulla receives input from the central chemoreceptors (stimulated by hypercarbia), and from the peripheral chemoreceptors in the carotid and aortic bodies (stimulated by hypoxia), to maintain normal blood gas levels under great variations in metabolic demand and carbon dioxide production. Voluntary control of respiration originates in the cortex and descends in the spinal cord to the respiratory muscles. With respiratory dysfunction the demand for work may exceed the ability to supply energy; thus respiratory muscle fatigue occurs with resulting hypoxia and hypercarbia or respiratory acidosis. With chronic respiratory acidosis, bicarbonate concentration increases to maintain near-normal pH, altering the "set point" of the control of respiration. Chronic hypoxia can lead to pulmonary hypertension and cor pulmonale if left untreated.

Etiology

Causes of chronic obstructive pulmonary disease (COPD) include

- Emphysema
- Chronic bronchitis
- Bronchiectasis
- Asthma

Causes of chronic restrictive pulmonary disease include

- Neuromuscular diseases with respiratory muscle weakness
  Duchenne muscular dystrophy
  Post-poliomyelitis syndrome
  Spinal muscular atrophy
  Congenital myopathies
  Amyotrophic lateral sclerosis (ALS)
  Myasthenia gravis
  Eaton-Lambert syndrome
- Distortion of the thoracic cage
  Kyphoscoliosis
  Ankylosing spondylitis
  Post thoracotomy
- Paralysis of respiratory muscles
  Traumatic quadriplegia
  Guillain-Barré syndrome

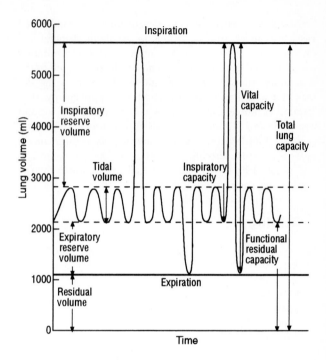

Figure 16-1. Diagram illustrating respiratory excursions during normal breathing and during maximal inspiration and maximal expiration. (From Guyton AC, *Textbook of Medical Physiology,* 7th ed., WB Saunders, 1986, p. 470.)

Lung Volume Definitions (See Figure 16-1 and Table 16-1).

- Forced Vital Capacity (FVC): amount of air moved when lungs are forcefully expanded after maximal expiration.
- Total Lung Capacity (TLC): amount of gas contained within the lungs at the end of maximal inspiration.
- Tidal Volume (TV): amount of gas moved in normal inspiratory effort.
- Functional Residual Capacity (FRC): amount of gas in lungs at the end of normal expiration.

Table 16-1. Characteristic Alterations in Pulmonary Function Tests

	Obstructive Pattern	Restrictive Pattern
Airflow (FEV$_1$/FVC, %)	↓	↔/↑
Airflow response to bronchodilators	↑/↔	↔
FRC	↑	↓/↔
TLC	↑	↓
RV	↑	↓/↑
Lung compliance	↔/↓	↓

- Residual Volume (RV): amount of gas in lungs at the end of maximal expiration.
- FEV$_1$: amount of air expelled in first second of FVC.
- Maximal Mid-expiratory Flow Rate (MMEF): average flow rate, between 25% to 50% of FVC.
- Maximum Voluntary Ventilation (MVV): the maximum volume of air exhaled in a 12-second period in liters per second.
- Maximal static inspiratory pressure (PImax): static pressure measured near RV after maximal expiration.
- Maximal static expiratory pressure (PEmax): static pressure measured near TLC after maximal inspiration.
- Minute Volume: tidal volume × rate of breathing per minute.

Evaluation

History

The medical history should include the following possible symptoms:

- Dyspnea

- Fatigue
- Orthopnea
- Decreased activity
- Morning headache
- Anorexia
- Dysphoria
- Poor sleep/vivid nightmares

Physical exam

The physical exam should document the following conditions:

- Tachypnea
- Shallow breathing pattern
- Inward (paradoxical) motion of abdomen with inspiration
- Accessory muscle activity during quiet breathing
- Prolongation of audible expiratory sounds
- Increased intensity of pulmonic second sound
- Tachycardia
- Dependent edema
- Clubbing
- Cyanosis

Diagnostic tests

The following diagnostic tests should be considered:

- Chest X-ray
- Electrocardiogram
- Hemoglobin/hematocrit
- Pulmonary function tests
- Pulse oximetry and end tidal CO_2 monitors
- Arterial blood gas
- Serum protein electrophoresis for alpha 1–antitrypsin
- Echocardiogram
- Sleep studies
- Others as indicated by underlying disease process

Table 16-2. Moser Classification of Functional Pulmonary Disability

Class	Assessment
Class 1	Dyspnea with strenuous activity
Class 2	Dyspnea on climbing stairs, but not with essential activities of daily living
Class 3	Dyspnea with some activities of daily living, but able to walk one block at a slow pace
Class 4	Dyspnea with minimal exertion; dependent on others for some activities of daily living
Class 5	Dyspnea at rest; requires assistance for most activities of daily living; essentially housebound

Adapted from Rondinelli RD, Hill NS. Rehabilitation of the patient with pulmonary disease. *In*: DeLisa JA, ed. *Rehabilitation Medicine: Principles and Practice.* Philadelphia: J.B. Lippincott, 1988, p. 691.

Functional Evaluation

Evaluate effect of pulmonary disease on morbidity, self care, vocational and recreational activities. Symptoms are classified according to functional impairment. See Table 16-2.

▨ Management

Medical

Preventive care plays an important role in stabilizing and preventing complications in chronic pulmonary disorders. Smoking cessation is by far the most important component of preventive care for these patients. Influenza and pneumococcal vaccines have been shown to reduce the incidence of infectious respiratory illnesses in this at-risk population. These patients should avoid exposure to irritants such as dust and chemicals at home and at the workplace. Treatment of other medical conditions as well as aggressive treatment of pulmonary infections is important in the medical management of patients with chronic respiratory disorders. Patients with COPD may benefit from the use of bronchodilators and corticosteroids delivered by metered dose inhalers, hand-held nebulizers or orally. Commonly used bronchodilators include beta–2 agonists (Albuterol, Metaproterenol), theophylline, and anticholenergics (Ipratropium).

Oxygen therapy should be used with caution in patients with chronic respiratory failure. Since hypoxic ventilatory drive predominates in these patients, oxygen therapy may exacerbate hypoventilation and place the patient in danger of respiratory arrest. Assisted ventilation can provide respiratory muscle rest, thus decreasing the energy expenditure of ventilatory muscles. Weaning protocol should include progressively increasing time off the ventilator with complete rest between work periods.

Forms of assisted ventilation include

- Negative pressure ventilators exert negative pressure on the chest wall, resulting in inspiration (iron lung, chest cuirass).
- Positive pressure ventilators displace the abdominal contents, assisting diaphragm movement (rocking bed, pneumobelt).
- Pressure limited positive pressure ventilators deliver air via a nose mask until a preset amount of pressure is reached; thus, the tidal volume will vary with airway resistance (continuous positive airway pressure, CPAP).
- Volume limited positive pressure ventilators deliver a preset volume of air with each breath; thus, constant ventilation is maintained by the minute. Portable models are available for home use. Air may be delivered via mouthpiece, nose mask, strapless oral-nasal interface (SONI), or tracheostomy.

Surgical Management

Tracheostomy is indicated for chronic positive pressure ventilation. Electrophrenic nerve pacing is appropriate for high

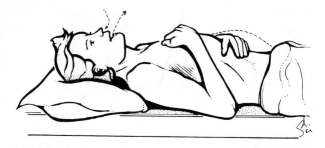

Figure 16-2. Diaphragmatic breathing technique. (Adapted from Rondinelli RD, Hill NS. Rehabilitation of the patient with pulmonary disease. *In* DeLisa JA, ed. *Rehabilitation Medicine: Principles and Practice.* Philadelphia: J.B. Lippincott, 1988, p. 696.)

cervical spinal cord injury (the patient must have intact phrenic nerves for pacing).

Rehabilitative Management

A multidisciplinary team including a physiatrist, social worker, physical therapist, occupational therapist, respiratory therapist, nutritionist, psychologist, and nurse work towards optimal medical management and functional independence for the patient, and address as well psychological and social issues.

Chest physical therapy

Breathing techniques
DIAPHRAGMATIC BREATHING. This technique involves retraining the patient to use the diaphragm while relaxing abdominal muscles during inspiration. The patient can feel the abdomen rise, while the chest wall remains stationary (see Figure 16-2).
PURSED LIP BREATHING. The patient's lips are pursed during expiration to prevent air trapping due to small airway collapse.

GLOSSOPHARYNGEAL BREATHING. The patient uses a piston-ing action of the tongue to project boluses of air into the lungs after taking a maximum breath.

Postural drainage. The use of gravity-assisted positioning can improve the mobilization of secretions. There are a variety of positions, designed for maximum drainage of each lung segment.

Manual percussion. Percussion or vibration of the chest wall can assist in the mobilization of secretions.

Controlled coughing. The patient sits leaning forward and initiates a timed, deliberate cough with enough force to mobilize mucus without causing airway collapse.

Assisted coughing. In this technique, pressure is applied to the abdomen during exhalation.

Physical therapy

* Assess endurance and provide an exercise program to progressively increase endurance while encouraging proper breathing techniques and body mechanics. Pulse oximetry monitoring may be indicated. Exercise is controversial in disorders such as post poliomyelitis and muscular dystrophy; with these disorders, avoid exercise to the point of fatigue.
* Provide an appropriate home exercise program.
* Instruct patient and family or caretakers in chest physical therapy and postural drainage techniques.
* Provide and train patient to use assistive devices as needed for mobility and functional independence.

Occupational therapy

* Assess and provide an exercise program for upper extremity range of motion and strengthening.
* Assess self care activities and provide training.
* Recommend adaptive equipment to increase independence and minimize energy expenditure.
* Evaluate home and work environment.

* Give suggestions to increase independence and energy conservation.

Respiratory therapy

Instruct patient and caregivers in the use of metered dose inhalers, nebulizers, supplemental oxygen, and home ventilator as needed.

Equipment

Nebulizer.   The nebulizer delivers medication suspended in liquid particles to lower airways and loosens secretions.

Suctioning.   Suctioning assists with clearing tracheal secretions.

IPPB.   Intermittent positive pressure breathing (IPPB) device provides positive airway pressure to augment inspiration and expand the lungs; these may be used with a nebulizer to deliver medication or saline solution.

Supplemental oxygen.   Supplemental oxygen is provided via nasal cannula, face mask, or trans-tracheal cannula.

Ventilator.   See previous descriptions of positive and negative pressure ventilators.

Wheelchair or walker.   A wheelchair or walker can be modified if needed for supplemental oxygen or portable ventilator.

Tracheostomy tube

CUFFED PORTEX.   This tube is soft and may result in less trauma to mucosa.

SHILEY FENESTRATED.   This tube with the inner cannula removed allows vocalization while off the ventilator.

JACKSON METAL (FENESTRATED).   This tube is for long-term use.

PASSY-MUIR VALVE.   This valve with the cuff deflated allows vocalization on or off the ventilator.

BAVONA (FOME-CUFF).   This high-volume/low-pressure cuff protects the airway with minimal trauma to mucosa; vocalization is not possible.

Table 16-3. Risks with Tracheostomy

Hemorrhage

Infection

Increased secretions

Lesions of tracheal mucosa from cuff or suction catheter

Thickening or mucus from inflow of dry air (always humidify air)

Stoma stenosis

Tracheomalacia

Tracheoesophageal fistula

Tracheal granulations

▓ Complications

Complications include

- Decreased ventilatory capacity with resulting activity limitations and decreased functional independence.
- Increased risk of infection secondary to decreased ability to clear secretions. There is a high risk of acute respiratory failure even with mild pulmonary infections because of low respiratory reserve.
- Respiratory arrest secondary to use of supplemental oxygen, as a result of suppression of hypoxic ventilatory drive in patients with chronic carbon dioxide retention.
- Pulmonary hypertension and cor pulmonale secondary to chronic hypoxia.
- Tracheostomy risks. Refer to Table 16-3.

▓ Outcome

Documented benefits of a comprehensive pulmonary rehabilitation program include a reduction in the average number of hospitalization days per year and subjective improvement in symptoms and quality of life. Rehabilitation goals and prognosis are determined by the underlying disease process, the psychological adjustment of the patient and family, and available financial resources.

▨ Suggested Readings

Bach JR. Alternative methods of ventilatory support for the patient with ventilatory failure due to spinal cord injury. *Journal of the American Paraplegia Society* 1991;14(4):158–174.

Bach JR, Alba AS, Garrison SJ. Pulmonary Rehabilitation. Arch Phys Med Rehabil 1990;71(4-S):s238–s243.

Coultas DB. The physician's role in smoking cessation. *Clinics in Chest Medicine* 1991;12(4):755–768.

Curran FJ, Colbert A. Ventilator management in Duchenne muscular dystrophy and post poliomyelitis syndrome: twelve years experience. *Arch Phys Med Rehabil* 1989;70:180–185.

Dail CW. Respiratory aspects of rehabilitation in neuro-muscular conditions. *Arch Phys Med Rehabil* 1965;46:655–676.

DeTroyer A, Estenne M. Functional anatomy of the respiratory muscles. *Clinics in Chest Medicine* 1988;9(2):175–193.

Dingemans LM, Hawn JM. Mobility and equipment for the ventilator-dependent tetraplegic. *Paraplegia* 1973;16:175–183.

Fishman AP, ed. *Pulmonary Diseases and Disorders.* 2nd ed. McGraw-Hill: New York, 1988.

Hodgkin JE, ed. *Pulmonary Rehabilitation: Guidelines to Success.* Butterworth: Stonehem, MA, 1984.

Kelly BJ, Luce JM. The diagnosis and management of neuro-muscular diseases causing respiratory failure. *Chest* 1991;99: 1485–1494.

Rondinelli RD, Hill NS. Rehabilitation of the patient with pulmonary disease. *In:* DeLisa JA, ed. *Rehabilitation Medicine: Principles and Practice.* Philadelphia: J.B. Lippincott, 1988.

Tobin M. Respiratory muscles in disease. *Clinics in Chest Medicine.* 1988;9(2):263–285.

Indira Lanig
William H. Donovan

17

Spinal Cord Injury

▓ Definition

Muscle paralysis is only one manifestation of the multisystem
dysfunction arising from spinal cord injury (SCI). Alterations
in function in other organ systems caused by SCI must be
constantly considered during all phases of management. The
most effective physician directing the care of a SCI patient
has a working knowledge of all the systems that can be
affected by the injury, and coordinates the medical, surgical,
and allied health professional care as indicated. This enables
the patient to maintain general medical health, maximize
functional capabilities, and successfully reintegrate into the
community after the initial phases of SCI.

▓ Anatomy

The spinal cord extends from below the foramen magnum
and tapers to an end opposite the L1 vertebral body. The
nerve roots of the cauda equina descend from the caudal
spinal cord, known as the conus medullaris. It is important to
recognize the relations of the spinal cord segments to the
vertebral bodies. For example, the eighth cervical cord segment lies opposite the sixth and seventh vertebral bodies,

Susan J. Garrison (Ed.): *Handbook of Physical Medicine and Rehabilitation
Basics*. First Edition. Copyright © 1995 J. B. Lippincott Company

with its roots exiting through foramina between the C7 and T1 vertebra. The T12 cord segment is usually located at the level corresponding to the tenth thoracic vertebral body. Below the L1 vertebral body, the spinal cord segments occupy a very short length of the cord; therefore, it is impractical to attempt to correlate them with their corresponding vertebral bodies. See Figure 17-1.

In the sagittal plane, the cord occupies approximately one-third to one-half of the spinal canal. The cord contains two enlargements, one extending from C2 to T2, with its greatest diameter at vertebral level C5/C6, and the other extending from T10 to T12. Normal spinal canal diameter averages 17mm +/− 5mm below C2.

The spinal column is at greatest risk for bony injury where a relatively mobile vertebral segment joins a less mobile segment, such as in the lower cervical region and at the thoracolumbar junction.

The cross-sectional topography of the spinal cord is illustrated in Figure 17-2. Incomplete spinal cord injuries occur when there is incomplete destruction of the laminated ascending and descending tracts.

The principal blood supply of the spinal cord is via the anterior spinal artery in the median fissure of the cord. This artery receives radicular reinforcement throughout its course. The midthoracic area is a relative watershed, and is therefore most vulnerable to ischemia.

▓ Epidemiology

The annual incidence rate of spinal cord injury in the United States is estimated to be approximately 30 to 32 cases per million population, or 8000 to 9000 new cases per year. This excludes those who die within 24 hours of injury. Prevalence is estimated to be 700 to 900 cases per million population (200,000 to 250,000 persons). Sixty-one percent of those injured are between the ages of 16 and 30 and 80% are between ages 16 and 45. Males are injured at a rate four times greater than females. The most common etiological factors are motor vehicle accidents (45%), falls (21.5%), gun-

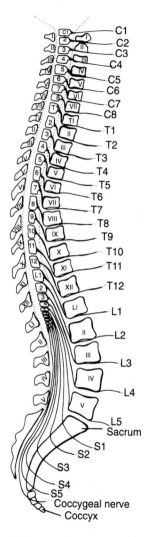

Figure 17-1. Diagram of the anatomical relationships of the spinal cord segments, vertebral bodies, and nerve roots. Note the disparity between spinal segmental level and localization of corresponding vertebrae. (Adapted from Carpenter MB, Sutin J: *Human Neuroanatomy.* Baltimore: Williams & Wilkins, 1983.)

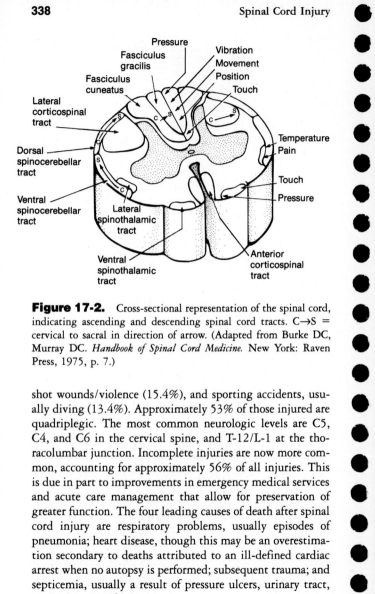

Figure 17-2. Cross-sectional representation of the spinal cord, indicating ascending and descending spinal cord tracts. C→S = cervical to sacral in direction of arrow. (Adapted from Burke DC, Murray DC. *Handbook of Spinal Cord Medicine.* New York: Raven Press, 1975, p. 7.)

shot wounds/violence (15.4%), and sporting accidents, usually diving (13.4%). Approximately 53% of those injured are quadriplegic. The most common neurologic levels are C5, C4, and C6 in the cervical spine, and T-12/L-1 at the thoracolumbar junction. Incomplete injuries are now more common, accounting for approximately 56% of all injuries. This is due in part to improvements in emergency medical services and acute care management that allow for preservation of greater function. The four leading causes of death after spinal cord injury are respiratory problems, usually episodes of pneumonia; heart disease, though this may be an overestimation secondary to deaths attributed to an ill-defined cardiac arrest when no autopsy is performed; subsequent trauma; and septicemia, usually a result of pressure ulcers, urinary tract, or respiratory infections.

In individuals over the age of 50, 30% to 50% of injuries

are due to falls, with underlying evidence of spinal spond-ylosis. Older patients tend to be female and quadriplegic.

Pathophysiology

The spinal cord is rarely anatomically transected or severed as a consequence of trauma. Extent of injury to the cord is estimated by the magnitude of neurological dysfunction as-sessed by serial clinical examinations. Acute trauma to the spinal cord initiates a cascade of physiological and biochemi-cal reactions that integrate synergistically to result in tissue damage. The current standard of care, as researched by the second National Acute Spinal Cord Injury Study (NASCIS II) in a 1985 multicenter clinical trial, involves administration of high doses of methylprednisolone. When given within 8 hours of injury, this appears to improve neurologic recovery in SCI patients significantly, by reducing free radical damage and lipid peroxidation. The protocol dose of methylpred-nisolone consists of a 30 mg/kg bolus, followed by 5.4 mg/kg per hour for 23 hours.

Mechanisms of Injury

Eighty-five percent of spinal cord injuries are caused by trau-ma. Other SCIs are a result of atraumatic pathology such as carcinoma, myelitis, ischemia, and multiple sclerosis. Such injuries are managed with rehabilitation principles similar to those for traumatic SCI.

Three basic mechanisms of injury, flexion, compression, or extension, can be deduced from the clinical history and the X-ray appearance of the spine. See Table 17-1. Combination mechanisms, including rotatory forces, occur often. In cases of pre-existing radiographic evidence of cervical canal steno-sis, hyperextension injuries may result in cord contusion without fracture demonstrated by radiography.

Spinal stability is evaluated using an anatomical three-column system. The anterior column consists of the anterior longitudinal ligament and anterior two-thirds of the annu-lus; the middle column consists of the posterior one-third of the annulus and the posterior longitudinal ligament; and the

Table 17-1. Schema of Injuries

Mechanism of Injury	X-ray Appearance
Flexion	Superior vertebral body lies anterior to the inferior one; evidence of compression forces anteriorally with resultant crushing of one of the involved vertebral bodies
Compression Axial loading forces are great enough to overcome the protective shock-absorbing qualities of the intervertebral discs	Normal or near normal alignment with loss of vertebral body height and dispersion of bony fragments, termed burst fractures
Extension/hypertension	Anterior separation of vertebral bodies with or without bone chips, or teardrop fractures just anterior to the vertebral body
	Compression fractures of posterior portion of vertebrae

posterior column is formed by the natural arch, ligamentum flavum, epiphyseal joint capsule, interspinous ligament, and supraspinous ligament. If two of three columns are disrupted, the lesion is intrinsically unstable.

■ Assessment

A systematic approach is required in assessment of SCI. Conduct evaluations of the neuromuscular, musculoskeletal, pulmonary, cardiovascular, genitourinary, gastrointestinal, and integumentary systems. Assess and document their functional status serially.

Neuromuscular System

Document the precise level of motor and sensory deficits, utilizing standard dermatomal and myotomal references during both acute and later stages. Interval changes in the neuromuscular exam can objectively reveal functional return or loss secondary to edema; post-traumatic cystic myelopathy, also known as syringomyelia; noncystic myelopathy, or tethering; and spinal stenosis during later phases of care.

Classify the injury by sensory levels, utilizing standards established by the American Spinal Association (ASIA). The key muscles for motor level classification are as follows:

- C5: elbow flexors
- C6: wrist extensors
- C7: elbow extensors
- C8: finger flexors
- T1: small finger abductors
- L2: hip flexors
- L3: knee extensors
- L4: ankle dorsiflexors
- L5: large toe extensors
- S1: ankle plantar flexors

Each muscle group is graded on a scale of 0 to 5. Refer to Chapter 1, Table 1-4. Key sensory points are as noted in Figure 17-3.

Determine the neurological level based on the results of motor and sensory examination. This level is determined by the most caudal segment that tests normal or intact for both motor and sensory function. By convention, a key muscle with at least a 3 grade is considered to have full or intact innervation, assuming that the key muscle group above is at least grade 4. An ASIA example is as follows: if no muscle activity is found in the C7 muscle, and the C6 muscle has a grade of 3, then the motor level is C6, provided that the C5 muscle is at least grade 4.

Use the ASIA Impairment Scale/Frankel's Classification System to document the degree of motor and sensory incompleteness. Document tendon and superficial reflexes sequen-

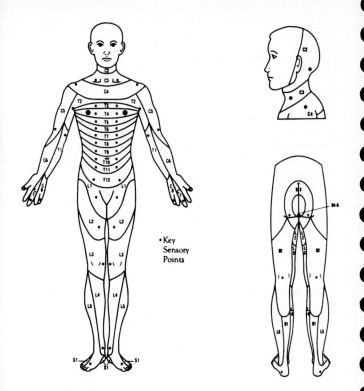

Figure 17-3. Dermatomal levels, with key. Sensory points as indicated. (From ASIA, International Standards for Neurological and Functional Classification of Spinal Cord Injury, 1992, used with permission.)

tially to assist in determining recovery from spinal shock (the initial areflexia and flaccidity seen acutely after spinal cord injury) or from root injury. The first reflex to recover after spinal shock is typically the bulbocavernosus reflex. This reflex is elicited by squeezing the tip of the penis or clitoris while a gloved finger rests in the rectum. The rectum will contract in response to this stimulus if the sacral segments of the spinal cord are intact.

In patients with quadriplegia, include a screening assessment of the muscles of respiration in the neuromuscular examination. Diaphragmatic breathing is typical. Shallow, rapid respiration utilizing the accessory muscles of respiration signals diaphragmatic compromise. Paradoxical inward movement of the intercostals is seen in patients without functioning intercostal muscles who are breathing only with the diaphragm. Diaphragmatic weakness or paralysis can be observed under fluoroscopy or double exposure chest X-rays.

Musculoskeletal System

Assessment of the musculoskeletal system includes a preliminary evaluation of spinal column stability, range of motion (ROM) in all joints, and muscle tone and strength. Document presence of musculoskeletal pain.

Evaluation of Spinal Stability

Obtain serial radiographs to monitor the extent of bone healing, as well as the alignment of the vertebrae during the first 6 to 12 weeks after injury. Radiographic evidence of vertebral bony healing is usually observed at 6 weeks in the cervical region and at about 8 to 10 weeks in the lumbar region. If there is a need for early mobilization and stabilization is questionable, obtain upright gravity-loaded films when the patient is to be mobilized in the sitting position. Consider more time for healing or surgical intervention if gravity creates any instability. In some cases, realignment of the halo vest posts and crossbars to obtain the desired alignment may allow continued healing.

Before the injury site is healed sufficiently to withstand the forces of muscle activity across the injured area, additional time with external orthotic support may be required. Typically, cervical injuries require an additional 6 weeks and lumbar another 8 to 12 weeks. After the appropriate period of time, obtain flexion/extension films in the upright position, with all support removed, to evaluate for late instability. This occurs in only a small percentage of cases.

Evaluation of Muscle Tone

Assess the degree of muscle tone and tailor range of motion, pharmacological, and functional treatment plans accordingly. Spasticity alone is not a reason for pharmacological intervention, unless it is painful or interferes with function or hygiene. Significant spasticity in the lower limbs can lead to the development of shearing forces while the patient is in bed, or the development of pressure ulcers while in the wheelchair. The heels, metatarsals, medial aspects of the knees, and popliteal areas can develop spasticity-induced pressure ulcers if proper assessment and interventions are not made. See Chapter 15, Pressure Ulcers. Contractures can usually be prevented in SCI patients by passive ROM (PROM) performed once or twice daily. In order to prevent adhesive capsulitis the shoulder may need to be placed in a 90-degree abducted position for 1 to 2 hours several times a day.

Musculoskeletal Pain

Pain can develop as a result of recent neuro-orthopedic trauma, surgery, posture, or compensatory body mechanics. Prompt systematic evaluation with prudent use of nonsteroidal antiinflammatory drugs (NSAIDs), analgesics, thermal modalities, and adjustments of posture and functional training activities should lead to timely resolution. Avoid use of heat over insensate areas due to the risk of burns.

Pulmonary System

The importance of optimal pulmonary management in the spinal cord-injured patient is underscored by studies that have shown a high incidence of morbidity from pulmonary complications in both the acute and chronic phases after injury. Respiratory dysfunction after spinal cord injury is secondary to impairments in ventilation and cough. The higher the level of injury, the more severe the impairments.

With levels of injury from T12 through T5, there is progressive loss of abdominal motor function that impairs forceful expiration and cough. With levels of injury from T5 through T1, the remainder of the intercostal volitional function is lost, causing further impairment. Cough is dramatically impaired in patients with low levels of quadriplegia from C8 through C4. At the C3 level, respiratory failure secondary to disruption of diaphragmatic innervation necessitates mechanical ventilatory support. Patients with new cervical injuries commonly experience a reduction of forced vital capacity (FVC) to between 24% and 31% of predicted normals secondary to paradoxical respirations during the acute phase. Over time, with the development of intercostal and abdominal spasticity, this can improve to 50% to 60% of the predicted normal.

In the initial assessment, include bedside pulmonary functions such as forced vital capacity, respiratory rate, and inspiratory forces. These parameters are helpful in assessing the risk of impending respiratory failure. Signs of impending failure include increasing respiratory rate in conjunction with decreasing tidal volume (rapid shallow breathing), a drop in forced vital capacity to a level less than 15 cc/kg bodyweight, a drop in inspiratory force (P_i) to less than 20 cm H_2O, and a neurological level of C3 or higher. Assess for possible associated trauma affecting pulmonary status such as hemothorax, lung contusion, and chest wall injuries. Concomitant head injury increases the risk of pulmonary complications secondary to aspiration, altered neurologic control of breathing, or the development of neurogenic pulmonary edema. In high-risk patients, obtain serial chest X-rays and arterial blood gases to detect atelectasis, pneumonia, hypoxia, and CO_2 retention at an early stage. See Chapter 16, Pulmonary Rehabilitation.

Cardiovascular System

During the early phases of the rehabilitation process, particular attention needs to be given to early detection of deep venous thrombosis (DVT) and the associated risk of pulmonary embolism. The reported incidence of pulmonary embolism ranges from 2% to 16% of patients within 2 to 3 months of their spinal cord injury. The most reliable clinical sign of DVT is asymmetric swelling of the involved limb in excess of 1 cm when compared with the opposite limb. Screening procedures include daily leg measurements, Doppler ultrasound, impedance plethysmography, and I-fibrinogen scanning. Scanning is of lesser value in the calf than in the thigh. The definitive study is venography, although this procedure is not without risk. The ventilation perfusion scan is useful in demonstrating thromboembolic phenomena, but the definitive diagnostic study is the pulmonary arteriogram.

Genitourinary System

During the early acute post-injury period, the bladder is typically areflexic. A closed system indwelling catheter may be used in the first several days while the patient is experiencing the initial recumbency-induced diuresis and while intravenous fluids are being administered. Upon discontinuing the indwelling catheter, initiate an intermittent catheterization program with fluid restriction, usually 100 cc/hour. Monitor catheterization volumes and keep them below 400 to 500 cc to prevent repeated overdistention that can result in delayed return of bladder reflex activity, the development of hydro-ureter, vesicoureteral reflux, or overflow incontinence. Evaluation of the genitourinary system during the first 2 weeks is usually limited to urinalysis, urine cultures to monitor for infection, and serum chemistries to monitor for evidence of renal insufficiency secondary to renal ischemia, medications, or rhabdomyolysis secondary to extensive soft tissue injuries.

During the first several weeks after injury, obtain baseline evaluation of the structure and function of the genitourinary system. The most sensitive measures of renal function, the glomerular filtration rate (GFR) and effective renal plasma flow (ERPF), can be evaluated by radionuclide renal scans. The intravenous pyelogram reflects renal anatomy and, to a lesser degree, renal function. The cystogram provides a means of evaluating bladder configuration, and most importantly, the integrity of the vesicoureteral junction.

Also obtain baseline urodynamic studies at this time to assess the three functional components of the lower urinary tract: the detrusor, the bladder neck mechanism, and the external sphincter. The basic urodynamic study should consist of electromyography (EMG) and pressure flow studies, and in patients with evidence of reflex voiding ability, a voiding cystourethrogram (VCUG). Order pressure flow studies to evaluate bladder compliance, resting and voiding intravesicular pressures, and voiding flow rates. External sphincter EMG performed simultaneously documents detrusor-sphincter dyssynergia at the level of the external sphincter. The VCUG dynamically reveals evidence of low-pressure or high-pressure vesicoureteral reflux, and can delineate the specific level of outflow tract obstruction. Urodynamic evaluation allows for functional classification of neurogenic bladder. See the management section of this chapter.

Gastrointestinal System

A paralytic ileus is usually present during the first 3 to 4 days after injury. Evaluation and management during this time focuses on precautionary measures taken to prevent secondary complications of the ileus, such as abdominal distention with respiratory compromise and/or aspiration of pooled gastric secretions; monitoring for evidence of stress-induced gastric ulcerations; and evaluation of patient's nutritional status. Preservation of nutritional stores during this stress-induced hypercatabolic state is very important.

Assessment of the gastrointestinal system during the transitional and chronic phases of SCI should include establishment and monitoring of a routinely performed bowel program, evaluation of problems suggestive of pathologic gastrointestinal pathology, and bodyweight assessment. A significant weight loss during the acute care phase can result in duodenal obstruction secondary to superior mesenteric artery syndrome. Cachexia increases the risk of skin breakdown. Obesity may impair transfers and mobility activities.

Integumentary System

Inspect skin overlying bony prominences for evidence of breakdown. Include the trochanteric areas, sacrum, ischia, occiput, elbows, and scapulae, as well as between the knees, and between the heels. Document any abnormalities. Monitor the status of the tracheostomy stoma; inflammatory reactions in this area can result in air leaks as well as other complications.

Functional Assessment

A rehabilitation program prescription by the physiatrist is based on well-known typical functional outcomes of patients with key levels of injury. Specify goals and activities to be emphasized during occupational and physical therapies. Review the goals and activities of nursing education. The spinal cord injury team members will typically collaborate on these goals under the direction of the physiatrist, who is at an objective vantage point to assess, integrate, and prioritize all aspects of the treatment plan. Modification of standard neurological level-specific goals will be necessary in the presence of co-morbidities such as concurrent traumatic brain injury, orthopedic problems, cardiopulmonary considerations, or advanced age. The degree of motor incompleteness, patient cooperation, and body habitus will also influence achievable goals. There are several functional assessment scales available for use in the rehabilitation setting. The most commonly utilized at this time is the Functional Independence Measure (FIM). Modifications specific to SCI individuals are commonly added to the core 18-item scale.

Table 17-2 summarizes functional expectations of patients with motor complete lesions at key levels. Commonly prescribed adaptive equipment and the average rehabilitation phase hospital stay (ARPHS) are described.

■ Treatment

After the initial assessment the spinal cord injury team, under the leadership of the physiatrist, formulates specific treatment plan goals with respect to medical management needs;

text continues on p. 352

Table 17-2. Functional Expectations Based on Level of Injury

Level of Injury	Functional Expectations
C4 and above	Independent mouthstick activity. Independent electric wheelchair propulsion with pneumatic or chin controls. Dependent in all other ADLs. Able to direct own care. Attendant required.
	Major adaptive equipment required: portable ventilator or other form of ventilatory system if indicated; related pulmonary toileting equipment; environmental control system; +/− mobile arm support. Electric wheelchair with manual backup.
	ARPHS*: 4–5 months and sometimes longer, secondary to the complex nature of the physical, psychological, and environmental support systems required.
C5	Self-feeding, facial hygiene and grooming, and writing accomplished with universal cuff, and setup/minimal assistance. Independent electric wheelchair propulsion with joy stick or chin control. Dependent in all other ADLs. Attendant/care provider required; living alone not practical.
	Major adaptive equipment required: Universal cuff +/− mobile arm supports, electric wheelchair with manual backup.
	ARPHS*: 3 to $3\frac{1}{2}$ months, usually no more than 4 months.

(continued)

Table 17-2. (*Continued*)

Level of Injury	Functional Expectations
C6	Independent feeding, facial hygiene/grooming, and writing with orthotic hand device. Independent locked elbow, horizontal transfers with or without assistance for management of legs. Modified manual wheelchair usually necessary for ramps and uneven terrain. Minimal to moderate assistance for energy-efficient completion of dressing, hygiene, bowel and bladder care; independent driving with hand controls and modified steering wheel.

Major adaptive equipment required: Reciprocal/tenodesis wrist orthotics; lightweight manual wheelchair with modified hand rims; electric wheelchair; care provider required for dressing and toileting.

ARPHS*: 3 to $3\frac{1}{2}$ months, usually no more than 4 months. |
| C7–C8–T1 | Independent in all ADLs with or without adaptive equipment. Lack of hand dexterity in C7 quadriplegia may make self-catheterizations difficult if not impossible. Independent driving with hand controls. Attendant not required, but may be helpful for time-efficient performance of dressing and toiletting activities, especially in patients with a C7 level of injury.

Major adaptive equipment required: lightweight manual wheelchair for shoulder joint preservation.

ARPHS*: 3 to $3\frac{1}{2}$ months, usually no more than 4 months. |

(continued)

Table 17-2. (*Continued*)

Level of Injury	Functional Expectations
T2–T6	Independent in all ADLs. Ambulation with knee ankle foot orthoses (KAFOs) and gait aids typically not realistic goals due to poor trunk control. Independent driving with hand controls.
	Major adaptive equipment required: Lightweight manual wheelchair.
	ARPHS*: $2\frac{1}{2}$ months, usually not more than 3 months.
T7–T12	Independent in all ADLs. The lower the level of injury, the greater the probability of upright ambulation with KAFOs and gait aids-usually exercise ambulation only. Independent driving with hand controls.
	Major adaptive equipment required: Lightweight manual wheelchair $+/-$ KAFOs and crutches/walker.
	ARPHS*: $2\frac{1}{2}$ months, usually not more than three months.
L1–L3	Independent in all ADLs. Upright ambulation with KAFOs and gait aids a realistic goal. Good pelvic control, hip flexors, and at least one fair to good knee extensor that will allow household and/or community ambulation. Wheelchair usually required for more efficient mobility. Able to drive with hand controls.
	Major adaptive equpment: lightweight manual wheelchair, KAFOs and crutches for appropriate candidates.
	ARPHS*: 2 to $2\frac{1}{2}$ months.

(*continued*)

Table 17-2. (*Continued*)

Level of Injury	Functional Expectations
L4–S1	Independent in all ADLs. Bipedal ambulation with bilateral ankle foot orthoses (AFOs) and gait aids. Driving may or may not require hand controls.
	ARPHS*: 1 to 1½ months.

*ARPHS: Average rehabilitation phase hospital stay

bowel, bladder, and skin care; functional skills, including patient education; and psychosocial support. The rehabilitation process begins with admission to the hospital and continues even after successful community reintegration. This involves outpatient physician follow-up visits, therapies, and potential subsequent inpatient rehabilitation admissions for learning additional functional skills, known as staged rehabilitation.

■ Management of Potential Complications

Respiratory System

The principle objective of early pulmonary management of SCI is to minimize the incidence of preventable secondary complications. Specific goals are as follows: prevent hypoxia, prevent and treat atelectasis, achieve and maintain adequate alveolar ventilation, minimize risk of aspiration, and provide aggressive pulmonary toileting to compensate for impaired cough and ineffective clearing of secretions.

Preventative Treatment

Typical components of pulmonary toileting efforts are as follows:

- assisted cough maneuvers or endotracheal suctioning
- respiratory therapy, including postural draining, incentive spirometry, and intermittent positive pressure breathing (IPPB) in conjunction with aerosolized bronchodilators and aminophylline to enhance diaphragmatic function and secretion clearance
- use of a rotating bed, in specific cases.

Intubation

Intubation to establish access for suctioning and bronchoscopy may be required for individuals in whom noninvasive pulmonary toileting proves ineffective. Preferably, intubation should be accomplished with at least a size eight tracheostomy tube to facilitate bronchoscopic examination as necessary. Tracheostomy should be performed early in individuals with injuries at C3 and above, who predictably continue to require long-term ventilatory support. To avoid tracheal injury, tracheal cuff pressures should be monitored and maintained below 25 cm H_2O. When the intubated patient is no longer at risk for aspiration, communication can be greatly enhanced by allowing a ventilator leak around the tracheostomy cuff and through the vocal cords. Ventilator tidal volumes and ventilator alarm sensitivities must be adjusted to accommodate the leak. Through the leak is initially created by simple cuff deflation, it may be more effectively accomplished later by insertion of a cuffless tracheostomy tube.

Assisted Ventilation

The most commonly used method of ventilatory support during the acute phase is positive pressure mechanical ventilation through tracheal intubation. To prevent atelectasis, use tidal volumes of 15 cc/kg of ideal bodyweight. PEEP above 5 cm H_2O can increase the risk of barotrauma. Instead, treat atelectasis with larger ventilator volumes. Suggested ventilator settings are as follows:

- Tidal volume: 15 cc/kg bodyweight
- respiratory rate: 12
- ventilator flow rate: adjusted to obtain P_i between 35 and 40 cm H_2O, and F_iO_2 to keep arterial oxygen saturations at 92% or above. Serially monitor spontaneous ventilation parameters, including forced vital capacity and maximum P_i in the ventilator-dependent patient, to assess potential for weaning.

Weaning

The appropriate technique of ventilator weaning is controversial. Federal Model Systems Spinal Cord Injury Centers favor the technique of progressive ventilator free breathing (PVFB) utilizing a T-piece. The patient is removed from the ventilator for progressively increasing times, alternating with a return to the ventilator for rest periods. However, basic criteria to begin the process include the following:

- clear chest X-ray
- adequate arterial blood gases (ABGs) on a ventilator F_iO_2 setting of 21%
- minimal secretions
- negative inspiratory force of at least -20
- forced vital capacity of at least 15 cc/kg bodyweight.

Avoid weaning too rapidly. Rapid weaning outstrips the muscular endurance of the diaphragm, resulting in a fatigue syndrome. The patient may then be incorrectly labeled as unweanable. Individualize the weaning process for each patient. Maintain the previous ventilator respiratory rate setting, usually 10 to 20, throughout the weaning process.

The following are general guidelines for the T-tube method of weaning:

- Always begin T-tubing in supine position.
- Begin T-tubing for a few to several minutes, 3 to 4 times per day. Gradually increase the times to tolerance, monitoring by pulse oximetry. Periodically check arterial blood gases after T-tube trials.

* Advance T-tubing by 15 to 30 minutes as tolerated every 2 to 3 days.
* Advance T-tubing to 24 hours with ABGs every 8 hours 3 times.
* After the patient is successfully off the ventilator for 24 hours, he/she may be placed back on the ventilator at night or every other night for a few nights to prevent diaphragmatic fatigue.
* Advance the patient as tolerated to 72 to 96 hours off the ventilator.

Problems that can arise during the weaning process include anxiety, air hunger, positional hypotension, mucus plugging, and fatigue.

Artificial Airway

Tracheostomy tube weaning begins by plugging the tube, with suctioning as needed. Once the patient tolerates plugging for several days, the tube can be removed when access to the trachea is no longer needed. In some cases, the tracheostomy site may heal over a period of several months. Keep the tracheostomy tube plugged and in place for a longer period (for example, through one winter season) in individuals with post-traumatic or previous intrinsic lung pathology.

Cardiovascular System

Orthostatic Hypotension

During the early phase of rehabilitation of patients with quadriplegia and high paraplegia, orthostatic hypotension can be significant. Management includes the following:

* apply elastic hose or wrappings to the lower limbs to minimize venous pooling;
* apply abdominal binders to assist respiration in the upright position; and

initiate the sitting program in a reclining-back wheelchair, approaching 90 degrees as tolerated.

When the patient can tolerate sitting at 90 degrees all day
without significant dependent edema or orthostatic symptomatology, remove the stockings. Refractory symptomatic
orthostatic hypotension may be treated by Ephedrine 25 mg
orally 30 to 40 minutes before arising in the morning and
every 6 hours as needed. Florinef 0.1 mg orally once daily
may also be used. Monitor serum potassium as well.

Deep Vein Thromboses/Pulmonary Emboli

The SCI patient is at increased risk for deep venous thrombosis (DVT) and subsequent pulmonary embolism (PE). All
SCI patients should be prophylaxed against DVT. Initial prophylaxis is provided by external pneumatic compression devices that are continued until mobilization is underway, in
addition to low-dose subcutaneous heparin, 5000 units every
8 to 12 hours. In patients considered at additional risk for
DVT, adjusted low-dose heparin or low-dose Coumadin may
be an appropriate alternative. Low molecular weight heparin,
with the advantages of twice-a-day subcutaneous dosing,
greater effectiveness, and a lower incidence of complications,
is the prophylactic treatment of choice. There is yet no clear
consensus in the Federal Spinal Cord Injury Model Centers
on duration of use or parameters appropriate to making such
a determination.

Once the clinical diagnosis of DVT is seriously considered, begin empiric anticoagulation with intravenous
heparin. Refer to Chapter 19, Stroke, for specific orders.
Discontinue heparin if DVT is rule out. Continue oral anticoagulation for 3 months in DVT without PE; for DVT with
PE, continue anticoagulation for 4 to 6 months.

Autonomic Dysreflexia

Autonomic dysreflexia, a syndrome seen in patients with
lesions above T6, can occur at any time post-injury except
during spinal shock. Onset is typically 1 to 4 months after

injury. It is characteristically associated with sudden onset headache, nasal congestion, bradycardia, hypertension, pilo-erection, and flushing or mottling above the level of injury. Typically precipitated by noxious stimuli below the level of the lesion, usually bladder distention, other causes include bladder stones, fecal impaction or bowel distention, and, rarely, distention of other viscera such as the appendix or gallbladder. Pressure ulcers, ingrown toenails, and dysmenor-rhea can also trigger dysreflexia. Hypertension is the major concern; seizures or death can occur as a result of cerebral hemorrhage.

Steps and management are as follows:

- Immediately sit the patient upright if supine.
- Use one of the following agents, listed in order of rapid-ity of onset and duration of action to lower blood pres-sure:
  a) Amyl nitrate 1 ampule inhaled;
  b) Nitroglycerin 1/150 sublingually;
  c) Hydralazine hydrochloride (Apresoline) 10 mg in-tramuscularly or by intravenous push over 30 sec-onds;
  d) Nifedipine (Procardia) 10 mg sublingually (puncture capsule first); may repeat in 30 minutes if hyperten-sion persists; or
  e) Clonidine (Catapres) 0.1 to 0.2 mg orally.
- Catheterize the bladder or check the patency of the in-dwelling catheter.
- If symptoms persist, search for other possible causes.
- If bladder irritation is the suspected etiology, instill 30 cc of Pontocaine 0.25% into the bladder.
- For fecal impaction, insert Nupercainal ointment or suppository. When symptoms subside, gently remove feces.
- If the patient is predisposed to recurrent episodes of dys-reflexia, chronic suppression can be obtained with phe-noxybenzamine hydrochloride (Dibenzyline) 10 mg orally two to three times daily, terazosin hydrochloride (Hytrin) 1 mg orally daily, or nifedipine (Procardia) 10 mg orally three to four times daily.

Genitourinary System

The goals of neurogenic bladder management are to promote preservation of the upper urinary tract, low storage and evacuation bladder pressures, and patient compliance by choosing a technique appropriate for his/her lifestyle, manual dexterity, and overall psychosocial situation. Decisions about the most appropriate long-term urological care plan are made after a systematic assessment of lower urinary tract function in addition to the above considerations. The ideal situation of a catheter-free, sterile urine is not always achievable. Routine management of characteristic types of neurogenic bladders is outlined in Table 17-3.

Management of detrusor-sphincter dyssynergia (DSD) can be directed either towards the detrusor or the sphincteric mechanisms. Factors to consider include the severity of the dyssynergia, the status of the upper tracts, the manual dexterity of the patient, the sex of the patient, and patient preference. Sphincterotomy should not be done prematurely. If the bladder neck is to be resected as well, counsel the patient on the possibilities of continuous dribbling incontinence or the loss of penile erectile function secondary to vascular phenomena. Sphincter ablative procedures should be avoided in female patients with DSD since a reliable external collecting device has yet to be developed. Fortunately, however, DSD does not tend to be as much of a problem in the female SCI population.

Avoid chronic indwelling catheters unless necessitated by the clinical or social situation. One example of appropriate long-term indwelling catheter utilization would be the female quadriplegic patient who lacks the manual dexterity to perform intermittent catheterization. If chronic indwelling catheters are utilized, maintain a high oral fluid intake (> 3 L/day). Use an anticholinergic medication, typically oxybutynin chloride (Ditropan) 5 mg orally twice daily, to decrease bladder reactivity to the catheter. Irrigate the catheter with normal saline periodically if the conduit becomes obstructed with sediment or mucous; change the catheter at least every 2 to 4 weeks. Keep the perineum very clean at all times to minimize migration of gram-negative organisms, normal bowel flora, up and around the catheter.

Table 17-3. Management of Bladder Function by Type

Type	Treatment	Rationale
Hyper-reflexic	Intermittent catheterization program (ICP) with use of anticholinergic medications: oxybutynin chloride (Ditropan) 5 mg orally 2–3 times/day; propantheline bromide (Probanthine) 5–30 mg orally 3–4 times/day; or dicyclomine hydrochloride (Bentyl) 10–20 mg orally 4 times/day.	Increases bladder storage capabilities between ICPs
Detrusor-sphincter Dyssynergia (DSD)		
a) Detrusor	Use anticholinergic agents to convert bladder to areflexic or hyporeflexic storage vessel	Intact sphincter used for continence
b) Sphincter	External sphincterotomy (male patient) with use of external collecting device	Prevents bladder distention and possible ureteral reflux
Areflexic bladder	Intermittent catheterization or catheter-free options a) Crede's maneuver: a method of emptying a flaccid bladder by exerting external pressure over the symphasis pubis b) Artificial urethral sphincter (if tone compromised)	Resting tone of external and internal sphincters remain intact; patient is continent

Regardless of the method of bladder drainage, chemoprophylaxis to decrease the incidence of symptomatic urinary tract infections is controversial. The literature demonstrates no clear evidence that long-term chemoprophylaxis reduces the rates of bacteriuria and symptomatology. However, for circumscribed periods of time during which chemoprophylaxis is felt to be prudent, one may use oral medications, bladder irrigations, or a combination of both. A few such options include:

- Methenamine mandelate (Mandelamine) 1 g + Vitamin C 1 g orally four times daily
- Renacidin 5% bladder irrigation after each catheterization
- Nitrofurantoin (Macrodantin) 100 to 200 mg orally daily
- Cotrimoxazole DS orally daily.

Do not implement these interventions until the evaluation of recurrent symptomatic bacteriuria eliminates renal calculi or poor technique as the etiology.

Gastrointestinal System

Initiate a formal bowel program after the acute-phase ileus has resolved and the patient has begun oral or nasogastric feedings. If ileus persists longer than 3 to 4 days, protect nutritional stores with hyperalimentation until oral intake is possible.

The goal of the bowel program is to train the bowel to evacuate at a set time each day, thereby preventing constipation or fecal incontinence. Performing the bowel program 30 to 60 minutes after a meal will make use of the gastrocolic reflex to assist with peristalsis. Digital stimulation will stimulate the anorectal reflex and peristalsis. Management of the typical reflexic neurogenic bowel consists of the following:

- a diet high in fiber to improve transit time
- stool softeners

- digital stimulation with or without suppositories
- judicious use of laxatives in selected patients.

The patient should perform the bowel program on the commode if sitting balance and tolerance permit. Gravity assists in evacuation. Patients who undergo two consecutive bowel programs with zero to negligible bowel evacuation results should be considered obstipated. Make adjustments to the bowel management program.

In conus or cauda equina injuries, neurogenic bowel management principles are somewhat different. In these lower motor neuron (LMN) injuries, the bowel is functionally areflexic and the external sphincter is typically hypotonic or patulous. A patulous anus provides no structural mechanism for continence. Therefore, in the management of LMN bowels, avoid softeners that increase the risk of bowel accidents. In the absence of extrinsic innervation to the bowel that allows for reflex evacuation, digital stimulation and cathartic suppositories are of limited use. The method of evacuation depends heavily on straining. Manual removal and, in some cases, enemas, are sometimes the only means of emptying the lower colon in such patients.

Integumentary System

The complication of pressure-induced ulcers is unnecessary and costly. Initially, turning schedules of every 2 hours are necessary to prevent tissue necrosis. Over time, with the proper mattress, some patients can build up a tolerance that allows for longer intervals between turning while in bed. Do not substitute mechanical beds for conscientious nursing care. Observe areas over bony prominences, as well as the perineum and intergluteal crease, where soilage or moisture can cause maceration.

Teach patients to perform or request assistance in weight shifting and pressure relief every 15 to 30 minutes while in the wheelchair. Many patients can tolerate a regular 4-inch foam cushion. Those with more fragile skin, or those with high ischial pressures documented by pressure pad evaluation, may benefit from gel or air cushions. Make decisions about wheelchair cushions based on skin-related concerns, as well as decisions about seating systems related to posture and pain issues. See Chapter 15, Pressure Ulcers, for management. Patient education in pressure relief is mandatory.

Musculoskeletal System

Spasticity

Depending on its severity, spasticity can be viewed either as an expected neuropathophysiologic occurrence after spinal cord injury or as a complication. It is a complication if it is painful, interferes with function, or gives rise to problems such as shear-induced or pressure-induced skin breakdown.

Manage increased tone by the following methods:

- Range of motion and sustained stretch activities.
- Pharmacologic interventions as follows:
  Baclofen (Lioresal) 5–10 mg three times/day starting dose; increase by 5 mg every 3 to 4 days until therapeutic response achieved. The usual effective dose is 10–20 mg four times/day. Generally do not exceed more than 120 mg a day.
  Dantrolene (Dantrium) 25–75 mg three to four times/day. This is an especially useful agent in patients who have a cortical supraspinal component to their spasticity, such as the patient with a concurrent traumatic brain injury.
  Diazepam (Valium). This agent is rarely utilized because of its central nervous system (CNS) depressant effects.
- In cases of refractory spasticity, consider implantation of an intrathecal baclofen pump or surgical rhizotomy.
- Five to 7% solutions of phenol can be useful in the control of spasticity during the perioperative/postoperative management of surgically closed sacral or ischial pressure ulcer. See Chapter 15, Pressure Ulcers.

Heterotopic Ossification

Heterotopic ossification (HO) is the formation of bone in soft tissue below the level of injury, most commonly around the hips, knees and elbows. Onset is typically observed 1 to 4 months after injury and is more common in complete injuries. The pathogenesis is unclear. Prevalence is typically cited as 20% to 30%. Clinically significant HO characterized by limitation of joint range of motion occurs in 10% to 20% of the SCI population.

HO may present clinically as unilateral swelling of the lower limbs and must therefore be included in the differential diagnoses, along with DVT, long bone fracture, soft tissue hematoma, and cellulitis. Radiographic evidence during the inflammatory phase is usually absent for 2 to 3 weeks after clinical signs appear. Three-phase bone scans can demonstrate increased uptake as early as 48 hours after initial onset, well before X-rays reveal the process. Elevation of serum alkaline phosphatase is not diagnostically reliable, especially in the presence of associated long bone fractures that may be healing, or in adolescents who are still growing.

Once HO has been detected, begin treatment with etidronate (Didronel) 20 mg/kg/day for 14 days, followed by 10 mg/kg/day for approximately 6 months. Indomethacin (Indocin), 25 mg orally three times/day, and radiation, used in preventing HO after total hip arthroplasty, have not yet been proven to effective treatment in the SCI population. Prophylactic treatment with etidronate (Didronel) during the first 3 months postinjury is advocated by some. However, if the heterotopic bone formation is not compromising joint movement or predisposing the patient to skin breakdown, omit etidronate (Didronel). Pseudoarthroses can be created in bridges of HO that form across joints. Aggressive PROM may be too painful for patients who are sensory incomplete. Some believe that aggressive manipulation can exacerbate HO.

Heterotopic bone tends to be hypervascular; it is not typically surgically removed unless extensive. Initiate etidronate (Didronel) therapy preoperatively; continue it for 6 to 12 months after surgery. Surgery is performed preferably after serial bone scans have shown progressively less uptake over time, indicating relative quiescence of the process.

Neuromuscular System

Post-Traumatic Cystic Myelopathy

The most common cause of late neurological deterioration is progressive post-traumatic cystic myelopathy. Focal cystic cavitation at the site of injury is a common feature of the glial scar formation process. In progressive cystic myelopathy, the cyst expands; progressive destruction of the central areas of the spinal cord occurs. The incidence is between 1% to 5%. Onset of symptoms can occur as early as several months post-injury to as late as 30 years post-injury. MRI is recommended for early detection. Pain is the most common presenting symptom, although modes of presentation vary. Dissociated sensory changes, characterized by loss of pain and temperature perception with relative sparing of light touch perception, is also common. With progression of the cyst, light touch and motor deficits occur. Other presenting symptoms include hyperhidrosis, changes in spasticity and, in patients with lesions above T6, new onset or escalation of autonomic hyperreflexia. Surgical intervention is indicated when symptoms are clearly progressive or if the functional consequences of the presenting symptoms are significant. Typically, surgery consists of cyst-subarachnoid shunting; the spinal cord, if tethered, may require surgical dissection from arachnoid scarring.

Deafferentation Pain

Central deafferentation pain is characterized by a variety of dysphoric sensations at, or diffusely below, the level of injury. It is described as burning, vice-like, twisting, stabbing, crushing, or ripping pain. It can be constant or paroxysmal. Some individuals have pain localized to a gluteal or saddle distribution; others report it as a sensation of a large mass or a stick in the rectum. Increased spasticity, urinary tract infections, dysmenorrhea, constipation, and/or pressure ulcers can cause acute exacerbations.

Pharmacologic interventions yield variable results and typically do not completely eliminate the pain. Commonly used options include amitriptyline (Elavil) 50 to 100 mg at bedtime, nortriptyline (Pamelor) 50 to 100 mg at bedtime, clonazepam (Klonopin) 0.5 to 1.0 mg two to three times/day, or combinations of these agents. When indicated, spasticity control is a component of pain management. Avoid use of narcotics. However, in a small percentage of patients, chronically disabling refractory deafferentation pain can be best treated with Methadone 5 to 10 mg orally two to four times/day.

A number of surgical interventions have been advocated for management of deafferentation pain. Unfortunately, they are generally ineffective. The dorsal root entry zone microcoagulation procedure has shown significant promise in providing immediate and long term relief from central deafferentation pain. The literature reports a 60% to 90% efficacy rate in eliminating small fiber deafferentation pain. The procedure will typically cause loss of sensation in the distribution of the surgical lesions. Loss of motor function can sometimes also occur in the transition zones. For this reason, individuals with quadriplegia are sometimes not considered appropriate candidates due to the risk of functionally significant sensory or motor loss.

Prognosis/Outcome/Follow-Up

Prognosis

SCI can produce a permanent disability regardless of whether it is complete or incomplete. As a rule, if one sees no recovery in a complete lesion (Frankel A) within the first 3 months, further recovery is not expected. If, however, the lesion is incomplete (Frankel B, C, or D) then additional recovery, either sensory or motor, may be possible up to a year or slightly more after injury. Beyond that time, further recovery is not likely.

Functional Outcomes

Physical, psychological and functional adaptation to SCI occurs over a period of time that extends far beyond discharge from an inpatient rehabilitation program. For this reason, comprehensive care of the SCI individual includes early and ongoing integration of vocational counseling, health and fitness education, and assistance with psychosocial adjustment, in addition to traditional medical management issues.

Follow-Up

In general, it is recommended the SCI individual undergo comprehensive assessments, preferably in a SCI system of care, every 1 to 3 years, or more frequently if problems develop. Assessments appropriate during the lifetime care of individuals with SCI include the following:

* weight
* blood pressure and pulse
* forced vital capacity
* biochemical and hematologic studies, including cholesterol/HDL/triglycerides
* urologic evaluation consisting of upper tract evaluation (renogram, ultrasound, or intravenous pyelogram); as well as lower tract evaluation (cystogram, post-void residuals, and cystoscopic examinations)
* motor and sensory evaluation
* equipment and functional assessments
* psychological evaluation
* nursing evaluation.

Age and gender-specific SCI follow-up includes the following. Annual pelvic examination and Papanicolaou smears with breast mammography screening study at age 35 years and then every 1 to 3 years is recommended for women. Annual prostatic evaluations with a digital rectal exam and prostate specific antigen (PSA) as indicated is recommended in men starting at age 45 years. Screening for colon cancer should be pursued per recommendation of the American Cancer Society.

▧ Suggested Readings

American Spinal Injury Association Standards for Neurological Classification of Spinal Cord Injury Patients. Atlanta: The Georgia Regional Spinal Cord Injury Care System, Shepherd Center for Treatment of Spinal Cord Injuries, Inc., 1992.

Balazy TE. Clinical management of chronic pain in spinal cord injury. *Clinical Journal of Pain* 1992;2(8):102–110.

Bloch RF, Basbaum M, eds. *Management of Spinal Cord Injuries*. Baltimore: Williams & Wilkins, 1986.

Carter RE. Respiratory aspects of spinal cord injury management. *Paraplegia* 1987;25:262–266.

Denis F. Spinal instability as defined by the three column spine concept in acute spinal trauma. *Clinical Orthopedics and Related Research* 1984;189:65–76.

Freehafer AA, Hazel CM, Becker CL. Lower extremity fractures in patients with spinal cord injury. *Paraplegia* 1981;19:367–372.

Holdsworth FW. Fractures, dislocations and fracture-dislocations of the spine. *J Bone Joint Surg* 1970;52A(8):1534f.

Lanig IS. The genitourinary system. *In* Whiteneck GG, Charlifue SW, et al., eds. *Aging with Spinal Cord Injury*. New York: Demos Publications, 1992.

Lanig IS, Lammertse DP. The respiratory system in spinal cord injury. *In* Kraft GH, Staas WE, Ditunno JF, eds. *Physical Medicine and Rehabilitation Clinics of North America: Traumatic Spinal Cord Injury*. Philadelphia: W.B. Saunders, 1992.

Lanig IS, Lammertse DP, Gerhart KA. *Durable Medical Equipment for the Patient with Spinal Cord Injury—A Task Force*

Report of the American Spinal Injury Association, 2nd ed. Chicago: 1993.

Merrit JL. Management of spasticity in spinal cord injury. *Mayo Clin Proc* 1981;56:614–622.

Stal S, Serure A, Donovan W, Spira M. The perioperative management of the patient with pressure sores. *Annals of Plastic Surgery.* 1983;11(4):347–356.

Whiteneck GG, Charlifue SS, Gerhart KA, Lammertse DP, et al. *Aging with Spinal Cord Injury.* New York: Demos Publications, 1992.

Whiteneck GG, Lammertse DP, Manley S, Menter RR, eds. *The Management of High Quadriplegia.* New York: Demos Publications, 1989.

Young W. Acute, restorative, and regenerative therapy of spinal cord injury. *In* Piepmeier JM, ed. *The Outcome Following Traumatic Spinal Cord Injury.* Mount Kisco, New York: Futura Publishing Company, 1992, pp. 173–197.

Zejdlik CP, ed. *Management of Spinal Cord Injury.* 2nd ed. Boston: Jones and Bartlett Publishers, 1992.

18

John Cianca

Sports Injury

This chapter introduces the basic principles of musculoskeletal medicine related to sports and human performance. It provides the essentials of the assessment and treatment of any injury that falls into this category. It is not a comprehensive review of treatment protocols or a discussion of all sports injuries.

▓ Factors that Lead to Injury

Injuries can be caused by either of two sets of factors. The first set are intrinsic factors, the second extrinsic factors. Intrinsic factors are those elements that are readily ascribable to the athlete. These include tissue weakness, inflexibility, or overload; biomechanical errors; and lack of conditioning. They also include overall body size, performance ability, and playing style.

Extrinsic factors include faulty equipment, externally driven forces such as other athletes or playing surfaces, and coaching, or the lack thereof. See Table 18-1.

Acute injuries are usually the result of sudden tissue overload and tensile failure. Chronic injuries occur most often from biomechanical and/or training errors. Chronic injuries may be insidious and slowly progressive, or may follow a waxing and waning course with acute exacerbations.

Susan J. Garrison (Ed.): *Handbook of Physical Medicine and Rehabilitation Basics.* First Edition. Copyright © 1995 J. B. Lippincott Company

Table 18-1. Factors that Lead to Injury

Intrinsic	Extrinsic
Tissue: weakness, inflexibility, overload	Faulty equipment
Biomechanical errors	Other athletes
Lack of conditioning	Playing surfaces
Body size	Coaching
Performance ability	Weather
Playing style	

Principles of Biomechanics

The musculoskeletal system is designed to affect the movement of the body. The means by which it does this is referred to as biomechanics. Movement is a function that is intricate, yet appears smooth and simple when performed efficiently with respect to biomechanical principles. Unfortunately, for most people refinement of movement patterns is at best trial and error, if it is attempted at all.

Few people understand or consider how or why their body moves a certain way; the outcome is all that matters. Biomechanical errors of movement are often not considered if the intended outcome is achieved. Therefore, people develop bad habits in movement and in static posture. This often results in injuries, particularly those that are more severe than would be expected given the nature of the circumstances.

There is little or no isolated movement in the body. Since ultimately all structures in the musculoskeletal system are connected, the entire body is affected by dysfunction in a particular area. The connection between the axial and appendicular skeleton occurs at the shoulder and hip; these are the critical points of energy transfer. The scapulae and both sides of the pelvis form the four cornerstones of the musculoskeletal system; through these areas, force to accomplish movement is transferred from the axial to the appendicular skeleton and vice versa. These are critical regions and thus areas where many biomechanical errors occur. As a result, many injuries have their origin in these regions.

People rely on distal limb function to accomplish tasks that are uniquely human. However, safe and efficient distal function is predicated on proximal control. Unless the cornerstones are correctly stabilized before distal function occurs, distal movements become inefficient, eventually leading to fatigue and injury.

A good example of this is the overhand throwing motion. Ground reactive forces are translated through the lower extremities and amplified as they pass through the hip into the spine. From here they are further amplified and transferred through the shoulder into the upper limb. The scapula and its musculature control this transfer, leading to useful force generation in the arm that is moved distally to the wrist, the fingers, and finally, the ball.

Scapular stability controls the efficiency of glenohumeral kinematics. As stability breaks down proximally, distal structures in the kinematic chain are subjected to greater strain and are more vulnerable to injury. The same phenomenon occurs in the lower limb at the sacroiliac joint.

Biomechanical analysis uncovers the layers of dysfunction present in a given movement pattern. Tissue injury complex refers to the area of the body that is disrupted and/or dysfunctional. Specifically, this would be the area of the body that is directly related to the presentation of symptoms. The clinical symptom complex is the constellation of symptoms that arises from an acute injury. This complex can involve pain, swelling, bruising, or any of the other descriptors that accompany the clinical injury. The functional biomechanical deficit refers to the combination of weakness and flexibility that leads to biomechanical errors in movement patterns. This is in essence a description of the factors that led to the tissue injury complex and the clinical symptom complex. The functional adaptation complex is a set of substitutions that are employed to compensate for the injured tissues' loss of function. These compensations are not optimal and tend to perpetuate and amplify already inefficient and unsafe movement patterns. This generally occurs in the more chronic situation. A clear example of this would be the limp that develops in a person with a chronic injury to a lower extremity. It allows the person to continue ambulating but in a faulty fashion that in itself can lead to further injury. Tissue overload complex refers to structures that are vulnerable because of overwork; as a result, subsequent injuries may develop. It is not unusual for this complex to be the precipitating cause of the presenting illness. Such tissues need to be treated and rehabilitated to ensure complete resolution of the problem.

■ Basic Physiatric Tenets of Sport Medicine

The eight basic tenets of sports medicine from the physiatric frame of reference are in Table 18-2. They are the essential elements in treatment of any musculoskeletal injury. Each is described below.

1. Control of Inflammation

The inflammatory process begins at the onset of injury. It is important in the initial stages of damage control and repair by the body; however, if left unchecked, it can impede and

---

Table 18-2. Basic Tenets of Sports Medicine

1. Control of inflammation

2. Pain control

3. Restoration of joint ROM and soft tissue extensibility

4. Restoration of muscular strength

5. Restoration of muscular endurance

6. Retraining in biomechanics

7. Maintaining cardiovascular fitness

8. Development of programs to maintain strength, flexibility, conditioning, and skills

---

prolong injury repair and rehabilitation. Effective control of inflammation begins at the time of the injury with compression at the injury site and prompt application of ice. Icing should be done for 15 to 20 minutes at least 2 to 3 times daily for the first 48 to 72 hours. If the injury is severe and is accompanied by ecchymosis and profound edema, ice should be applied as frequently as every hour for 15 to 20 minutes during the first 24 to 48 hours. Be careful to protect the skin from thermal injury by application of a towel or cloth. If using ice massage, the layer of water that forms between the skin and the ice should be sufficient to protect the skin from injury. Compression of the injury, along with rest and elevation, decreases swelling. The use of anti-inflammatory agents is an effective and sometimes powerful adjunct in the control and reduction of inflammation. Nonsteroidal anti-inflammatory drugs (NSAIDS) are the first line of pharmacologic intervention. Local and systemic glucocorticoids are often very effective, but these should be used judiciously and reserved for refractory and/or severe inflammation.

2. Pain Control

Pain also begins with the injury and progresses during the ensuing 24 to 48 hours. It is during the initiation of the pain process that intervention is critical. If pain is left uncontrolled, limitation of movement can become prolonged and severe. However, pain is an indicator of injury severity; absolute ablation of pain can be counterproductive, by providing a false sense of security to the patient. It is important that the patient be comfortable, yet still aware that there is an injury present.

Musculoskeletal injury pain control can be accomplished in several ways. Limiting inflammation reduces tissue distension, thus making the injured area less tender. Compression and rest decrease inflammation and promote healing of the injured tissue. Icing limits pain by reducing reactive muscle hypertonus and providing superficial analgesia. Ice also causes vasoconstriction, which slows hemorrhage and decreases metabolic activity, thereby decreasing inflammation and pain.

NSAIDS are effective in pain control by reducing inflammation as well as decreasing pain. Refer to Chapter 2, Acute Pain. Modalities such as transcutaneous electrical nerve stimulation (TENS) serve as a counterirritant and therefore block perception of pain. Limitation of weight-bearing and the use of splints, braces, and taping serve to protect the injured area by limiting potentially unstable movement and controlling edema. This allows rest of the injured area and prevents the perpetuation of pain.

Pain and inflammation control is an interrelated process essential to the initiation of healing and rehabilitation. Once pain and inflammation are controlled, the next phase of rehabilitation can begin. This initial phase is the foundation of later phases and provides for repair of damaged tissue.

3. Restoration of Joint Range of Motion and Soft Tissue Extensibility

Pain-free full joint active range of motion (AROM), as well as soft tissue extensibility surrounding the joint, must be restored prior to initiating strengthening or endurance exercise. AROM prevents joint contracture and resulting functional limitation. Failure to reach full AROM prior to strengthening may lead to reinjury and/or biomechanical error.

Passive techniques are first used (PROM), followed by active assisted (AAROM) and then AROM. PROM does not require muscle activation and therefore can be used very early in the rehabilitation process. It can help reduce edema as well as promoting early return of joint function. The muscles and supporting structures are allowed to rest, resulting in less pain and edema.

4. Restoration of Muscular Strength

Once painfree full AROM is restored, strengthening can begin. It is initiated with isometric exercises and progresses through manual resistance, elastic tubing (Theraband), isotonic, then isokinetic and finally functional testing. Isometric exercises protect injured joints and antagonist muscles since they do not cause movement. They can actually be started before restoration of full range of motion because of the lack of movement production. Elastic tubing exercises are an excellent way of introducing strengthening via AROM since they provide minimal, yet constant resistance. There are several grades of tubing resistance, typically categorized according to color by the specific manufacturer. Isotonic exercise involves the use of machines or free weights that provide greater amounts of resistance and also require more skill in integrating other body parts to varying degrees in any given exercise. Isokinetic strengthening incorporates changing rates of speed in the movement arm, making the exercise more functionally based. Functional testing utilizes the actual activity to be performed; it is therefore the most challenging to the recovering athlete because strength is required in specific movement patterns. Coordination is much more important in these exercises.

Resistance exercise consists of sets of repetitions. Sets that consist of 15 to 30 repetitions are used to develop muscular endurance. Sets that consist of 10 repetitions or less are used to enhance power. Generally speaking, there should be a day of recovery between resistance workouts to allow muscles to rebuild. If muscle soreness lasts beyond 24 hours after exercise, the next resistance session should be delayed until the soreness has abated.

5. Restoration of Muscular Endurance, Including Unloading

This tenet is reached with strengthening. Generally speaking, low-weight, high-repetition weight sets develop muscular endurance. Isometric sets can also increase a muscle's endurance. Variable resistance aerobic equipment is useful in developing muscular endurance in limb muscles, as well as promoting cardiovascular fitness. Water exercise therapy, such as swimming or aqua running, is very useful in maintaining fitness and enhancing endurance, especially in injuries that necessitate weight-bearing restrictions. This type of treatment is called unloading. It can also be land-based, through the use of pulleys and harnesses to counter the effect of body weight to varying degrees.

6. Retraining in Biomechanics; Activity-Specific Movement Patterns

At this stage of treatment the patient has regained full ROM and functional strength in the affected area. Muscular endurance has also returned and injured tissue is responsive to the demands of sustained activity. Retraining the athlete in a sports-specific fashion has several advantages. The adage "practice makes perfect" is quite correct. The more a specific skill is performed, the more ingrained it becomes, in a process known as engram formation. The need for correct technique is obvious. The muscle is repetitively taken through motion and force requirements when a specific task is performed. Sport-specific retraining allows for proper biomechanical function, thereby preventing the development of substitution patterns that can lead to re-injury. By the end of the program the athlete has become more efficient in the activity, resulting in a safer, more effective performance.

7. Maintaining Cardiovascular Fitness

As an injury is treated, generalized conditioning can be advanced as soon as the athlete is able to tolerate sustained activity. This may be almost immediately if the affected area can be protected or rested during aerobic activity. Cross-training is a valuable addition to rehabilitation programs for this reason. As the injured area recovers, it can be incorporated into the fitness program. Eventually, the athlete functions at full capacity in an aerobic program; cardiovascular fitness can be improved and subsequently maintained. (Refer to Chapter 7, Cardiovascular Conditioning Exercise and Cardiac Rehabilitation).

8. Development of Programs to Maintain Strength, Flexibility, Conditioning, and Skills

These programs are integrated into the rehabilitation program as soon as active teaching is completed in a given area. At this point the athlete assumes responsibility for ongoing function beyond the rehabilitation program. It is an absolutely essential step in the return to safe, effective, independent function. Flexibility, strength, and aerobic fitness all need to be incorporated into maintenance programs.

■ Phases of Rehabilitation

See Figure 18-1.

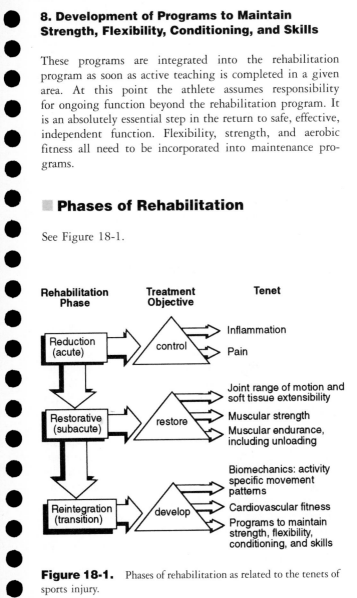

Figure 18-1. Phases of rehabilitation as related to the tenets of sports injury.

Reduction (Acute) Phase

This phase includes inflammation and pain control; it centers on the control of the acute signs and symptoms of an injury. In an acute injury such symptoms include pain and inflammation as a result of local tissue injury. This injury can involve macro and/or micro trauma. The PRICE principle— protection, rest, ice, compression, and elevation—is an effective means of implementing intervention. Such measures should be used as soon as possible following injury.

In a chronic injury signs and symptoms are not as apparent; however, protection, rest, and icing are still important measures. Much of the damage is at a micro level and is due to repetitive overload and secondary compensations that lead to inefficient and faulty biomechanics. This in turn can lead to further tissue injury and/or dysfunction.

Restorative (Subacute) Phase

This phase includes the restoration of joint range of motion and soft tissue extensibility and restoration of muscular strength and endurance, including unloading. The injury is now subacute in nature, having been treated when acute in the reduction phase. Therapy is designed to prepare tissues for return to integrated function in a specific task. Flexibility (ROM) is restored first, followed by strength, and then endurance. The tenets can overlap somewhat, but generally it is best to advance rehabilitation through these tenets sequentially.

This phase may take the greatest amount of time and effort in therapy. Advancement to the next phase is predicated upon successful restoration of flexibility, strength, and endurance. For this reason it is important to maintain cardiovascular fitness by means that still allow for restoration of injured tissue. For instance, if there is an ankle injury that precludes weight-bearing during the restoration phase, fitness can be maintained by an arm ergonomer or by aqua running, which is nonweight-bearing.

Encourage the patient to take a more active role in recovery. The transition toward self-care is an important step in prompt return to independent function, and can best be accomplished by development of a home exercise program that mimics or supplements what has been taught in therapy. It then becomes the patient's responsibility to comply with the exercise program.

Finally, this phase serves as an initiation of the transition to coordinated tissue function. As flexibility is restored, strengthening begins. As strength returns, endurance training can be instituted. By the completion of this phase, the patient is ready to begin retraining in sport-specific tasks.

Reintegration (Transition) Phase

This phase consists of graded retraining in function. It begins with low-speed sport-related drills. Once a task is accurately performed, repetitions are increased and then the speed of performance of the reps is increased. The drills are then grouped into sessions. Once sessions are mastered in a similar fashion as the individual drills, the athlete is advanced to sport-specific maneuvers or activities.

When the athlete has mastered the skills necessary to perform the sport in safe and efficient form, practice of the activity on a regular basis begins. Concomitantly, cardiovascular fitness that has been developed is maintained. These two activities merge as the athlete begins performance of the sport for extended periods of time. At this point, rehabilitation moves into maintenance programs, and the athlete progresses to independent function in activities. Thus, rehabilitation is completed. The maintenance program is the most important aspect of the entire rehabilitative process, as it assures ongoing independence and prevention of re-injury.

■ History and Physical Examination

History

Include a description of the current dysfunction and any similar previous occurrences. A thorough pain description should be obtained, including the location, frequency and intensity of the pain. Pain descriptors pertaining to pain quality, radiation and time of occurrence are appropriate. A rating of the pain such as from 1 to 10 can be helpful as a means of evaluating pain intensity from visit to visit. Attempts to elucidate what relieves, exacerbates, or worsens the pain are also important.

Obtain a description of the events leading up to and occurring during the actual injury. The mechanism of injury is the process of mechanical disruption or compromise that causes the injury. Ask questions that help recreate the scene. Have the patient describe what was happening when the injury occurred, and describe in what position the injury began. See Table 18-3 for common sports-related injuries. If there was outside force, attempt to quantify its magnitude and from what direction it came. Record any other descriptors, such as an audible pop or snap, that might contribute to an understanding of the injury.

Once the mechanism of injury has been identified, the tissue or structures involved should be more obvious. This helps direct the physical exam and contributes to an understanding of the severity of the injury. However, often there is no discrete point of injury; therefore a mechanism of injury is not as clear. In these cases, it is still helpful to have the athlete describe activities that seem to exacerbate the injury. This helps develop a functional picture of the injury.

It is also very useful to know about previous injuries, as they can shed light on pre-existing dysfunctions or methods of biomechanical compensation. Frequently the current injury is directly related to previous injuries, or indirectly a result of trauma from other activities.

Recent treatments can also provide clues to the process. These might include other physician visits, allied health interventions, or self-administered treatment. This information can also help to direct the treatment plan once the injury has been clearly defined.

Physical Examination

The area in question must be clearly visible. Have as much of the body exposed as necessary, but protect the patient's modesty; clothe the patient in a pair of shorts and a T-shirt or jog

Table 18-3. Common Injuries in Selected Physical Activities

Sport	Injury
Running	Plantar fasciitis
	Iliotibial band friction syndrome
	Patellofemoral dysfunction
	Hamstring tightness
	Low back pain
	Ankle sprains
	Achilles tendinitis
	Shin splints
	Stress fractures
Racquet sports	Lateral epicondylitis
	Rotator cuff impingement
	Muscle strains
Football	Mild head injury
	Ligamentous injury to the knee
	Dislocations and fractures
	Muscle strains
	Joint dislocations (shoulder, knee)
Basketball	Ankle sprains
	Muscle strains
	Jumper's knee (patellar tendinitis)
	Ligamentous injuries to the knee
Throwing Sports	Rotator cuff impingement
	Lateral epicondylitis
	Shoulder instability

(continued)

Table 18-3. (*Continued*)

Sport	Injury
Skiing	Mild to severe head injury
	Shoulder dislocation
	Clavicular fracture
	Knee ligament injuries
	Lower limb fractures
	Skier's thumbs
	Patellofemoral dysfunction

bra to begin the exam. As the exam progresses, these articles can be removed as indicated.

Begin the exam with visual inspection of posture, noting the condition of the axial skeleton. Inspect the area of complaint for deformities, erythema, or asymmetry. Compare this area to the other side of the body, if appropriate.

Palpate contiguous structures and proceed centrally to the area of injury. Initially, palpate lightly to obtain a general feel for the tissue and the surrounding structures, then deeper and more localized, noting areas of tension or asymmetry.

The passive portion of the exam consists of manual muscle testing, range of motion testing, neurologic assessment, and provocative testing to elicit tissue dysfunction.

Dynamic assessment is necessary to obtain a functional diagnosis. It involves biomechanical evaluation during movement pertinent to the injury.

Assimilation and Differential Diagnosis

Formulate a differential diagnosis after considering the data and a biomechanically reasonable hypothesis. Identify all involved structures and their roles in the injury process so that the underlying cause, as well the presenting injury, can be corrected.

Utilize the components of soft tissue injury as outlined earlier in this chapter for a broader and more in-depth understanding of the biomechanical process of injury as it relates to particular athletes. This contributes to the formation of a differential diagnosis. The differential diagnosis then sums up all the clinical entities that contribute to or involve pathologies in any of the five components of soft tissue injury. More traumatic acute processes or injuries may not have this depth of involvement, and may be described and understood by simpler terminology. In the end, the differential diagnosis becomes an aid in the process of treating any given injury.

▨ Therapy Prescription

Writing a prescription for physical therapy should be a precise means of communication from the physician to the therapist. Simply writing "evaluate and treat" nullifies the time and effort of the physician's evaluation, and gives the therapist no helpful information in the attempt to treat the patient. It is ineffective and inadequate communication.

A proper physical or occupational therapy prescription contains the complete diagnosis, with elaboration of the involved structures. It also specifies the types of methods called for and the area to be treated. The prescription gives a time frame for implementation of the therapies, and indicates the frequency and duration of therapy. Finally, it includes special instructions for restrictions and variations in treatment. Table 18-4 is an example of a prescription for sports medicine.

Pursue conservative treatment at the onset and for as long as progress continues. Reserve surgical intervention for those cases that are obviously unstable (such as an anatomical defect as a result of trauma), have demonstrated no progress, or have reached an endpoint in conservative therapy.

▨ Types of Therapies

Sports medicine therapies are shown in Table 18-5. In addition, modalities such as heat or cold, typically used for other

Table 18-4. Example of a General Sports Medicine
Prescription

Diagnosis: Right supraspinatus impingement with
underlying scapular instability.

Treatment: (Note: A, B, and C are prescribed sequentially as
the athlete advances through the three phases of rehabilitation
over several weeks to months.)

A. *Acute*: Treat supraspinatus muscle with phonophoresis and
range of motion; progress to strengthening program for all
rotator cuff muscles.

B. *Restorative*: Begin scapular stabilizer muscle program with
myofascial release techniques for the superior trapezius and
levator scapulae. Strengthen the middle and inferior scapular
muscles, including the rhomboids, middle and lower
trapezius, and the serratus anterior to promote balanced
muscular stabilization of the scapula. Concurrently stretch the
anterior chest wall, including the pectoralis major and minor.

C. *Reintegration*: As pain subsides and range of motion returns,
re-educate the shoulder girdle muscles in proper firing
sequence for upper extremity activities such as throwing.

Frequency/duration: Please treat 2–3 times weekly for one
month.

Special instructions: Please treat one on one during the
acute phase of treatment and thereafter as closely as possible.
Keep me updated with problems as they arise and with
patient progress. The patient will see me again in 4 weeks.

Next Physician Visit: 4 weeks.

rehabilitative problems, may be indicated. Refer to Chapter
2, Acute Pain.

■ Special Populations

The pediatric population undergoes much of the same injury
processes as adults; however, there are specific issues that
need to be addressed. The pediatric patient tends to lack

text continues on p. 387

Table 18-5. Typical Sports Medicine Therapies

Therapy	Description
Myofascial Release	Deep massage to an area in order to free layers of tissue from movement restrictions, alleviating pain and promoting unified tissue function
Unloading	A method of relieving a portion of the patient's body weight (by means of pulleys or by water) to lessen the impact to a certain area during exercise, allowing the patient to exercise within the parameters of weight-bearing restriction
Stretching	Performed in either dynamic or static fashion
	Passive: Uses only external force
	Active Assisted: Uses a combination of external and internal forces
	Active: Uses force provided by the participant alone
	Proprioceptive neuromuscular facilitation (PNF): The muscle antagonist is activated, then passive stretch occurs.
Strengthening	A program of muscle contractions
	Concentric: A shortening contraction
	Eccentric: A lengthening contraction
	Isometric: Activating the muscle without movement
	Isotonic: Moving a uniform load by muscle contraction
	Isokinetic: Moving a varying load by muscle contraction at a uniform speed

(continued)

Table 18-5. (*Continued*)

Therapy	Description
Proprioceptive	Exercises promoting position sense without visual input to enhance joint function.
Manual therapies	Articulation: A technique of rhythmic oscillation applied to a joint which attempts to restore neutral mechanics to that joint
	Muscle energy: The patient develops force through activating muscles used by the therapist to influence the bony structure to which the muscles are attached
	High-velocity/low-amplitude: A quick but forceful thrust applied externally by the therapist; used cautiously, particularly in older or frail patients
Alternative therapies	Pilates: Exercise that promotes rhythmic movement through proximally-based strength, flexibility, and coordination
	Feldenkrais: Use of movement to increase kinesthetic awareness, enabling more graceful, safer movement
	Alexander technique: Focuses on kinesthetic awareness, particularly of the head and neck, to improve posture during movement
	Water exercise therapy: Unloading that relies on submergence in water, that can accomplish greater levels of unloading than land-based therapy

(*continued*)

Table 18-5. (*Continued*)

Therapy	Description
	Plyometrics: Activities using rapid eccentric muscle contraction to facilitate a more powerful concentric contraction
	Work hardening: Therapy designed to reacclimatize the worker to the work environment in a safe, efficient fashion
	Open kinetic chain activities: Distal aspect of the exercised limb is nonweightbearing
	Closed kinetic chain activities: Distal aspect of the exercised limb is weight-bearing during exercise, more functionally based than open chain activities

stability and strength in tissues that are undergoing rapid growth. Typically, injury results at the sites of maximal growth. The epiphyseal regions of bones are particularly vulnerable. The apophyseal areas, where muscles attach to bone, are also at risk for overload or overuse injury. Children are particularly susceptible to injury during or just after a growth spurt, because of a lag in development of soft tissue tensile strength. Overuse and overload injuries diminish as children gain strength and stability in soft tissue structures and as epiphyses close. Acute injuries to growth plates typically require orthopedic attention. Utilize the recovery period as an opportunity for education in biomechanics, because during these formative years proper technique can be taught and integrated into the child's movement patterns. Therefore, emphasize proper technique and movement re-education during the restorative phase of rehabilitation.

Women comprise a group of patients who have unique sports medicine issues, specifically the role of exercise as related to pregnancy, the menstrual cycle, and the prevention of osteoporosis.

The geriatric athlete also has special concerns, because aging tissues lose their resiliency to injury, becoming weaker and less pliable. As a result there is less room for error in exercise. Injuries take longer to rehabilitate and must be rehabilitated in a less vigorous fashion. Counsel the geriatric athlete about these issues. The same general rehabilitation principles that apply to younger adults also apply to the geriatric population, but the time frame of recovery tends to be longer.

■ Patient Education

The doctor-patient-therapist relationship is a dynamic working alliance. It demands the respect of all three parties. The doctor/patient relationship is one where mutual responsibility is the rule. The doctor acts as the educator, to empower the patient in coming to a new understanding of the workings of the body. The patient must assume the responsibility for regaining health and then maintaining it. The therapist enters the picture to help the physician in the education process, by using therapeutic techniques to educate the patient in the reattainment of health. In working with the therapist, the patient takes on the responsibility of becoming an active participant in health care, first by attending therapy, then by actively participating in the process of moving through acute therapy into a home-based program. The physician and therapist should work together in one conjoined care plan.

One-on-one therapist-patient interactions are best, especially in the acute phase of therapy. Having multiple therapists for one patient tends to lead to variation in treatment methods, which can be less effective, disconcerting to the patient, and decreases to patient compliance.

Patient education and empowerment are the goals of this triad of treatment. As one becomes educated, the ability to make decisions and eventually to take action in a productive fashion increases. The patient regains control of the condition as understanding of the situation and its implications grows. The doctor and the therapist are the facilitators of this process. The patient ultimately determines if the situation will change, assuming the doctor and the therapist have fulfilled their roles.

■ Follow-Up and Discharge

Once the therapeutic program has begun, regular follow-up with the physician is needed to monitor progress and to make adjustments in the program. During these follow-up visits, the therapist's notes should be available for review. The patient should also provide an impression of progress. In this way, the physician can monitor the patient's progress and evaluate the effectiveness of the patient-therapist interaction.

Follow-up visits become less frequent as the rehabilitation program continues. However, additional visits may be necessary if complications arise. In general, though, the patient eventually visits with the doctor only for evaluation of progress. At this point, discharge from physician care should be considered.

■ Suggested Readings

Cailliet R. *Shoulder Pain.* 2nd ed. Philadelphia: F.A. Davis, 1981.

Herring SA. Rehabilitation of muscle injuries. *Med Sci Sports Exer* 1990;22:4:453–456.

Hoppenfeld S. *Physical Examination of the Spine and Extremities.* Norwalk, CT: Appleton Century Cross, 1976.

Kibler WB. Clinical aspects of muscle injury. *Med Sci Sports Exer* 1990;22:4:450–452.

Reid DC. *Sports Injury Assessment and Rehabilitation.* New York: Churchill Livingstone, 1992.

Saal JA. Rehabilitation of the injured athlete. *In* DeLisa JA, Gans B, eds. *Rehabilitation Medicine: Principles and Practice.* 2nd ed. Philadelphia: J.B. Lippincott, 1993, pp. 1131–1164.

Saal JA. Dynamic muscular stabilization in the nonoperative treatment of lumbar pain syndrome. *Orthopedic Review* 1990;19:8:691–700.

Strauss RH. *Sports Medicine.* Philadelphia: W.B. Saunders, 1984.

Team Physician Course, Part I. Dallas, Texas: American College of Sports Medicine, February 9–23, 1994.

19

Susan J. Garrison

Stroke

Definition

A stroke, or cerebrovascular accident (CVA), is an infarction of the brain in which ischemia or hemorrhage causes disruption of function. Characterized by sudden onset focal neurological deficit, hemiparesis is the hallmark of stroke. The terms CVA and stroke are generally used interchangeably. To avoid confusion, use a description such as right CVA with left hemiparesis.

Anatomy

Symptoms of stroke may arise from the anterior circulation, involving the carotid artery and its main branches; the anterior and middle cerebral arteries; or the posterior circulation, including the vertebral basilar and posterior cerebral arteries. Eighty percent of strokes occur in the carotid distribution, resulting in weakness of one side of the body, involving the face, arm, or leg in any combination. CVAs in the posterior circulation, known as brain stem strokes, are generally a result of thrombosis and occlusion of small, penetrating arterioles arising directly from the vertebrobasilar arteries. The clinical picture of a brain stem stroke is more complex, due

Susan J. Garrison (Ed.): *Handbook of Physical Medicine and Rehabilitation Basics*. First Edition. Copyright © 1995 J. B. Lippincott Company

to the more compact arrangement of important neurological structures in that location when compared to the cerebral hemispheres.

Epidemiology

The most common serious neurologic problem in the world, in the United States stroke is second only to head trauma as the leading cause of neurologic disability. CVA ranks behind heart disease and cancer as the third commonest cause of death in the western world. Approximately 500,000 new CVAs occur annually in the United States; about two-fifths of these are fatal. Eighty percent of those hospitalized for stroke sustain such limited neurological deficit that rehabilitation is not necessary. However, 20% of patients hospitalized for stroke require some type of rehabilitative services.

The incidence of stroke has fallen despite an aging population. This decrease is attributed to emphasis on healthy lifestyles, better management of hypertension, use of antiplatelet agents, and management of other cardiac diseases. However, the prevalence of stroke, the number of those who have sustained previous stroke, continues to increase as the population ages.

Etiology/Pathophysiology

There are four major forms of vascular disease of the brain (see Table 19-1). Thrombotic strokes are usually due to atherosclerotic stenosis or occlusion of the carotid or middle cerebral artery. The deficit may be preceded by transient ischemic attacks (TIAs) or evolve over time, since thrombotic occlusion occurs gradually. Embolic strokes, in contrast, occur abruptly as platelets, cholesterol, fibrin, or other blood components float in the circulation until they occlude small distal cortical vessels. Strokes occurring in the setting of myocardial infarction are usually a result of cardiac emboli. Lacunar strokes are very small infarctions, less than 1 cm^3, occurring where small perforating arterioles branch directly

Table 19-1. Forms of Vascular Disease of the Brain

Thrombotic	40%
Embolic	30%
Lacunar	20%
Hemorrhagic	10%
	100%

off large vessels. Hemorrhagic stroke is the most catastrophic. Regions of the brain affected are similar to those affected in lacunar stroke, including the basal ganglia, internal capsule, and brainstem.

Assessment/Evaluation

Perform a thorough neurological evaluation, including history and physical examination at the time of presentation. Repeat it frequently to assess further neurologic deficit. Document risk factors. Routine diagnostic evaluations may include computerized axial tomography (CAT scan) of the head, electroencephalogram (EEG), magnetic resonance imaging (MRI), carotid Doppler studies, cardiac evaluation, including 2-D echocardiograms as well as electrocardiogram (EKG), and routine bloodwork with clotting times. These studies are undertaken to determine cause of the stroke, so that risk factors may be addressed. See Table 19-2.

Typical patterns of deficits occur that may aid in localization of ischemic stroke. Lesions of the anterior cerebral artery usually result in paralysis and cortical hypesthesia of the contralateral lower limb, with mild involvement of the contralateral arm (Figure 19-1). There may be impaired judgement and insight, incontinence of bowel and bladder, apraxia of gait, and sucking and grasping reflexes of the contralateral side.

Middle cerebral infarction typically produces contralateral hemiplegia. Usually, the arm is more affected than the leg. Sensation is impaired in the same areas as motor loss (cortical

Table 19-2. Risk Factors for Stroke

Age

Hypertension

Cardiac impairment

Previous CVA

TIAs

Diabetes

sensory deficit, or cortical hypesthesia). Blindness in one half of the visual field (hemianopsia), inability to recognize persons and things (agnosia), or difficulty in communicating (dysphasia) may occur. See Figure 19-2.

Posterior cerebral artery lesions result in mental change with memory impairment, inability to recognize or comprehend written words (alexia) or people and things (visual agnosia). The third cranial nerve may be paralyzed. Cortical blindness (unawareness by the patient that he cannot see) or hemianopsia may occur. See Figure 19-3.

Brain stem strokes either leave minor deficits, or are so severe that recovery is rare. Typical brain stem deficits include swallowing, visual, and balance problems.

Functional Evaluation

Several functional evaluation scales have been devised for use in stroke and other disabilities. The most widely accepted is the Functional Independence Measure (FIM). The FIM involves seven levels of function within six areas, including self-care, sphincter management, mobility, locomotion, communication, and social cognition.

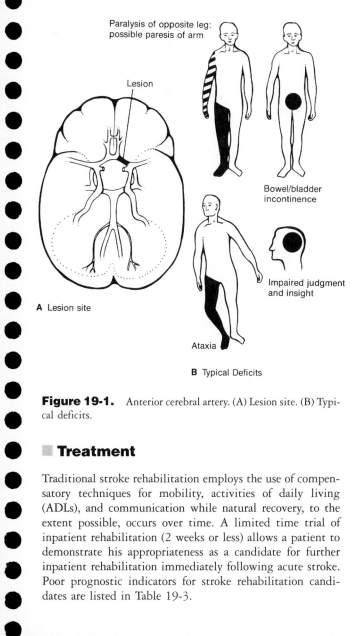

Paralysis of opposite leg: possible paresis of arm

Lesion

A Lesion site

Bowel/bladder incontinence

Impaired judgment and insight

Ataxia

B Typical Deficits

Figure 19-1.   Anterior cerebral artery. (A) Lesion site. (B) Typical deficits.

▓ Treatment

Traditional stroke rehabilitation employs the use of compensatory techniques for mobility, activities of daily living (ADLs), and communication while natural recovery, to the extent possible, occurs over time. A limited time trial of inpatient rehabilitation (2 weeks or less) allows a patient to demonstrate his appropriateness as a candidate for further inpatient rehabilitation immediately following acute stroke. Poor prognostic indicators for stroke rehabilitation candidates are listed in Table 19-3.

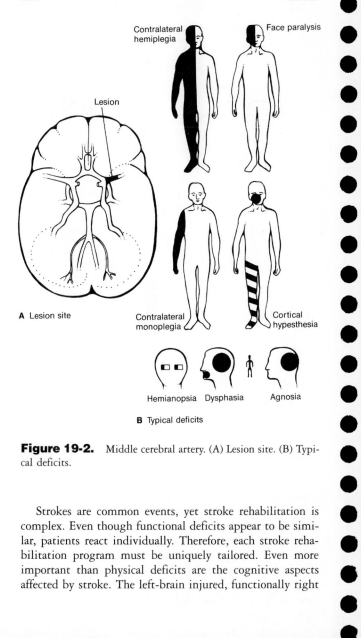

Figure 19-2. Middle cerebral artery. (A) Lesion site. (B) Typical deficits.

Strokes are common events, yet stroke rehabilitation is complex. Even though functional deficits appear to be similar, patients react individually. Therefore, each stroke rehabilitation program must be uniquely tailored. Even more important than physical deficits are the cognitive aspects affected by stroke. The left-brain injured, functionally right

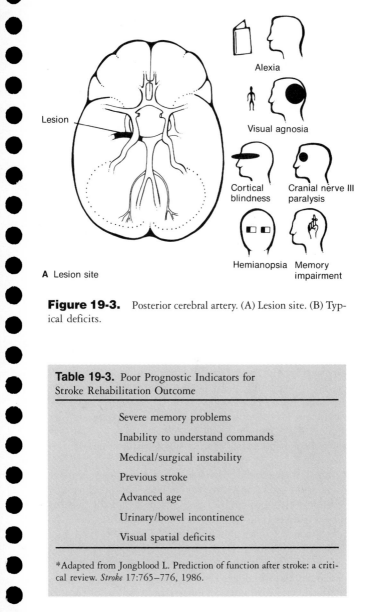

A Lesion site

Figure 19-3. Posterior cerebral artery. (A) Lesion site. (B) Typical deficits.

Table 19-3. Poor Prognostic Indicators for Stroke Rehabilitation Outcome

Severe memory problems

Inability to understand commands

Medical/surgical instability

Previous stroke

Advanced age

Urinary/bowel incontinence

Visual spatial deficits

*Adapted from Jongblood L. Prediction of function after stroke: a critical review. *Stroke* 17:765–776, 1986.

Table 19-4. Characteristics of Right and Left
Hemiplegic Patients

Right Hemiplegic (Left-Brain Injured)	vs.	Left Hemiplegic (Right-Brain Injured)
Communication impairment		Visual/motor perceptual problems
Learns by demonstration		Loss of visual memory
Will learn from mistakes		Left side neglect
May require supervision due to communication problems		Impulsive
		Lacks insight/judgment, requires supervision

From Garrison SJ, Learning after stroke: left versus right brain injury.
Topics in Geriatric Rehabilitation 1991;6:3:45–52.

hemiplegic patient is much different with respect to communication and learning than the right-brain injured,
functionally-left hemiplegic patient. See Table 19-4. These
differences must be recognized and addressed in treatment.

Rehabilitation of the stroke patient begins in the acute
care setting. Timely intervention maximizes potential recovery and prevents problems due to immobility. See Chapter
10, Immobility. Post-stroke rehabilitation of the uncomplicated, medically stable patient is generally as follows. See
Table 19-5. However, medical problems at any stage may
slow the rehabilitation process (see Complications in this
chapter).

Medical treatment of stroke consists of evaluation of the
cause of the stroke and correction of underlying problems, if
possible. One aspirin a day is the current accepted treatment
for the patient who has sustained a thrombotic stroke. Di-
pyridamole (Persantine) has not been shown to be efficacious.
Ticlopidine (Ticlid), 250 mg orally twice daily, is indicated
in thrombotic stroke if aspirin is not tolerated. Embolic stroke
patients should undergo thorough cardiovascular examinations, and be anticoagulated, long-term, if indicated. Lacunar

Table 19-5. Basic Guidelines for Post-Stroke Rehabilitation*

Day 1–3 (Bedside)
Avoid positioning on affected limbs

Relieve common pressure areas, such as heels and sacral area

Document reflexes, tone, and muscular strength

Begin PROM & AAROM, daily by OT/PT or nurse

Dangle out of bed

Sit in chair

Document bowel/bladder function

Identify communication deficits

Implement dietary modifications

Assess social situation

Days 3–5 (To Therapy Department)
Send to PT/OT department by wheelchair

Use wheelchair cushion; avoid doughnut cushion

Evaluate ambulation potential in parallel bars

Baseline evaluations by PT/OT

Provide sling if shoulder subluxed

Remove indwelling catheter; begin timed voiding

Days 7–10 (Acute Inpatient Rehabilitation)
Transfer activities (wheelchair to mat; wheelchair to bed)

Pre-gait activities

Admission to acute rehab unit

ADL practice: a.m. care and dressing

Psychological evaluation

Strategies for communication

Swallowing addressed by speech/dietary therapy

Learning independence at wheelchair level

(continued)

Table 19-5. (*Continued*)

2–3 Weeks (Acute Inpatient Rehabilitation)
Upgrade gait: assistive device/AFO

Team/family conference regarding prognosis and discharge planning

Therapeutic home evaluation

Upgrade from bedside commode to bathroom

3–6 Weeks (Acute Rehabilitation Discharge)
Family member/caretaker learns home program

Self-medications taught

Independent in dressing, grooming

Independent in wheelchair transfers and mobility

Bathroom and kitchen evaluations complete

Upgrade diet

Communication needs addressed

10–12 Weeks (Outpatient Physician Office Follow-up)
Review functional abilities

Discuss safety issues (falls)

Renew/adjust outpatient therapy orders

Renew medications

Obtain follow-up with other physicians, as indicated

Assess need for further patient/family counseling

---

*See Chapter 1 for specific orders and description of rehabilitation team.

and hemorrhagic stroke patients with elevated blood pressures may require antihypertensive medications.

There is little surgical intervention for acute stroke. Ipsilateral carotid endarterectomy is indicated for patients who have TIAs or mild or recovered strokes, who have angiography-documented carotid stenosis of 70% or more.

▪ Complications

Any patient who has sustained a stroke is at risk for further complications due to immobility, as well as from problems relating to his or her general medical condition.

Deep Venous Thrombosis

Deep venous thrombosis (DVT) of the legs occurs in approximately 30% to 50% of stroke patients. It may not be detected clinically in the paralyzed leg. The risk of pulmonary embolism (PE) with DVT is approximately 10%. The lower extremities should be examined daily for discoloration, edema, or pain upon movement. Noninvasive Doppler studies are diagnostic. Prevention includes antiembolic stockings, protection of the affected extremity, proper positioning, and ambulation as soon as appropriate. Use of mini-dose heparin is advocated. If DVT is suspected clinically, the patient should be adequately anticoagulated with heparin. A hemorrhagic stroke with onset longer than 3 weeks will generally be anticoagulated. Typical orders are as follows:

1. Obtain stat baseline PT/PTT.
2. Place 25,000 units of heparin in 500 cc D_5W (each cc with 50 units heparin).
3. Begin infusion by minidrip infusion pump at 20 cc per hour (1000 units heparin/hr.).
4. IV bolus 5000 units heparin now.
5. PT/PTT 4 hours after infusion begun—please call me with results.
6. Daily PT/PTTs.

PTT should be maintained at $1\frac{1}{2}$ to 2 times control.

On day three of heparin, start oral anticoagulation with coumadin. When diagnostic testing confirms DVT, the patient should be at bedrest, the affected leg elevated on pillows with warm compresses. There should be no movement of the limb; PT, OT, and speech therapy should be given

at bedside. Oral anticoagulation should precede return to full
rehabilitation activities. In specific cases, placement of an
inferior vena cava filter may be considered. Coumadin therapy usually continues for 3 months.

Seizures

Seizures, more common following embolic than thrombotic
strokes, occur in 10% to 15% of stroke patients. One half of
these occur in the acute period. Phenytoin (Dilantin) is the
drug of choice when seizures occur. Lethargy is a sign of
overmedication. Do not treat prophylactically for seizures.
The typical amount of phenytoin (Dilantin) is 300 to 400 mg
orally per day, which may be given as a single dose.

Depression

Post-stroke depression is believed to relate to catecholamine-
containing neurons partially damaged by focal brain injury.
It appears to be more common in left hemisphere than right
hemisphere injury. The depression may not become apparent
until 6 months to 2 years following injury. Signs include
poor cooperation, management problems, inconsistent recovery, or increasing neurological deficit. Listen to the patient's
words rather than watching his or her behavior. Interview the
family. Psychological/psychiatric support should be given.
All patients who are depressed should be given a trial of antidepressant medication. Amitriptyline (Elavil) or trazodone
(Deseryl) are commonly used in full antidepressant dosages.
Nortryptyline (Pamelor) has the lowest anticholinergic side
effects of the tricyclic antidepressants. Cardiac problems or
prostatic hypertrophy may preclude the use of these specific
medications due to anticholinergic activity; others with fewer
side-effects should be employed. Sertraline (Zoloft) has also
been shown to be effective clinically. Suicidal ideation merits
immediate psychiatric intervention.

Dysphagia

Evaluation and management of dysphagia may prevent aspiration pneumonia and helps ensure adequate nutrition. Swallowing problems, usually the result of the absence of or severe delay in the swallowing process, may be seen following brain stem stroke as well as unilateral cerebral lesions. Warning signs of swallowing impairment in the stroke patient include confused mental state, dysarthria, complaint of obstruction, weight loss, nasal regurgitation, and mouth odor. Dysphagia evaluation may be made at the bedside by the speech pathologist. A modified barium swallow may document abnormalities in the swallowing process. Treatment includes therapy to improve oral motor control and stimulate swallowing (thermal stimulation), as well as modification of the diet. Thickened liquids and altered consistency of food may be helpful. Nasogastric feeding is recommended for patients at severe risk of aspiration. For those for whom little recovery is anticipated over 2 to 3 months, gastrostomy feeding with constant drip or bolus feeding is used. Bolus feeding should be avoided in any stroke patient who is at risk of aspiration, as stomach distension, regurgitation, and aspiration may occur.

Nutritional Status

Poor nutritional status is common in patients who are chronically ill or undergo prolonged hospitalizations. In addition to dysphagia, upper extremity paralysis, visual field neglect, communication impairment, and depression may decrease caloric intake. Calorie counts, weight records, total protein, serum albumin, and other laboratory indices of nutritional status should be monitored.

Incontinence

Urinary incontinence is common following stroke, but is usually transient. A voiding trial (offering the patient the urinal, or bedside commode upon awakening, every two hours, and prior to sleep) will often solve the problem. Adult diapers can be used *only* in therapy to prevent accidents. Treat all significant urinary tract infections (UTIs). Repeat UTIs should be evaluated urologically. Fecal incontinence is generally related to immobility, change in diet, or fecal impaction. Continued incontinence of urine and feces may be indicative of bilateral or brain stem lesion, and therefore be incurable.

Shoulder Hand Syndrome

Shoulder hand syndrome (SHS), a type of reflex sympathetic dystrophy (RSD), is a well-recognized post-stroke complication, though rare in carefully monitored patients. Characterized by painful active and passive range of motion at the affected shoulder, pain on extension of the wrist, edema over the metacarpals and fusiform edema of the digits with pain on passive flexion of metacarpal phalangeal (MCPs) and proximal interphalangeal (PIPs), SHS is commonly seen in the second to fourth month post-stroke. The diagnosis is made clinically. Routine X-rays show osteoporosis; delayed isotope scans may reveal increased uptake. Early recognition is necessary for appropriate treatment. The affected hand should be observed daily. Careful attention to positioning of the extremity is necessary to decrease edema and thereby decrease pain. Use of a compression glove may help decrease edema. The goal is to decrease pain so that passive stretching can be done, to further decrease edema. This may be accomplished through application of a cold pack prior to stretching. Avoid contrast baths or application of warm water, that may increase blood flow and thereby increase edema. In severe cases, a short course of oral steroids may be helpful. Use pillows, overhead sling, regular sling, arm trough, or lapboard with elbow pad. Low doses of amitriptyline (Elavil) (25 to 100 mg orally at bedtime) may be helpful for the patient who cannot sleep due to shoulder pain at night. In severe prolonged cases, stellate ganglion blocks may be considered. Throughout SHS, the rehabilitation program should continue. If the problem recurs, the patient should undergo a second course of treatment.

Shoulder Subluxation

Shoulder subluxation, due to muscular weakness of the affected rotator cuff muscles and lack of tone, is a common finding post-stroke. It is unclear whether subluxation itself leads to shoulder pain. The use of a standard sling is controversial. The ambulatory patient with a flaccid upper limb should use a sling when ambulating, but should use an arm trough on the wheelchair. Nonambulatory patients should use a lapboard when seated.

Spasticity

Spasticity results from loss of cortical inhibitory influences. Fortunately, it changes over time, as there is as yet no good medical therapy for cortically induced spasticity. Diazepam (Valium) should be avoided, as it is a central nervous system depressant. Dantrolene (Dantrium), which works directly at the skeletal muscle level, may result in overall weakness and thereby impair muscular function. Baclofen (Lioresal), which acts mainly at the spinal cord level, may also lead to drowsiness. Local nerve blocks may be helpful in specific cases.

Other Complications

Other post-stroke complications include overmedication, poor endurance secondary to cardiac complications, and falls. All medications should be reduced to the minimum. Avoid use of long-acting sedative-hypnotics, such as flurazepam (Dalmane), which accumulate over time. Use chloral hydrate 500 mg orally at bedtime for sleep. Patients with known cardiac problems should be on appropriate medications. Nitroglycerin, if needed, should be available to the patient in therapy. Monitor blood pressures routinely. Observe for possible digitalis toxicity. Prevent falls by use of gait belts, restraints when necessary, close observation, and good transfer techniques.

The patient who has had a stroke is at increased risk for another. Note any new neurological problem, especially refusal to eat, loss of speech, or focal motor deficit. Document the findings and investigate the cause.

Prognosis/Outcome/Follow-Up

Recovery from stroke is a natural process; rehabilitation techniques provide compensatory skills for functional deficits. In a typical pattern of recovery, muscular strength returns in a proximal to distal fashion, arm independent of leg. This accounts for the ability of most post-stroke patients to ambulate eventually. When this typical pattern is not observed, the diagnosis of stroke must be questioned. In addition, other post-stroke injuries such as fractured hip or brachial plexus injury must be ruled out.

At onset, when the totally paralyzed limbs are areflexic, the affected extremities are said to be flaccid. Within 48 hours, deep tendon reflexes usually return. Over time, this progresses to spasticity and eventually to normal muscle tone. Muscle weakness resolves through synergy patterns to isolated movement. This process of recovery may stop at any phase.

From a functional standpoint, prognosis is related to prolonged flaccidity, late return of reflexes, late onset of motor movement, and lack of hand movement. Lack of sensory function is extremely debilitating in terms of activities of daily living and ambulation. A patient who has voluntary muscular movement but no sensation will not use the affected limb functionally.

Communication disorders and swallowing functions usually improve over months. Speech therapy will often be continued over a period of 1 to 2 years in severely aphasic patients who show improvement.

The "typical" left hemiplegic will require a 3 to 4 week stay in acute care rehabilitation. The right hemiplegic, with severe communication/swallowing problems, may require 4 to 6 weeks of inpatient rehabilitation.

All therapies should be continued at a less intense frequency (2 to 3 times per week) after discharge from acute care rehabilitation for a period of 1 to 4 months, or until the patient reaches established goals. Some patients initially require home care and advance to outpatient therapies as mobility improves. Outpatient physician follow-up visits should be scheduled every month or two to assess progress and renew therapy prescriptions. A patient who is nonambulatory due to hip weakness at the time of acute rehabilitation discharge may be considered for staged rehabilitation; when hip strength improves, he/she may be readmitted to learn ambulation. The patient who loses previous gains may also require readmission for assessment and remediation of problems.

On all office visits, equipment checks are made. Patients are instructed to keep the appropriate wheelchair prescribed while an inpatient to use for long-distance ambulation for up to several months.

■ Suggested Readings

Brandstater ME, Roth EJ, Siebens HC. Venous thromboembolism in stroke: literature review and implications for clinical practice. *Arch Phys Med Rehabil* 1992;73:S379–391.

Garrison SJ. Geriatric stroke rehabilitation. *In* Felsenthal G, Garrison SJ, Steinberg FU, eds. *Rehabilitation of the Aging and Elderly Patient.* Baltimore: Williams & Wilkins, 1994, pp. 175–186.

Garrison SJ. Learning after stroke: left versus right brain injury. *Top Geriatr Rehabil* 1991;6:3:45–52.

Garrison SJ, Rolak LA. Rehabilitation of the stroke patient. *In* DeLisa JA, Currie D, Gans B, et al., eds. *Principles and Practice of Rehabilitation Medicine,* 2nd ed. Philadelphia: J.B. Lippincott, 1993.

Goodstein RK. Overview: cerebrovascular accident and the hospitalized elderly—a multidimensional clinical problem. *Am J Psychiatry* 1983;140:2:141–147.

The Healing Influence (videotape). Santa Fe, NM: Danamar Products, 1991.

Hurd MM, Farrell KH, Waylonis GW. Shoulder sling for hemiplegia: friend or foe? *Arch Phys Med Rehabil* 1974;55: 519–522.

Jongblood L. Prediction of function after stroke: a critical review. *Stroke* 1986;17:765–776.

Moskowitz E. Complications in the rehabilitation of hemiplegic patients. *Med Clin North Am* 1969;53:541–558.

Orif R, Heiner S. Orthoses and ambulation in hemiplegia: ten year retrospective study. *Arch Phys Med Rehabil* 1980;61:216–220.

Robinson RG, Kubos KL, Starr LB, et al. Mood disorders in stroke patients: importance of location of lesion. *Brain* 1984;107:81–93.

Tepperman PS, Greyson ND, Hilbert L, et al. Reflex sympathetic dystrophy in hemiplegia. *Arch Phys Med Rehabil* 1984;65:442–447.

Catherine Bontke
Cindy Ivanhoe
Madhura Patel

20

Traumatic Brain Injury

▉ Definition

Traumatic brain injury (TBI) can be defined as head injury
with evidence of brain involvement. The trauma causing the
injury may be blunt, such as a blow to the head, or penetrating, as in missile injuries. Injury can also be caused by movement of the brain within the skull. Damage may be manifested by loss of consciousness, post-traumatic amnesia
(PTA), skull fractures, or evidence of intracranial injury on
neuroimaging. Varying degrees of motor and cognitive deficits may result, depending on the severity of damage, secondary complications, and associated injuries. These deficits
range from mild traumatic brain injury to severe cognitive
and physical impairment. Often, cognitive deficits play a
predominant role in producing functional disability.

▉ Epidemiology

In this country, TBI is the leading cause of death and disability for the 1 through 40 year age group. It is estimated that
as many as 1.5 million people a year sustain brain injuries. Of
these, 50,000 to 70,000 injuries will be classified as moderate to severe. The peak incidence of TBI occurs between the

Susan J. Garrison (Ed.): *Handbook of Physical Medicine and Rehabilitation
Basics.* First Edition. Copyright © 1995 J. B. Lippincott Company

ages of 15 to 24 years, with males injured two to three times more often than females. There is another rise in the incidence rate in the over-75 age group. Most persons with traumatic brain injury are single and from lower socioeconomic groups. There is often a history of alcohol abuse, drug abuse, and/or psychiatric care. One third of TBI patients have had a previous head injury.

Motor vehicle accidents are the leading cause of TBI in adolescent and adult populations. There is a high correlation of positive blood alcohol levels at the time of injury. Falls are responsible for approximately 55% to 65% of TBI in the pediatric population, and are the second most common cause in adolescent and adult populations.

■ Anatomy/Pathophysiology

Primary brain damage as a result of TBI occurs at the moment of impact. Refer to Figure 20-1. Secondary damage occurs as a result of the subsequent pathologic complications arising from the intra- and extracranial damage.

Primary Brain Damage

Linear acceleration and deceleration result in the relative movement between the rigid skull and the soft, incompressible brain. Contusions occur over the frontal lobes and the anterior tips of the temporal lobes; the occipital lobe is damaged less frequently. Hemorrhagic contusions can vary in extent from a superficial layer of blood (a subpial hemorrhage), to one which involves the whole depth of the cortex, causing necrosis and edema. The contusions may be bilateral and asymmetrical. Localized contusions under the area of impact are seen with depressed skull fractures and gunshot wounds.

Rotational acceleration causes movement between the different components of the brain, resulting in diffuse axonal injury (DAI), thought to be due to shearing of nerve fibers in

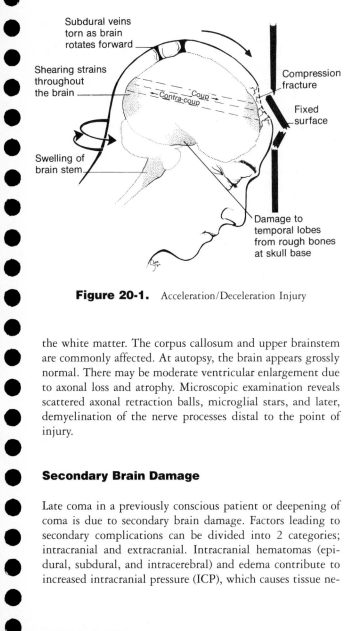

Subdural veins
torn as brain
rotates forward

Shearing strains
throughout
the brain

Coup
Contra-coup

Compression
fracture

Fixed
surface

Swelling of
brain stem

Damage to
temporal lobes
from rough bones
at skull base

Figure 20-1. Acceleration/Deceleration Injury

the white matter. The corpus callosum and upper brainstem are commonly affected. At autopsy, the brain appears grossly normal. There may be moderate ventricular enlargement due to axonal loss and atrophy. Microscopic examination reveals scattered axonal retraction balls, microglial stars, and later, demyelination of the nerve processes distal to the point of injury.

Secondary Brain Damage

Late coma in a previously conscious patient or deepening of coma is due to secondary brain damage. Factors leading to secondary complications can be divided into 2 categories; intracranial and extracranial. Intracranial hematomas (epidural, subdural, and intracerebral) and edema contribute to increased intracranial pressure (ICP), which causes tissue necrosis and obstruction of intracranial veins. Pressure is increased, thereby compromising cerebral blood flow. Watershed areas (boundary zones between adjacent major vascular territories) and the basal ganglia, hippocampus, and purkinje cells of the cerebellum are most vulnerable to ischemia. Increased ICP can also cause various herniation syndromes (transtentorial uncal herniation and cingulate gyrus herniation) leading to compromised brainstem function, cranial nerve palsies, and contusion. Subarachnoid hemorrhage can lead to vasospasm and ischemia. The arachnoid villi which normally absorb cerebrospinal fluid (CSF) may become blocked by cellular debris, leading to a further rise in intracranial pressure.

The most common extracranial factor which contributes to secondary brain injury is hypoxemia. This may be caused by the head injury itself or by associated injuries. Hypotension, anemia, hyponatremia, and other metabolic abnormalities must also be monitored and appropriately managed.

■ Assessment

At the Time of the Injury

The Glasgow Coma Scale (GCS) is most commonly utilized to categorize patients' level of consciousness at the initial neurologic examination in the field and emergency room. It assesses the patient's ability to open the eyes, speak, and make motor responses to standard stimuli. The patient's condition is then categorized as mild (GCS 13–15), moderate (GCS 9–12) or severe (GCS 3–8) head injury. See Table 20-1.

Brainstem dysfunction in a comatose patient is evidence of great force at impact; the prognosis is worse. Pupillary responses, eye movements, and oculovestibular reflexes as well as signs of autonomic dysfunction, posturing, and movement disorders are helpful in determining prognosis. Document detailed neurologic evaluations and repeat sequentially.

Table 20-1. Glasgow Coma Scale

Indicator	Category of Response	Grade
Eye Opening	Spontaneous	4
	To voice	3
	To pain	2
	None	1
Verbal Response	Oriented	5
	Confused	4
	Inappropriate words	3
	Incomprehensible words	2
	None	1
Motor Response	Obeys command	6
	Localizes pain	5
	Withdraw (pain)	4
	Flexion (pain)	3
	Extension (pain)	2
	None	1

At Rehabilitation Admission

Record the following information:

History

- Loss of consciousness
- Initial Glasgow Coma Scale (GCS)
- Length of coma
- Secondary complications such as hypoxia or hyponatremia
- Associated injuries
- Diagnostic studies
- Surgeries

Social History

* Premorbid personality
* Family support
* Financial issues
* Educational level
* History of substance abuse

Physical Examination

* complete
* emphasize neurological examination
  a. mental status
  b. motor movement

Cognitive function is evaluated by a variety of tests, usually administered by neuropsychologists and speech pathologists, as in Table 20-2.

◼ Treatment

General

Different TBI programs have varying criteria for admission. Patients may be accepted for coma management, or they may need to be able to follow one or two step commands. Some programs accept patients while they are still ventilator-dependent. Generally, the rehabilitation length of stay averages from 2 to 8 months, depending upon the patient's needs and specific rehabilitative program.

Coma Management Programs

Coma management programs have increased in number in the last few years. They are often available through skilled nursing facilities or hospital-based brain injury programs. The goals are to facilitate arousal from coma, prevent compli-

Table 20-2. Tests for Cognitive Functioning

Visual Perception	Visual form discrimination
	Facial recognition test
	Judgment of line orientation
	Line bisection
	Right left orientation
Description	Patient is shown visual stimuli and asked to identify them, discriminate them from others, or judge spatial relationships.
Visual Construction	Block design and object-assembly subtests of the Wechsler Adult Intelligence Scale-Revised (WAIS-R), Rey Complex Figure copy
Description	Patient is shown a visual stimulus and asked to copy it.
Memory	Wechsler Memory Scale-Revised
	Recognition Memory Test
	California Verbal Learning Test
	Rey Complex Figure Recall
	Continuous Visual Memory Test
	Continuous Recognition Memory Test
	Rey Auditory Verbal Learning Test
Description	Patient is presented with unfamiliar information and asked to memorize it and recall it after a delay. Tests are designed for verbal or visual memory.
Problem-Solving	Category Test
	Wisconsin Card Sorting Test
Description	Patient is presented with problems to solve that may require abstract reasoning.

(*continued*)

Table 20-2. (*Continued*)

Cognitive Speed	Symbol Digit Modalities Test
	Visual Reaction Time
	Paced Auditory Serial Addition Test
Description	Patient performs a paced task, with performance measured in terms of speed and/or accuracy.
Motor Performance	Grip strength
	Finger tapping
	Grooved pegboard
Description	Patient performs tasks requiring strength, speed, and dexterity. Performance of right and left hands is compared.

cations of immobility, and educate and train families. Sensory stimulation programs have yet to be proven effective, but are useful for monitoring responsiveness and involving family members. Medications can be adjusted to minimize clouding of the patient's already impaired sensorium. A few medications are proposed to increase arousal and recovery of consciousness. Methylphenidate (Ritalin), dextroamphetamine, pemoline (Cylert), and fluoxetine (Prozac) may improve arousal through their dopaminergic serotonergic activity. In the same manner, anti-Parkinson drugs such as amantadine (Symmetrel), bromocriptine (Parlodel), and carbidopa/levodopa (Sinemet) may be beneficial.

The Rehabilitation Team

The professionals who comprise the rehabilitation team vary, but usually include a physiatrist, neuropsychologist, social worker, occupational therapist, physical therapist, speech and language pathologist, rehabilitation nurse, audiologist, orthotist, respiratory therapist, and vocational and therapeutic recreation counselors. An education liaison is involved for children and adolescents with TBI. When necessary, other medical consultants may play a role. The team assesses the patient's strengths and deficits and sets appropriate short- and long-term goals.

Functional Evaluation

A comprehensive rehabilitation evaluation is necessary for appropriate goal-setting. Types of evaluations performed vary by individual patient abilities. There is often overlap in the evaluations, but in general, team member responsibilities are listed in Table 20-3.

Post-Traumatic Amnesia (PTA)

When admitted for rehabilitation most patients are follow- ing one-step commands, but are confused and in a state of post-traumatic amnesia (PTA). PTA is defined as the length of time until the return of continuous memory. At this stage, patients are often confused and agitated, as they try to make sense of an environment that they no longer understand. Tranquilizers often increase the patient's confusion and can thereby increase agitation. If behavioral interventions and reassurance are not adequate, pharmacologic interventions may become necessary. Use of an antidepressant, psycho- stimulant, or mood stabilizer in an agitated patient is prefer- able to a tranquilizer or neuroleptic medication.

Other Treatment Issues

Swallowing evaluations at bedside and/or in radiology should be performed (Figure 20-2). The patient may require inser- tion of a gastrostomy tube to insure proper nutrition with minimal risk of aspiration. When possible, initiate intermit- tent catheterization if the patient is not continent of urine.

Table 20-3. Functional Evaluation of TBI Patient by Rehabilitation Team Member

Team Member	Activities	Rationale
Neuropsychologist	Employs battery of psychological tests, which vary according to patient's level of functioning.	To assess intellectual functioning, judgment, attention, concentration, language and memory for incorporation into aspects of the patient's program.
Physical Therapist	Identifies gross movement patterns (synergy).	Head control is influenced by muscle weakness, abnormal reflexes, and tone.
Occupational Therapist	Assesses through functional tasks: evaluates postural reflexes, tone, coordination, and range of motion (ROM). Records reactions to pain, tactile, auditory, gustatory, and olfactory stimuli.	To evaluate sensorimotor status.
Speech Pathologist	Evaluates language, communication, speech, cognition, hearing, swallowing; uses battery of tests, including: Woodcock-Johnson Psychoeducational Battery Ross Information Assessment Processing Detroit Test of Learning Aptitude	There is no standard battery of speech tests for the TBI population.
Recreational Therapist	Designs a program of leisure activities to help carry over skills from other therapies; aids in reintegration into community	

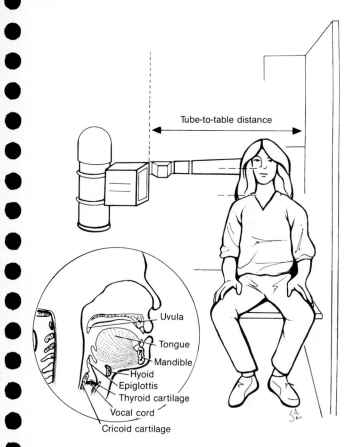

Figure 20-2. Modified barium swallow ("cookie swallow") procedure, performed under fluoroscopy.

Many patients have tracheostomies performed. Monitor respiratory status, with the goal of promoting pulmonary hygiene and eventual tracheal tube removal.

■ Complications

Swallowing

Swallowing disorders or dysphagias after brain injury are usually the result of damage to the brainstem or anterior cortical areas. Evaluation includes an assessment of reflexes (cough, bite, gag, rooting, suck); head, tongue, and jaw control; taste; and pulmonary function. The patient may pocket oral contents or demonstrate drooling and choking. Use of video fluoroscopy, also known as the "cookie swallow" or modified barium swallow, documents the presence or absence of aspiration and allows a more accurate determination of food consistencies that the patient can safely swallow. See Figure 20-2.

Seizures

Approximately 5% of all TBI patients develop posttraumatic seizures. The risk is greatest in patients who have depressed skull fractures, acute intracranial hematomas, or early seizures (occurring within the first week after injury). Patients are often started on phenytoin (Dilantin) or phenobarbital in the acute neurosurgical setting because these drugs are easily administered parenterally and have been in use for a long time. Recent literature suggests that prophylaxis is probably not necessary after the first 2 weeks. There is a trend to treat only patients who have had seizures. Carbamazepine (Tegretol) and valproic acid (Depakene) have the fewest cognitive and behavioral side effects. The most significant side effect of carbamazepine (Tegretol) is bone marrow suppression. If the leukocyte count falls below 3000 cells with less than 50% neutrophils, this medication should be discontinued.

Post-Traumatic Hydrocephalus

Symptoms range from deep coma to the triad of dementia, ataxia, and incontinence. Presentation may be atypical, with emotional disturbances, seizures, spasticity, or subtle cognitive changes. Diagnosis is based on radiographic evidence on CT scan. When there is a question as to the significance of CT findings, monthly CT scans may be helpful. Patients with cerebrospinal fluid (CSF) pressures greater than 276mm of water usually benefit from ventriculoperitoneal shunting. If there is a question as to the usefulness of a proposed shunt, an adapted version of the CSF tap test can be performed, as follows: perform gait assessment and three psychometric tests before and after a lumbar puncture, removing 50 cc of CSF. Improvement on two or more of the four parameters implies a favorable outcome from shunting.

Spasticity

Spasticity following traumatic brain injury is influenced by postural changes, body positioning, and labyrinthine and tonic neck reflexes. Spasticity is useful in preventing osteoporosis and deep vein thrombosis. It also maintains muscle bulk and assists patients with marginal motor strength in transfers and standing. Spasticity does not need to be treated unless it causes pain, interferes with hygiene, limits function, or causes contractures.

Management using physical modalities includes the application of cold or heat, stretching, splinting, inhibitive casting (application of serial casts), positioning, functional electrical stimulation (FES), relaxation, and motor reeducation. Motor point blocks or nerve blocks are preferable to systemic medications that have CNS depressant effects. When medications are necessary, dantrolene (Dantrium) is the drug of choice. Acting directly on skeletal muscle, it decreases the release of calcium from the sarcoplasmic reticulum.

Heterotopic Ossification

Heterotopic ossification (HO) is ectopic bone formation around joints. Risk factors include coma longer than 2 weeks, spasticity, long bone fractures, or decrease in range of motion. Incidence ranges from 11% to 76%. The most commonly involved locations are the shoulder, elbow, and hip. Diagnosis is usually made when there are clinical findings of limited range of motion, pain, and swelling. An elevated alkaline phosphatase level is suggestive of HO, but is nonspecific in patients with multiple trauma. Triple phase bone scans are most sensitive for early diagnosis of HO. Nonsteroidal anti-inflammatory drugs (NSAIDs) are sometimes used acutely to decrease pain and swelling. Continue aggressive range of motion. Etidronate (Didronel) 20 mg/kg in a single daily dose for 3 months, followed by 10 mg/kg daily for 3 months, may inhibit bone formation. The most common side effects are gastrointestinal, but usually do not mandate cessation of the medication. Long-term treatment with etidronate can lead to osteomalacia.

Endocrine

The syndrome of inappropriate antidiuretic hormone secretion (SIADH) is most frequently seen. This results in dilutional hyponatremia and is therefore managed with fluid restriction. SIADH generally resolves during the acute neurosurgical phase of treatment. Diabetes insipidus (DI) is less commonly seen. It results in a failure of ADH secretion with resultant diuresis of dilute urine and hypernatremia. Treat DI with vasopressant tannate and oil or intranasal 1-desamino-8-D-arginine vasopressin (DDAVP). Menstrual irregularities are frequent and pregnancy must be ruled out. Menstruation usually resumes by 6 months post-injury. Studies suggest that up to 20% of persons with severe brain injuries have one or more disturbances of anterior pituitary hormones; the significance is unknown.

Injuries and Fractures

Up to 89% of patients have one or more extracranial injuries which must be identified early to minimize long-term disability. Always evaluate patients for cervical spine injuries. Peripheral nerve injuries may result from initial trauma, compression due to positioning, or HO.

Autonomic Disturbances

Systemic hypertension, which may result from high intracranial pressure and catecholamine release, is frequently seen. Increased cardiac output and tachycardia are also common in the acute care setting. Focal injuries near the hypothalamus can result in hypertension. Beta blockers, indicated in the hyperdynamic state, may later impair the patient's cognitive functioning. Hypotension is usually orthostatic. Central fevers, while uncommon, are seen in patients with lesions of the anterior hypothalamus or generalized decerebration. Hypothermia, secondary to lesions of the posterior hypothalamus or due to endocrine dysfunction, may occur.

Respiratory Complications

Pneumonia is common, as is bacterial colonization of tracheostomy sites. Decannulation is indicated when the need for mechanical ventilation has resolved, the proximal airway is intact, there is no further need for pulmonary toilet, and the patient can swallow safely. Abnormalities seen prior to decannulation include vocal cord paralysis, tracheal stenosis, subglottic stenosis, glottic stenosis, and tracheomalacia. These may be due to intubation, head injury, or a combination of the two.

Gastrointestinal Complications

The head injured patient is hypermetabolic, with high caloric needs. Patients receive tube feedings or hyperalimentation; observe for changes in weight and serum albumin level.

The risk of gastrointestinal bleeding secondary to stress ulcers is increased and histamine H_2-receptor antagonists are
frequently prescribed. Ranitidine (Zantac) or famotidine
(Pepcid) are preferable to cimetidine (Tagamet), which may
cause behavioral disturbances. Metaclopramide (Reglan), frequently used to improve gastric motility, is related to the
phenothiazines; it can cause sedation, extrapyramidal symptoms, restlessness, and movement disorders. Decrease gastric
reflux by using a feeding jejunostomy tube, specific positioning, and small bolus or continuous tube feeding rather than
simply medicating with metadopramide (Reglan).

Genitourinary Complications

Neurogenic bladder is rare following head injury. If present,
there is usually uninhibited detrusor hyperreflexia. Use an
external collecting device for males and diapers for females. A
hyporeflexic bladder with resultant overdistension may also
occur. Bladder training should begin once the patient is
aware of his or her surroundings. There is a high incidence of
urinary tract infection in patients arriving on the rehabilitation unit, usually secondary to prior instrumentation. Obtain
a screening urinalysis, culture, and sensitivity at the time of
rehabilitation admission.

Hematologic Complications

Coagulopathies occur in the acute care setting; they rarely
persist into the rehabilitation phase. Anemias, as a result of
profound blood loss, are sometimes treated by iron supplementation or transfusion. Other problems are frequently the
iatrogenic result of medications.

■ Prognosis

The majority of patients who remain unconscious 1 month
following brain injury will either recover or die within the
first year. Consciousness is usually regained within 3 months.

Twenty to 30% of patients who do not regain consciousness will die within the first year. Age is a powerful predictor of outcome; the pediatric population demonstrates a better outcome than the adult. Common negative prognosticators include a low GCS, impaired eye movements and pupillary responses, surgical mass lesions, and unconsciousness longer than 3 months.

Psychosocial aspects of patients' lives also influence outcomes. Emotional disturbances and changes in behavior frequently accompany TBI. A lack of self-awareness and the disinhibition that often accompany brain injury can lead to increasing isolation from friends and family. It is generally easier for family members to accept their loved one's physical disability than change in personality.

A number of scales and tests exist that provide valuable information about the degree of a patient's injury. Numerous physical findings are interpreted as good or bad prognosticators. However, patients have varying combinations of factors contributing to disability; accurate predictions are difficult.

The Glasgow Coma Scale is the most widely used scale for assessing and categorizing brain injury (see Table 20-1). The scale provides broad quantification of responsiveness, but does not evaluate subtle changes that occur in patients progressing from coma. The Disability Rating Scale and the Rancho Los Amigos Levels of Cognitive Functioning scale are also insensitive measures in unconscious patients.

The Coma/Near Coma Scale rates the patients reaction to pain, verbal commands and sensory modalities. Coma is divided into 4 levels as follows:

- Extreme coma: No response to any stimulation
- Marked coma: Inconsistent responses to one modality without any verbalization or ability to follow commands
- Moderate coma: Inconsistent responses in 2 to 3 modalities with nonverbal vocalization
- Near coma: Consistent responses in 2 modalities and/or follows commands inconsistently

▪ Outcome

The Glasgow Outcome Scale is widely used for categorizing late outcome after traumatic and nontraumatic coma. It reflects the patient's social dependency by placing him or her in one of the following categories: vegetative state, severe disability, moderate disability, and good recovery.

The vegetative state describes the finding of wakefulness without awareness. A patient in coma will either die, awaken, or become vegetative. In the vegetative state, the patient resumes sleep-wake cycles. He/she may blink in response to threat and his/her eyes may move from side to side, seemingly following family members or staff. This phenomenon of "tracking" is frequently misinterpreted by observers as awareness of the environment. Patients may also exhibit primitive postural reflexes, including limb movements. These findings, which represent brain stem functioning, often make it difficult for observers to accept that the patient has no awareness of the environment. In the work of Jennett and Teasdale, no patient classified as vegetative 3 months after injury ever gained independence. Ten percent regained consciousness but remained dependent.

Severe disability describes patients who are dependent on another person for some activities of daily living in a 24-hour period. The impairment may be physical, communicative, or cognitive. It can include patients who are ambulatory, but unsafe due to impulsive, disinhibited behavior. Moderate disability describes patients who are able to care for themselves and perform some degree of occupational activity. Patients who can return to work and participate in a social life comprise the good recovery category. Patients may still demonstrate residuae of their injuries, but these do not significantly affect their daily level of functioning.

▪ Follow-Up

Following discharge from acute rehabilitation, patients with TBI may be treated in comprehensive outpatient services, day treatment, transitional or skilled living facilities or home. Goals are for them to eventually participate in a rewarding lifestyle, within functional limitations. This may include supported or sheltered employment. For many TBI survivors, some degree of dependence on others remains the reality. Ideally, there should be access for continued support. The difficulties are dynamic and continue to present physical, social, cognitive, and behavioral challenges to patients and families. While many patients require minimal follow-up, others will always require frequent medical rehabilitative support.

▉ Suggested Readings

Berrol S, ed.: *Traumatic Brain Injury.* Physical Medicine and Rehabilitation Clinics of North America. Philadelphia: W.B. Saunders, 1992.

Bontke CF, Boake C: Traumatic brain injury rehabilitation. *Neurosurg Clin North Am* 1991;2(2).

Bontke CF: Medical advances in the treatment of brain injury. *In* Kreutzer JS, Wehman P, eds. *Community Integration Following Traumatic Brain Injury.* Baltimore: Paul H. Brookes, 1990.

Bontke CF: Medical Complications related to traumatic brain injury. *In* Horn LJ, Cope DN, eds. *Traumatic Brain Injury.* Philadelphia: Hanley and Belfus, 1989, pp. 43–58.

Cope DN: Head injury rehabilitation: benefit of early intervention. *Arch Phys Med Rehab* 1982;69:433–437.

Horn LJ, Cope DN: *Traumatic Brain Injury. State of the Art Reviews.* Philadelphia: Hanley & Belfus, 1989.

Mackay LE, Bernstein BA, Chapman PE, et al.: Early intervention in severe head injury: long-term benefits of a formalized program. *Arch Phys Med Rehabil* 1992;73:635–641.

Rappaport M, Herrero-Backe C, Rappaport ML, Winterfield KM: Head injury outcome up to ten years later. *Arch Phys Med Rehab* 1989;70:885–892.

Rosenthal M, Griffith ER, Bond MR, Miller JD, eds.: *Rehabilitation of the Adult and Child with Traumatic Brain Injury.* 2nd ed. Philadelphia: F.A. Davis, 1990.

Sandel ME: Rehabilitation management in the acute care setting. *In* Horn LJ, Cope DN, eds. *Traumatic Brain Injury.* Philadelphia: Hanley and Belfus, 1989, pp. 27–41.

Temkin NR, Dikmen SS, Wilensky AJ, et al.: A randomized, double-blind study of phenytoin for the prevention of post-traumatic seizure. *N Engl J Med* 1990;323:497–502.

Whyte J, Glenn MB: The care and rehabilitation of the patient in a persistent vegetative state. *Journal of Head Trauma Rehabilitation* 1986;1(1):39–53.

Index

Abdominal muscles, immobilization effects on, 191

Acceleration/deceleration injury, of brain, 410, 411f

Acetylcholine receptors, dysfunction of, in myasthenia gravis, 227–228

Acid maltase deficiency, myopathy in, 226

Acidosis, respiratory, 323

ACTH, in multiple sclerosis, 215

Active assisted range of motion exercise, in sports injury, 374

Active range of motion exercise, in sports injury, 374

Activities of daily living
of burn patient, 99
in cancer rehabilitation, 111–112
in cardiac rehabilitation, 131, 135, 136t
in immobilization, 194
vs. spinal cord injury level, 349t–352t
in toxic myopathy, 221

Acupuncture, electro-, 22–23

Acute pain. *See under* Pain

ADFR therapy, in osteoporosis, 242

Adhesive capsulitis, shoulder, in spinal cord injury, 344

Adrenocorticotrophic hormone (ACTH), in multiple sclerosis, 215

Aerobic exercise, in cardiac conditioning, 120
in sports injury, 376

A-fibers, in pain transmission, 14f, 15

Agnosia, in stroke, 394, 396f–397f

Air cushions, for wheelchairs, 308t

Air flotation bed, 305, 306t
problems with, 317

Albuterol, in chronic obstructive pulmonary disease, 328

Alcohol, toxic myopathy from, 220–222

Alexander technique, in sports injury, 386t

Alexia, in stroke, 394, 397f

Alfentanil, pharmacokinetics of, 160t–161t

Alkalosis, metabolic, in immobilization, 190

Amantadine, in brain injury coma, 416

Ambulation
after amputation, energy requirements of, 35–36, 37t
assistive devices for
in chronic respiratory disease, 331
in rheumatoid arthritis, 71
of burn patient, 99
in Duchenne muscular dystrophy, 261–262
in multiple sclerosis, 214
in spinal cord injury, 351t–352t
in spinal muscle atrophy, 203
in stroke, 407

American Burn Association, burn classification of, 89, 91t

American Spinal Association, motor level classification of, 341

Amitriptyline
in brachial plexus injury, 293
in pain management, 24, 32t, 159
in spinal cord injury, 365
in stroke, 402, 404

Amnesia, after brain injury, 417

Amputation, 34–60
above-knee, 48–55, 52f, 55t
anatomic aspects of, 34–35
below-knee, 37t, 43–48, 46f, 49t
in cancer, 115
definition of, 34
energy requirements in, 35–37, 37t, 48–49
epidemiology of, 35
etiology of, 35–36, 35t
evaluation in, 36–38, 37t

429

434

Index

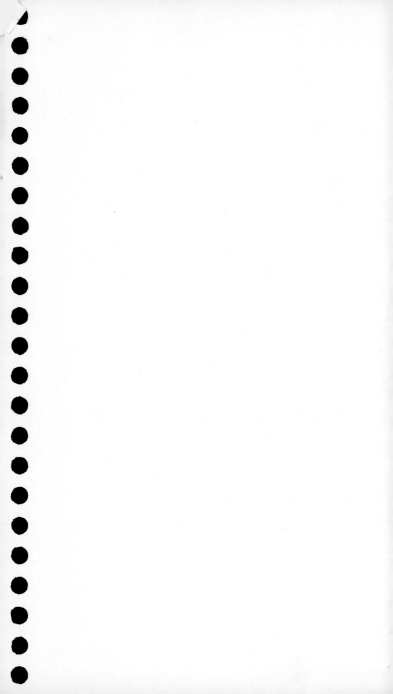

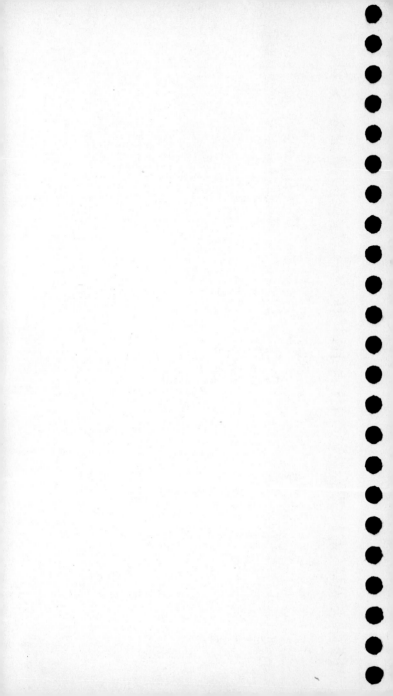